Recent Advances in

Anaesthesia and Analgesia

Edited by

A. P. Adams MB BS PhD FRCA FANZCA DA
Professor of Anaesthetics, University of London; Honorary Consultant
Anaesthetist, Guy's, King's and St Thomas' Hospitals, London, UK

J. N. Cashman BSc MB BS BA MD FRCA
Consultant Anaesthetist, St George's Hospital, London, UK; Honorary Senior
Lecturer, University of London

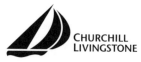

CHURCHILL
LIVINGSTONE

EDINBURGH LONDON NEW YORK PHILADELPHIA SYDNEY TORONTO 1998

CHURCHILL LIVINGSTONE
An imprint of Harcourt Brace and Company Limited

Robert Stevenson House, 1–3 Baxter's Place, Leith Walk, Edinburgh EH1 3AF, UK

First published 1998

ISBN 0-443-05988-8
ISSN 0309-2305

British Library Cataloguing in Publication Data
A catalogue record for this book is available from the British Library

Library of Congress Cataloging in Publication Data
A catalog record for this book is available from the Library of Congress

Medical knowledge is constantly changing. As new information becomes available, changes in treatment, procedures, equipment and the use of drugs become necessary. The authors and publisher have, as far as possible, taken care to ensure that the information given in this text is accurate and up-to-date. However, readers are strongly advised to confirm that the information, especially with regard to drug usage, complies with current legislation and standards of practice.

The
publisher's
policy is to use
**paper manufactured
from sustainable forests**

Produced by B A & G M Haddock
Printed in Singapore through Addison Wesley Longman China Limited

Recent Advances in

Anaesthesia
and Analgesia

Recent Advances in Anaesthesia and Analgesia 19
Edited by A.P. Adams and J.N. Cashman

ISBN 0443 053065
ISSN 0309 2305

Contents

Preface

How do anaesthetics work? This question has puzzled us for over 150 years ever since the concept of modern general anaesthesia was born. Numerous theories and hypotheses have been proposed. An intriguing account of the molecular and cellular mechanisms of general anaesthesia is provided by Professor Kress from Vienna. Much more is known about the mode of action of the neuromuscular blocking drugs (muscle relaxants) and several new agents have been introduced. Professor Bowman provides a state-of-the-art account of the physiology of neuromuscular transmission which he has integrated with the pharmacological behaviour of these drugs.

Ventricular fibrillation is the leading cause of death and more than a quarter of a million people die from sudden unexpected death each year in Europe. The majority of such deaths are associated with acute myocardial ischaemia. The chapter on ventricular ventilation and transthoracic defibrillation by Professor Bossaert provides the latest opinion on such matters. He provides a detailed discussion of the initiation of ventricular fibrillation and its epidemiology together with mechanisms of defibrillation which include an analysis of the waveforms which may be used; he also discusses automatic external defibrillators.

Anaesthesia and surgery of patients who have suffered a recent head injury, but who are not undergoing neurosurgical procedures, is still problematic. Any patient with even a mild or moderate head injury is still a risk of complication from anaesthesia and surgery – adverse complications pose risks for several weeks, even after a mild head injury and may result from any kind of anaesthetic technique. There are problems with the interruption of both clinical and physiological monitoring of the neurological condition and the risk of exacerbating the effects of the head injury because of anaesthesia and surgery. Dr Walker provides a comprehensive account of the management of such patients from the anaesthetist's viewpoint. He also considers resuscitation and anaesthesia for emergency surgery to control bleeding and goes on to provide pertinent advice concerning the provision of pain relief in the head-injured patient.

The general public rightly continues to be concerned about reports in the media concerning awareness during general anaesthesia. Indeed, this matter of the greatest importance to all concerned. Dr Michael Wang is a clinical psychologist who is well known to have an interest in such matters: he considers the concepts of learning, memory and awareness during anaesthesia and his account is an important one for all anaesthetists.

Another matter that has been the subject of much recent media attention is whether the fetus can experience pain or unpleasant sensations. There had been a marked change in medical practice in the provision of analgesia for neonates undergoing major surgery. Furthermore, doctors are now able to correct some congenital abnormalities *in utero*. Many publications dealing with pain or fetal development have largely ignored the subject of fetal pain and thus it is important that this question is asked again. Dr McCullagh provides a fascinating chapter where he explores his subject from an extrapolation from studies of experimental animals to the human fetus. He also analyses direct studies of human fetal function and emphasises that structure frequently provides a useful indication of functional capability.

Critically ill and severely injured children are not always treated by the right people in the right place. The media has reported several instances where seriously ill children have been transported long distances within the UK, often because of a lack of intensive care beds. Drs Alexander and Macrae have addressed this crucial subject. Their chapter considers the aims and organisation of the transport of seriously ill children between hospitals, communications, the mechanics and equipment involved and the importance of prior stabilisation of the child by the referring hospital.

It is now time that the concept of the `Golden Hour' is updated. This is the name which has been given to the period which elapses between an injury and definitive surgical care and which is a critical factor in determining the survival rate of victims. Drs Roberts and Beale provide a useful account of developments concerning this concept. Improvements in the structure of trauma management have resulted in a more thorough approach to these patients. Haemorrhage and head injury are the leading causes of mortality in this group and frequently co-exist.

Monitoring of cardiac output is a vital aspect of the management of very ill patients requiring anaesthesia and intensive care. New developments using non-invasive techniques are particularly welcome and Drs Montgomery and Singer have provided an intriguing overview of the methods currently available. Such techniques facilitate early identification and prevention, or faster correction, of circulatory derangement before a significant tissue oxygen debt has been allowed to develop,

Anaesthetists and intensivists are bombarded by pharmaceutical houses regarding the merits of new drugs to support a failing circulation. Drs Grant and Nimmo have written a detailed and succinct account of circulatory support using inotropes in critically ill patients. They consider both the aims and the monitoring of such therapy and the effects of such drugs on the body as a whole; no single drug appears adequate to correct haemodynamics in all cases of shock and in many instances combination drug therapy has to be used.

Nitric oxide is the wonder drug of this decade. However, its use is not without problems and it is now time to consider carefully how inhaled NO should be used and when it should not be used. Readers are brought right up-to-date with this subject by Dr Singer and Professor Evans.

The provision of adequate pain relief to patients, especially those receiving controlled ventilation of the lungs, in intensive care units is a matter of concern. Dr Lawson considers this important subject.

Increasingly we are being made to ration health care and to introduce greater economies into our clinical practice. The editors' regard anaesthesia as being excellent value for money – it can be argued that it is too cheap – and, indeed, the cost of an anaesthetic is peanuts compared with the sums of money spent on expensive drugs, chemotherapy, radiation treatment, transplantation, and so on. Dr Hitchcock gives us a sensible account of the economics of anaesthesia.

London   A.P.A
1998   J.N.C

Contributors

Shirley M. Alexander MB ChB MRCP
ECMO Research Fellow, Cardiac Intensive Care Unit, Great Ormond Street
Hospital for Children NHS Trust, London, UK

Richard J. Beale MBBS FRCA
Senior Lecturer, Departments of Intensive Care and Anaesthetics, Guy's
Hospital, London, UK

Leo L. Bossaert MD
Departement Geneeskunde, Universitaire Instelling Antwerpen, Antwerpen,
Belgium

William C. Bowman PhD DSc FIBiol FRSE FRSA HonFRCA
Head, Department of Physiology and Pharmacology, University of
Strathclyde, Glasgow, UK

Timothy W. Evans BSc MD PhD FRCP EDICM
Professor of Intensive Care Medicine, Unit of Critical Care Medicine,
Imperial College School of Medicine, Royal Brompton Hospital, London, UK

Ian S. Grant FRCP FFARCSI
Consultant Anaesthetist and Director of Intensive Care, Western General
Hospital, Edinburgh, UK

Mark Hitchcock BSc MBBS DCH FRCA
Director of Day Surgery and Consultant Anaesthetist, Addenbrooke's NHS
Trust, Cambridge, UK

Hans Georg Kress MD
Head, Department of Anaesthesiology and General Intensive Care B,
University of Vienna, Vienna, Austria

Andrew D. Lawson FFARCSI FANZCA
Consultant in Pain Management, Magill Department of Anaesthetics, Chelsea
and Westminster Hospital, London, UK

Christopher P. Leng FRCA
Senior Registrar, Magill Department of Anaesthetics, Chelsea and Westminster Hospital, London, UK

Duncan J. Macrae BMSc MB ChB FRCA FRCPH
Consultant in Paediatric Intensive Care, Cardiac Intensive Care Unit, Great Ormond Street Hospital for Children NHS Trust, London, UK

Peter M^CCullagh MD BS DPhil MRCP
Senior Fellow, Developmental Physiology Group, Division of Molecular Medicine, The John Curtin School of Medical Research, The Australian National University, Canberra, Australia

Hugh Montgomery MBBS BSc MD FRCP
Lecturer in Intensive Care, Bloomsbury Institute of Intensive Care Medicine, University College London Medical School, Rayne Institute, London, UK

Graham R. Nimmo MD MRCP FFARCSI
Consultant Physician, Acute Receiving Unit, Intensive Care Unit, Western General Hospital, Edinburgh, UK

Peter C. Roberts MB BS FRCA
Department of Intensive Care and Department of Anaesthetics, Guy's Hospital, London, UK

Mervyn Singer MBBS MD MRCP
Senior Lecturer in Intensive Care, Bloomsbury Institute of Intensive Care Medicine, University College London Medical School, Rayne Institute, London, UK

Suveer Singh BSc MB MRCP
British Heart Foundation Clinical Training Fellow, Unit of Critical Care Medicine, Imperial College School of Medicine, Royal Brompton Hospital, London, UK

Douglas A.J. Walker MA DPhil BM BCh FRCA
Consultant Neuroanaesthetist, Department of Neuroanaesthesia, Institute of Neurological Sciences, Southern General Hospital, Glasgow, UK

Michael Wang BSc MSc PhD CPsychol AFBPsS
Clinical Director, Department of Clinical Psychology, University of Hull, Hull, UK

Lukas Weigl PhD
Research Assistant, Department of Anaesthesiology and General Intensive Care B, University of Vienna, Vienna, Austria

Hans Georg Kress   Lukas Weigl

The molecular and cellular mechanisms of general anaesthesia

What is general anaesthesia?

Soon after Morton's public demonstration of the use of ether in 1846, the term 'anaesthesia' was suggested by the physician and writer Oliver W. Holmes to describe this special state of 'insensibility' and tolerance to surgery. After the development of local and regional anaesthetic techniques, the more precise term 'general anaesthesia' has come into use. The uniform appearance of this state supported for a long time the antiquated, but still persisting, idea of one common anaesthetic action correlated to lipophilicity and shared by all the different, relatively inert, chemical agents (unitary hypothesis).

Used in a traditional way, the term general anaesthesia describes a broad spectrum of distinguishable physiological states, which are comparable to those brought about by diethyl ether (e.g. hypnosis, amnesia, analgesia, paralysis, attenuation of the stress response) and are considered suitable for human surgery. The introduction of intravenous anaesthetics has made it quite clear that some of these desirable effects are not obligatory components of general anaesthesia, and thus do not define it (e.g. the inclusion of muscle relaxation in the definition of anaesthesia is illogical and confusing).[1] Since the suppression of the sensory perception of a noxious stimulus is the only pharmacological action common to all general anaesthetics, anaesthesia may be defined more precisely as a state in which, as a result of reversible, drug-induced unconsciousness, noxious stimuli can neither be perceived nor recalled.[1] This definition also implies that anaesthesia is the true effect, and that drugs which are able to reversibly induce such a state as their primary effect are to be considered general anaesthetics by definition.

Prof. Dr Hans Georg Kress MD, Head, Department of Anaesthesiology and General Intensive Care B, University of Vienna, Währinger Gürtel 18–20, A-1090 Vienna, Austria

Dr Lukas Weigl PhD, Research Assistant, Department of Anaesthesiology and General Intensive Care B, University of Vienna, Währinger Gürtel 18–20, A-1090 Vienna, Austria

Where do general anaesthetics act in the brain?

On the basis of the aforementioned definition, general anaesthetics apparently exert their specific actions in the central nervous system (CNS); however, there is no consensus as to the CNS structures and neuronal circuits which are critical to anaesthesia.[2,3] It is consciousness which is notoriously difficult to define and to localize within the CNS, as it seems to be determined by the activity of the brain in general, and the cerebral cortex and brain stem in particular.[2,3] Normal cerebral activity requires intact thalamic, hypothalamic, limbic and reticular structures as well as cortical functions. Thus, the higher centres of the brain, the cortex and the so-called reticular formation would appear to be prime anaesthetic target structures.

Based on the concept of brain stem nuclei conducting the sleep/wakefulness cycle, a selective vulnerability of the reticular formation was suggested as the neuronal basis of general anaesthesia. Increased inhibition and decreased excitation were seen as actions of anaesthetics on the reticular control of sensory neurones. Indeed, the reticular influence on brain stem, basal ganglia, cerebellar and motor cortical neurones could explain the reduction of volitional movements during anaesthesia; furthermore, the disruption of the transfer of ascending sensory information across the thalamic sensory relay synapse might produce decreased or garbled input to the cerebral cortex, resulting in the loss of consciousness.[2]

Beside the fact that the activity of the reticular formation alone does not account for variations in the level of consciousness, most studies revealed a more or less global depression of CNS activity, and no distinct area of particular anaesthetic susceptibility could be found in the brain so far.[3] Positron emission tomography (PET) studies failed to detect circumscribed spots of enhanced or diminished activity during general anaesthesia.[4,5] However, the metabolic situation, at the precise moment when consciousness was lost, could not be examined because of the limited time resolution of the PET method. Interestingly, relative cortical metabolism was significantly more depressed during propofol anaesthesia than during isoflurane anaesthesia, which argues for a different pattern of how global metabolism and neuronal activity were reduced by various agents.[4,5]

Lipid or protein?

Since the lipophilicity of general anaesthetics enables them to dissolve in all cellular and subcellular membranes and compartments, each neurone possesses a host of potentially relevant molecular sites of action. No specific chemical group is required for anaesthetic activity, and a structure-activity relationship, usually seen with bioactive chemicals, is also absent. Thus, no further conclusion can be drawn on potential targets and their molecular nature, except that the anaesthetic target site(s) or the environment where general anaesthetics act must have both polar (hydrophilic) and non-polar (lipophilic) properties.[6] Both the fact that general anaesthesia is produced by such a wide variety of structurally unrelated, relatively inert, chemical agents and the remarkably strong relationship between anaesthetic potency and lipid solubility (Meyer-Overton rule) have been misinterpreted as principal actions of general anaesthetics on membrane lipids, and have led to the predominant belief in a unitary mechanism of anaesthesia.[3,6]

The more the lipid theories had to be abandoned and the complex biology of the neurone has been understood, the more proteins have been realized to represent plausible targets of general anaesthetics. The extremely steep dose response curves, empirically found for the clinical phenomenon of general anaesthesia, also suggest the involvement of more than one single mechanism in the state of anaesthesia.[6,7] Thus, it is widely accepted today that direct and/or lipid-mediated interactions of anaesthetics with membrane proteins contribute substantially to the development of the state of general anaesthesia. The burdens of 'unitarism' and 'lipid theories' having been shaken off, it is no longer necessary to be hampered by a narrow thinking restricted to lipid **or** protein categories. For too long, progress had been hindered rather than promoted by a dogmatic discussion that makes no sense as long as the critical anaesthesia-sensitive processes have not been identified on a cellular level.

CELLULAR AND MOLECULAR ACTIONS OF GENERAL ANAESTHETICS

Where do general anaesthetics act at the neurone?

As the basic functional unit of the brain is the neurone and as the overall pattern of neuronal activity is governed by functional connections between them, the anaesthetic state may be considered a direct consequence of a modulation of information processing in neuronal networks.[2,3,8] In the CNS, each neurone is interconnected with thousands of other neurones via excitatory and inhibitory chemical synapses.

A model neurone (Fig. 1) consists of an input region, an integrating region, a conducting and an output region. It receives information from the dendrites and the cell body (input region). Cellular information processing involves the passage of numerous inputs to the triggering region of the axon hillock, where an action potential (AP) may or may not be triggered (integrating region). From there, APs spread unidirectionally along the axon (conducting region) to the presynaptic terminals where the respective neurotransmitters are released into the synaptic cleft (output region). Whether or not a neurone fires, therefore, depends on the location, the size and the shape of the incoming synergistic or antagonistic synaptic potentials. Small changes in one of these determinants may alter the firing pattern of whole regions in the brain causing fundamental changes in mental abilities.

Based on this simplified model of a neuronal circuit (Fig. 1), the anaesthetic state may be produced by effects on neurones or axons, on excitatory or inhibitory transmission, or any combination of these.[3,7–9] Inhibition suppresses the activity of parallel neuronal pathways or prevents an activated cell from being overstimulated. In both cases, an inhibitory interneurone gets an excitatory input which is used to relay an inhibitory input to the postsynaptic cell, thus excitation is required for inhibition (Fig. 1).

Although we are far from understanding the mechanisms of anaesthetic action in sufficient detail, there is a broad consensus as to the predominant role of synaptic transmission (excitatory and inhibitory) for the anaesthetic state (Fig. 2).[3,6–9] General anaesthetics have been shown to act principally on synaptic processes,[8] but, as discussed below, a potential role of signal integration and axonal conductance cannot be ruled out.[9,10]

Voltage-gated Na⁺ and K⁺ channels

During the past 10 years, molecular cloning of voltage-gated ion channels has given insights into the primary structure of these molecules and the hetero-logous expression of these peptides in combination with advanced electro-physiological methods, such as patch clamping and single channel analysis, have been used as powerful tools for the investigation of anaesthetic effects.

Na⁺ channels

Na⁺ channels provide the basis for integration of synaptic potentials in the axon hillock where the AP is generated (Fig. 1). Any impairment, inhibition or potentiation of these channels should lead to altered neuronal firing patterns.[11] Changes in the shape of an AP, as a consequence of altered channel behaviour, may also influence calcium influx at presynaptic terminals resulting in altered transmitter release and synaptic transmission (Fig. 2). Mammalian CNS Na⁺

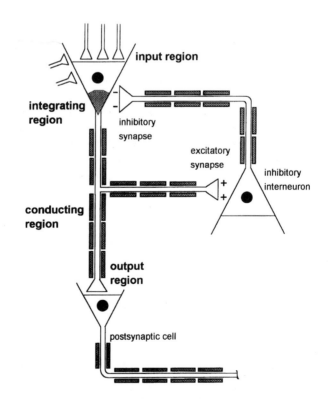

Fig. 1 Schematic diagram of a model synaptic relay. Further explanations are given in the text.

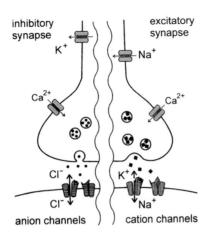

inhibitory synapse

excitatory synapse

K+

Na+

Ca2+

Ca2+

Cl−

K+

Cl−

Na+

anion channels

cation channels

Fig. 2 Schematic diagram of major mechanisms involved in inhibitory or excitatory synaptic transmission. Inhibitory postsynaptic potentials (IPSPs) are generated by increased Cl− conductivity through ligand-gated channels. By analogy, excitatory postsynaptic potentials (EPSPs) are induced by ligand-gated cation channels. Transmitter release from presynaptic vesicles is triggered by Ca^{2+} influx through voltage-operated Ca^{2+} channels that are activated by action potentials (stimulus-secretion coupling).

channels have been shown to be sensitive targets for volatile anaesthetics.[12] Rat brain IIA channels expressed in Chinese hamster ovary (CHO) cells were suppressed by clinical concentrations of the volatile anaesthetics halothane, sevoflurane, isoflurane, desflurane, diethyl ether and enflurane. This suppression was more pronounced at physiological membrane potentials, and about 50% of the sodium current was suppressed at a resting potential of –60 mV.[12] In contrast, halothane had no, or only minor, effects on Na+ currents of bovine chromaffin cells.[13] Only concentrations well beyond the clinical range (> 1.42 mM) resulted in a potential-independent reduction of Na+ inward currents.

Ion flux through veratridine modified Na+ channels of neuroblastoma cells and voltage-gated Na+ channels of synaptosomes (a subcellular fraction of pinched off nerve terminals), were inhibited by propofol, with half-maximal inhibition (IC_{50}) at 31 µM and 8.9 µM, respectively.[14,15] Propofol and pentobarbitone have been reported to affect human brain Na+ channels in anaesthesia-relevant concentrations in planar lipid bilayers, where a voltage-independent reduction in channel open time could be seen.[16] Racemic ketamine had no apparent effect at clinically relevant concentrations in this system.[17]

Nevertheless, as already shown at the beginning of this century, the impulse conduction in mammalian or amphibian axons remains largely unaffected by most anaesthetics at clinical dose.[18,19] This may be due to the high 'safety factor' which ensures AP propagation even at depressed Na+ channel function.[20] Due to this safety factor, the inhibition of Na+ channels should primarily lead to changes in neuronal firing threshold and less to an impairment of AP propagation. Indeed, such an elevation of the neuronal firing threshold was produced by volatile anaesthetics.[21]

K+ channels

Action potentials are terminated by repolarizing K^+ currents. K^+ channels determine the length and shape of an AP, influence the firing frequency and set the resting potential of the neurone. Thus, K^+ channels are essential for propagation and processing of signals within neuronal networks (Fig. 2).

Inhibition of Kv2.1 delayed rectifier channels by ketamine and halothane was reported.[22] Other investigators found an inhibition of voltage-gated K^+ channels at high concentrations of ketamine.[23] Supraclinical concentrations of i.v. anaesthetics have been shown to inhibit axonal K^+ channels of frog sciatic nerve.[19] Summarizing these data, general anaesthetics apparently inhibit, rather than activate, voltage-gated K^+ channels in the neurone. This is in contrast to what would be expected to produce decreased neuronal excitability.

K^+ channels, which are not voltage gated and mainly determine the normal resting potential, may contribute to the anaesthetic action. Such channels are the inward rectifier and a potential-independent flickering K^+ channel that have been shown to be blocked by general anaesthetics; but again only supraclinical concentrations were effective.[24,23] Calcium-activated K^+ channels in cultured rat glioma C6 cells were inhibited by clinical concentrations of four volatile anaesthetics. As suggested by the authors, the anaesthetic inhibition of these channels may contribute to general anaesthesia by interfering with the spatial buffering of K^+ ions performed by these non-neuronal cells.[25] In ganglia of *Lymnaea stagnalis*, a pulmonate snail, a K^+ current was found to be triggered by anaesthetics and was, therefore, named $I_{K(An)}$.[26] When activated, this conductance was able to terminate spontaneous firing of certain neurones. Although the existence of such channels in mammals is absolutely unclear, the large group of K^+ channels remains a potential target of general anaesthetic action worthy to be investigated in the future.

Voltage-operated Ca2+ channels (VOCC)

Voltage-operated Ca^{2+} channels (VOCC) represent the predominant cellular Ca^{2+} entry mechanism and their functional properties and spatial distribution are major determinants of neurotransmitter release.[27,28] T type channels appear to be involved in regulating the rhythmic bursting activity and action potential firing patterns.[29] N, Q and P type channels are thought to be mainly responsible for neurotransmitter release, but also some contribution of the L type channel cannot be ruled out.[30] T and P type channels are mainly expressed in the cell bodies, whereas channels of the L, N and Q types can be detected in axonal terminals of neurosecretory cells.[31] This heterogeneity highlights the complex regulation of Ca^{2+}-dependent stimulus-secretion coupling that is still not very well understood.

In different cell lines T, L and N type channels experience a reduction by volatile anaesthetics.[13,32–34] Methohexitone and methoxyflurane produce a Ca^{2+} current decrease of 20–30% at relevant concentrations, but halothane and etomidate have only minor effects at clinical concentrations.[35] In accordance with these findings is the decreased Ca^{2+} influx in cultured rat hippocampal neurones with methohexitone following depolarization of the cells, but in this system halothane, isoflurane and enflurane showed less pronounced effects. T, L, N and probably P type channels of rat hippocampal pyramidal neurones

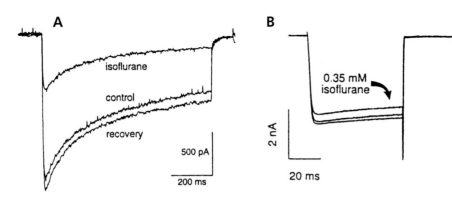

Fig. 3 **(A)** Isoflurane reversibly inhibits whole cell calcium currents composed of T, L and N type channels in hippocampal neurones. Cells were exposed to buffer solution equilibrated with isoflurane (2.5% atm). With permission from *Anesthesiology*.[37] **(B)** P type Ca^{2+} channels of dissociated cerebellar Purkinje neurones were found to be relatively insensitive to a variety of general anaesthetics including isoflurane. Note the lower concentration of isoflurane (0.35 mM vs approx. 1.4 mM) compared to (A). With permission from *Anesthesiology*.[38]

proved sensitive to isoflurane, but only minor effects of various anaesthetics on P type channels of Purkinje neurones were found when low clinical concentrations of anaesthetics were administered (Fig. 3).[37,38]

As long as the role of the various subtypes in the process of synaptic transmission remains unclear, however, it is difficult to assess the involvement of VOCC in the state of anaesthesia.[6,7,27,28]

Synaptic transmitter release and re-uptake

Various degrees of reduction in presynaptic release of excitatory transmitters have been described that may contribute more or less to the anaesthetic state, depending on the respective drug.[8] Anaesthetic effects on the secretion of the inhibitory amino acid GABA were controversially discussed.[3,8] Recently, a study using synaptosomes from rat striatum showed that halothane and isoflurane differentially act on the presynaptic cholinergic regulation of the release of dopamine and GABA.[39] These results suggest that the complex cholinergic control of synaptic inhibition may also represent an important presynaptic target for volatile anaesthetics which may influence synaptic inhibition in an indirect manner.

Investigations of cerebrocortical synaptosomes provided direct evidence for a presynaptic effect of halothane, isoflurane, enflurane and propofol, but not pento-barbitone, on glutamate release evoked by Na^+ channel-dependent stimuli.[15,40] This was interpreted as a blocking effect on presynaptic Na^+ channels, but a Ca^{2+} channel-mediated mechanism cannot be completely ruled out. Glutamate release has also been shown to be depressed from mouse hippocampal cells though the underlying molecular mechanism remains unclear.[41]

Released neurotransmitters are cleared from the synaptic cleft either by cleavage of the transmitter molecule (e.g. acetylcholine) or by re-uptake into the presynaptic terminal. Both processes result in the termination of synaptic transmission and may, therefore, theoretically be regarded as potential targets of general anaesthetics. Recent studies have demonstrated an increased uptake of glutamate,[42,43] but not of GABA, in the presence of volatile anaesthetics.[43] Interestingly, the glutamate transporter is stimulated by protein kinase C (PKC) and PKC has been shown to be activated by halothane.[44,45] Other carrier mechanisms that have been investigated so far were inhibited rather than stimulated by general anaesthetics.[46–48] A mechanism potentially relevant to the state of anaesthesia could be the resulting desensitization of the postsynaptic receptor. Desensitization of the receptor could reduce the ability to evoke postsynaptic potentials and would, thereby, alter synaptic transmission.

Choline uptake, which is the rate limiting step in ACh resynthesis, was also impaired at high concentrations of volatile anaesthetics.[49] This may lead to a presynaptic depletion of neurotransmitters and could finally result in an impairment of synaptic transmission. The potential role of these effects for anaesthesia remains to be elucidated.

Ligand-gated ion channels

Ligand-gated channels of the postsynaptic membrane have a common overall design as revealed by molecular cloning. Based on the homology of sequences, ligand-gated channels can be divided into two super families: glutamate receptors (NMDA [N-methyl-D-aspartate] and non-NMDA receptors) and nicotinic acetylcholine, 5-hydroxytryptamine, GABA and glycine receptors.

Nicotinic acetylcholine receptor (nAChR)

The nicotinic acetylcholine receptor of the neuromuscular junction is the most thoroughly studied ligand-gated ion channel.[50] Thus, it is not surprising that a major part of experimental work on anaesthetic mechanisms has been done with this receptor. However, the relevance of such studies to the potential mechanisms of anaesthesia is limited, as the subunit composition of the muscle receptor differs from that found in the brain. In fact, neuronal nAChRs seem to be more sensitive to anaesthetics than the muscle isoforms.[51,52] Nevertheless, the muscular nAChR is considered a reasonable molecular model of direct interactions of anaesthetic molecules with receptors. Forman and colleagues[53] found that specific mutations in the pore forming M2 domain enhanced the sensitivity of the receptor to isoflurane, suggesting a discrete binding site of the anaesthetic molecule at the channel protein. The stereospecific action of isoflurane on the neuronal nAChR of *Lymnaea stagnalis* is in accordance with this finding.[54] The binding of halothane to the hydrophobic interior of a synthetic tetra-α-helix bundle protein also suggests a possible interaction of volatile anaesthetics with the pore of ion channels, but direct photoaffinity labelling of a nAChR from *Torpedo* showed the incorporation of halothane not in the pore but at the lipid-protein interphase of the transmembrane sequences.[55,56] Allosteric modulation of the channel, rather than competitive inhibition, could then account for impaired channel function.

Volatile anaesthetics (enflurane, isoflurane, halothane and methoxyflurane) as well as the i.v. anaesthetics (ketamine and propofol) significantly decreased the open time of acetylcholine-activated nAChRs without altering single

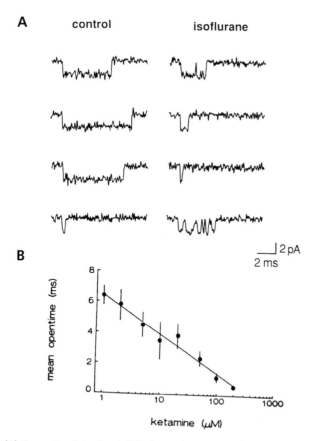

A   control   isoflurane

⌐⌐ 2 pA
2 ms

B

Fig. 4 (A) Currents of single nAChR channels measured with the patch clamp method. Currents were activated by 250 nM acetylcholine. Isoflurane (1.1% atm) induced shorter channel openings that appeared grouped together in bursts. Similar changes were observed with halothane. Downward deflections of the traces show channel openings. (With permission from Wachtel RE, Wegrzynowicz ES. Ann NY Acad Sci 1991; 625: 116–128.) (B) Reduction of mean open times of the nACh channel by increasing concentrations of ketamine. (With permission from Wachtel RE. Anesthesiology 1988; 68: 563–570.)

channel conductivity (Fig. 4).[57,58] This effect occurred at clinical concentrations and may be explained by an open channel block, with the anaesthetic molecules binding to the open pore of the receptor and obstructing the channel. Immediately after binding, the anaesthetics dissociate away from the pore again, allowing ions to pass through the open channel. Ether reduced the apparent current amplitude of nAChR channels, whereas isoflurane induced flickering (Fig. 4A); propofol, as well as ketamine, decreased the channel open time (Fig. 4B). A proposed 'unitary' mechanism for this phenomenon can be deduced from the open channel block hypothesis, which postulates that various anaesthetics act on different time scales.[59] Ether is assumed to be a fast blocker, but the time resolution of standard electrophysiological techniques is assumed to be insufficient to completely resolve single channel blocking events. In this respect, propofol would be a slow and isoflurane an intermediate channel blocker. The model requires the direct binding of the anaesthetic molecules to the channel and thus supports the idea of a specific anaesthetic interaction with certain receptor sites.

Subunit composition obviously affects the sensitivity of nAChRs to anaesthetics. When expressed in *Xenopus* oocytes, the muscle isoform of the nAChR is relatively insensitive, whereas neuronal isoforms are not.[52] In this experimental approach, the neuronal nAChRs are approximately 30 times more sensitive to volatile anaesthetics (IC_{50} is 0.1–0.3 MAC for halothane, isoflurane and sevoflurane) and 10 times more sensitive to propofol ($IC_{50} = 1.3$ µM) than the muscle form. In bovine chromaffin cells, which express a neuronal form of the nAChR, the carbachol-induced catecholamine secretion was inhibited by halothane with an IC_{50} close to one MAC.[60]

Whether or not the sensitivity of heterologously expressed neuronal nAChRs may be relevant to anaesthesia has to be proven in more physiological preparations, and the discrepancy of the experimental findings with other in vitro systems still awaits clarification. Moreover, the relative role of nAChR in the CNS is still a matter of debate, but the physiological importance of these receptors is underscored by their wide distribution within the CNS.[61,62] Another, maybe even more important, aspect of these studies is the fact that a specific interaction of general anaesthetics with a distinct functional membrane protein could be clearly shown. Although this does not prove a direct interaction with receptor protein as the principal mechanism of general anaesthetics, these findings at least point to it as a more than theoretical possibility.

Glutamate receptors

One of the major excitatory neurotransmitters in the mammalian brain is the amino acid glutamate. Its receptors can be divided into four subgroups, three of them being ionotropic receptors, one belonging to the seven helix receptor family which couples to G proteins. According to their agonist sensitivity, ionotropic glutamate receptors are classified into kainate and AMPA (also designated as non-NMDA receptors) and the NMDA receptor.

These channels conduct Na^+ and K^+, while the NMDA receptor channel also conducts Ca^{2+} ions. In contrast to AMPA receptors, the NMDA receptor has a binding site for Mg^{2+} which blocks the channel at the resting potential of the cell, but dissociates and gives free passage to cations when the cell becomes depolarized. NMDA receptors always exist in the neighbourhood of other excitatory ion channels. Their physiological role resembles more that of a voltage-operated Ca^{2+} channel than that of an excitatory receptor channel, as they do not contribute substantially to the generation of EPSP. Especially NMDA receptors are thought to play an essential role in long term potentiation and learning.

The AMPA and kainate receptors are weakly inhibited by volatile anaesthetics, but show a remarkably high sensitivity to ethanol. The inhibition of receptors expressed in *Xenopus* oocytes occurred at concentrations of ethanol as low as 100 mM.[63] It is of note that this study also showed that inhalational anaesthetics slightly reduced AMPA currents in *Xenopus* oocytes, but enhanced the response to kainate. In contrast, other investigators found that both kainate and AMPA receptors from brain mRNA expressed in the same system were inhibited by two MAC of enflurane to about 30%.[64] This

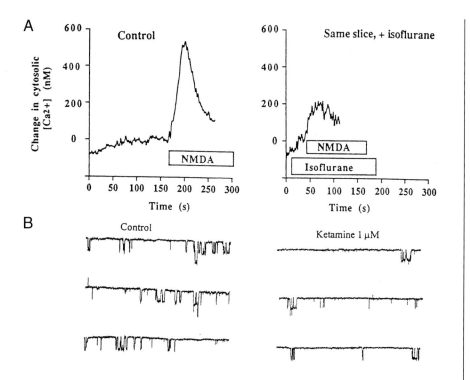

A

Fig. 5 (A) NMDA-evoked Ca^{2+} influx in rat cortical neurones. Isoflurane (1.16 MAC) reduced cytosolic Ca^{2+} rise by 60%. With permission from *Anesthesiology*.[74] **(B)** NMDA-evoked single channel inward currents from cultured hippocampal neurones. Inhibition by ketamine. With permission from *Anesthesiology*.[72]

discrepancy may reflect a different subunit composition of expressed receptors, but also possible influences of other proteins that were co-expressed in this model system.

In summary, the studies of recombinant receptors suggest that the sensitivity of AMPA and kainate receptors to anaesthetics does not play a primary role in anaesthetic action. Ketamine, for instance, does not inhibit the monosynaptic reflex which is mediated by non-NMDA glutamate receptors in the isolated rat spinal cord.[65] The fact that the MAC of halothane could be reduced by about 60% in rats when a selective AMPA receptor antagonist was co-administered during anaesthesia is not sufficient to argue for a role of this receptor in the state of anaesthesia, since the observed effects might be the net result of two independent actions supplementing each other.[66]

NMDA receptor blockade by ketamine is well established and the anaesthetic effect of this phencyclidine derivative is believed to be mainly a result of inhibition of excitatory pathways.[65–71] Two distinct mechanisms have been postulated by which ketamine may block NMDA channels: (i) blocking the open channel and, thereby, reducing channel mean open time without influencing channel conductance; and (ii) a decrease in the frequency of channel openings by an allosteric mechanism, when ketamine gains access to the channel via a hydrophobic pathway (Fig. 5B).[72] Blocking concentrations of ketamine are reported in the range 0.43–10 µM, which can easily be achieved during anaesthesia.[72] Antagonist blocking sites have been investigated by using site-directed mutagenesis, and the NMDA binding site responsible for blocking the pore was found to be near the Mg^{2+} site at the putative transmembrane domain.[73]

Whereas there is no doubt about the specific interaction of ketamine with the NMDA receptor, its implications on the mechanism of ketamine anaesthesia are still under debate.[69,71] Recently, the NMDA receptor was also shown to be a target for other general anaesthetics. Isoflurane (1.16 MAC) inhibited the glutamate and NMDA-evoked Ca^{2+} rise in murine cortex slices (Fig. 5A).[74] In single channel experiments, 1 MAC isoflurane decreased the open probability of the channels to about 80%.[75] Enflurane at high concentrations (2–3 MAC) is also able to inhibit NMDA-induced currents, whereas pentobarbitone had no effects in mice.[7,64] Thus, with the exception of ketamine, a potential involvement of NMDA receptors in general anaesthesia remains more or less speculative. NMDA receptors, however, may contribute to the analgesic effects of certain general anaesthetics.[27,28]

GABA$_A$ receptor

The inhibitory GABA$_A$ and glycine receptor channels conduct Cl^- ions that prevent the membrane from reaching threshold potential because of the low equilibrium potential of Cl^- (–60 to –70 mV). Inhibitory channels transiently change the passive membrane properties of the cell by reducing its membrane resistance and, therefore, shortcut a synaptic potential (shunting action of inhibition).

As inhibition of synaptic transmission in the mammalian CNS is mainly mediated by GABA$_A$ receptors, one would expect GABA-ergic transmission to be potentiated by anaesthetics. In fact this is true for virtually all anaesthetics tested so far. In addition, the half-maximal effects on GABA stimulated $^{36}Cl^-$ flux significantly correlate with anaesthetic potencies.[76] The degree of potentiation of GABA-induced Cl^- currents, however, is not uniform, and ketamine has less effect than barbiturates, benzodiazepines, and even volatile agents (Fig. 6A).[64] In recent years, the stimulating effect of volatile anaesthetics on this receptor protein have been demonstrated in more detail.[77–79] Anaesthetics increase inhibitory postsynaptic currents by increasing the open time and the frequency of channel openings rather than by affecting single channel conductivity (Fig. 6B).[80] The affinity of GABA to the receptor seems to be increased by anaesthetics leading to higher sensitivity of the receptor for its natural agonist. As a result, the channel opens at lower concentrations of GABA. In vitro investigations on channels expressed in *Xenopus* oocytes showed that currents induced by high concentrations of GABA largely remained unchanged;[81] with enflurane, even a slight inhibition occurred at saturating GABA concentrations. Thus, depending on the GABA concentration, an enhancement in GABA activity could be observed at clinical concentrations of general anaesthetics.

Increased GABA affinity would result in prolonged occupation of the GABA receptor during stimulation of an inhibitory synapse. In accordance with these findings, volatile anaesthetics have been shown to prolong inhibitory postsynaptic currents up to 400% in cultured rat hippocampal

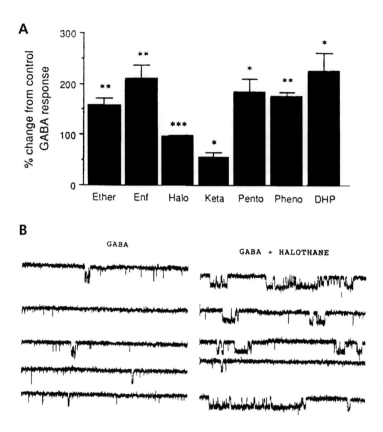

Fig. 6 **(A)** Enhancement of GABA-activated Cl⁻ currents in *Xenopus* oocytes expressing mouse cortical mRNA. Ether, 39 mM diethyl ether; Enf, 1.78 mM enflurane; Halo, 0.81 mM halothane; Keta, 365 μM ketamine; Pento, 30 μM pentobarbital; Pheno, 300 μM phenobarbital; DHP, 300 nM 3α-OH-5α-dihydroprogesterone. Concentration of volatile anaesthetics is 1.8–2.0-fold of MAC. GABA was 5–10 μM. With permission from *FASEB Journal*.[64] **(B)** Single channel currents recorded from GABA$_A$ receptor channels activated by 10 μM GABA. Halothane at a concentration of 2 MAC increased GABA-activated channel activity by prolonging the open times and promoted bursting activity without changing the single channel current (Yeh JZ et al. Ann NY Acad Sci 1991; 625: 155–173).

neurones.[82] The increased duration of postsynaptic potentials is thought to make an important contribution to the state of anaesthesia, and also the lack of effect observed with certain non-anaesthetic fluorinated hydrocarbons suggests a role of GABA in general anaesthesia.[63] The influence of subunit composition on receptor sensitivity to general anaesthetic actions is remarkably small. To date at least six α, four β, four g, one δ, one ε and three ρ subunits have been found in mammalian CNS, with each subunit exhibiting a distinct pattern of cerebral distribution. The α to ε subunits probably form heteropentameric complexes in different combinations giving functional GABA$_A$ receptors. In contrast, ρ subunits form homo-oligomeric channels, which resemble GABA$_C$ receptors in their properties and are insensitive to the anaesthetics pentobarbitone, alphaxalone, or propofol. No distinct type of subunit is obligatory for the action of anaesthetics on the heteromeric GABA$_A$ receptors.[63] However, a newly described ε subunit has been reported to confer anaesthetic resistance to $GABA_A$ receptor molecules containing α and β subunits, but these findings still need further confirmation.[84]

A potential role of $GABA_A$ receptors in mediating actions of various anaesthetic drugs was also supported by pharmacogenetic studies: mice bred selectively for sensitivity or resistance to diazepam also showed analogous changes in their sensitivities to halothane or phenobarbitone. Diazepam-sensitive mice expressed GABA receptors that also showed augmented Cl^- flux in the presence of the two general anaesthetics.[85] A different pharmacogenetic approach was used by Homanics and colleagues who tried to assess the role of the $\alpha6$ subunit of the GABA receptor for anaesthesia.[86] Interestingly, gene knock out of this subunit did not affect the animals' response to various anaesthetics. However, the interpretation of such experiments may be hampered by unforeseen compensatory mechanisms that could account for the observed lack of effect on anaesthetic sensitivity. Nevertheless, valuable insights can be expected from the genetic approach in the future, not only with respect to anaesthesia but also to the physiological relevance of certain gene products for the state of consciousness.

Second messenger pathways

Second messenger pathways are substantially involved in synaptic transmission and may, therefore, represent potential targets for general anaesthetics. To date, however, only second messenger calcium ($[Ca^{2+}]_i$) has proven to be sensitive to the action of general anaesthetics, whereas inconclusive results have been reported on G proteins, protein kinase C and cyclic nucleotides.[6,27,28]

Intracellular free calcium

In the neurone, calcium mediates not only synaptic transmitter secretion (stimulus-secretion coupling) but regulates also the activities of certain Ca^{2+}-dependent potassium channels, key enzymes (phospholipase A_2, phospholipase C), and protein kinases. The low intracellular Ca^{2+} concentration is maintained by extrusion from the cytoplasm with the help of ATP-driven Ca^{2+} pumps (membrane Ca^{2+}-ATPase) and the Na^+/Ca^{2+} exchanger which is driven by the Na^+ concentration gradient. Since cytoplasmic calcium comes either from outside the cell or from intracellular sources, its complex regulation can be described as the net result of inward (transmembrane influx, intracellular release) or outward cytoplasmic shift (cellular extrusion, uptake into intracellular stores).[27,28] Both calcium shifts have been shown to be more or less sensitive to general anaesthetics supporting the view that intraneuronal calcium homoeostasis may be a potential mechanism of anaesthetic action ('calcium hypothesis').[27,28,36]

In neurones, intracellular Ca^{2+} release is triggered by inositol 1,4,5-trisphosphate (IP_3) which is produced by the membrane-associated enzyme phospholipase C. This phosphoinositol pathway represents a major mechanism of signal transduction in neurones and is, therefore, a potential target site of anaesthetics. Most general anaesthetics enhance the spontaneous leak from IP_3-sensitive calcium stores in neural tissues and glial cells.[87] Receptor-stimulated calcium release from IP_3-sensitive stores, however, was reported to be inhibited by volatile anaesthetics and octanol in certain neurosecretory cells, but this was not a constant finding with other neuronal cell lines (e.g. PC12).[6,27,28,34] Conflicting data also exist on the direct effects of anaesthetics on IP_3 generation. Whereas neuronal inositol pathways were well preserved or even enhanced in the presence of volatile anaesthetics, in non-neuronal tissues both stimulatory and inhibitory actions of halothane and alkanols have been observed.[6,28] Thus, a direct role of IP_3 for anaesthetic-induced effects on cytoplasmic calcium release is unclear.

In recent years, the effects of general anaesthetics on plasma membrane Ca^{2+}-ATPase came into focus, when its suppression by some anaesthetics could be shown.[88,89] Beside the fact that Ca^{2+}-ATPase is considered only a fine tuner of cytoplasmic Ca^{2+} concentration, because it is not a fast, high capacity system able to transport large amounts of Ca^{2+}, its actual role in setting basal intracellular Ca^{2+} level in the neurone still remains to be defined.[36] Although favoured by its protagonists as a cellular mechanism of general anaesthesia, inhibition of Ca^{2+}-ATPase does not fulfil the criteria of a major molecular mechanism of general anaesthetics.[36]

Also the fast, high capacity process of transmembrane Na^+/Ca^{2+} exchange, which was affected by volatile agents in cardiac cells, remained largely unaffected in synaptosome preparations.[88] Similarly, the Ca^{2+}-ATPase mediated uptake of cytosolic calcium into intracellular calcium stores of synaptosomes and intact neurosecretory cells was not influenced by halothane, isoflurane, ketamine or octanol.[28,36]

As proposed by the 'calcium hypothesis of anaesthesia', key target proteins of the neurone may be influenced by alterations of cytoplasmic calcium caused by general anaesthetics.[36] The resulting elevation of the resting $[Ca^{2+}]_i$ could: (i) activate Ca^{2+}-dependent K^+-channels, which would hyperpolarize the cell membrane; and/or (ii) augment $GABA_A$ receptor-mediated inhibition. Both effects could contribute to the state of anaesthesia.[27,28] However, there is not sufficient evidence for such a role of intracellular calcium in anaesthesia. Unlike the case in non-neuronal tissues, an increase in resting $[Ca^{2+}]_i$ is not a constant finding with volatile anaesthetics in neurones. Moreover, increased $[Ca^{2+}]_i$ is not required for the modulatory action of anaesthetics on the $GABA_A$ channel.[81] Thus, a major role of increased cytoplasmic calcium as a mechanism of anaesthesia remains uncertain.[6,27,28,36]

Key points

- To date, no unique pivotal macroscopic or microscopic site of general anaesthetic action has been identified within the brain.

- Synaptic transmission, rather than axonal impulse conduction, is affected by general anaesthetics.

- Anaesthetics are found to be selective in their actions at a cellular and molecular level.

- General anaesthetics differ in their effects on distinct neuronal processes and even their isomers do so. Thus, a non-specific 'unitary mechanism' is unlikely.

Key points (continued)

- There is, however, a broad consensus as to a drug-specific pattern of multimodal cellular and subcellular actions that would finally result in the state of anaesthesia.

- The role of second messenger pathways for general anaesthesia remains unclear, though intraneuronal Ca^{2+} homoeostasis is affected by many agents ('calcium hypothesis of anaesthesia').

- Certain voltage-operated Ca^{2+} channels, but also other voltage-gated ion channels, may be involved in anaesthetic inhibition of transmitter release.

- Ligand-gated ion channels ($GABA_A$, nicotinic acetylcholine, and glutamate receptors) are most promising candidates for postsynaptic, anaesthesia relevant neuronal target sites.

- Based on current evidence, proteins and not lipids are considered the primary targets of general anaesthetics. But it is premature to look for a definite answer.

ACKNOWLEDGEMENT

The excellent secretarial help of Ms Ulrike Kropp is gratefully acknowledged by the authors.

References

1. Prys-Roberts C. Anaesthesia: a practical or impractical construct? Br J Anaesth 1987; 59: 1341–1345
2. Angel A. Central neuronal pathways and the process of anaesthesia. Br J Anaesth 1993; 71: 148–163
3. Richards C D. The mechanisms of general anaesthesia. In: Norman J, Whitwam J. (eds) Topical Reviews in Anaesthesia, Vol. 1. Bristol: John Wright, 1980: 1–84
4. Alkire M T, Haier R J, Barker S J, Shah N K, Wu J C, Kao Y J. Cerebral metabolism during propofol anesthesia in humans studied with positron emission tomography. Anesthesiology 1995; 82: 393–403
5. Alkire M T, Haier R J, Shah N K, Anderson C. Positron emission tomography study of regional cerebral metabolism in humans during isoflurane anesthesia. Anesthesiology 1997; 86: 549–557
6. Franks N P, Lieb W R. Selective actions of volatile general anaesthetics at molecular and cellular levels. Br J Anaesth 1993; 71: 65–76
7. Franks N P, Lieb W R. Molecular and cellular mechanisms of general anaesthesia. Nature 1994; 367: 607–614
8. Richards C D. The synaptic basis of general anaesthesia. Eur J Anaesthesiol 1995; 12: 5–19
9. Urban B W. Order despite a multitude of molecular anaesthetic actions. Eur J Anaesthesiol 1995; 12: 1–4
10. Elliott J R, Urban B W. Integrative effects of general anaesthetics: why nerve axons should not be ignored. Eur J Anaesthesiol 1995; 12: 41–50
11. Urban B W. Differential effects of gaseous and volatile anaesthetics on sodium and potassium channels. Br J Anaesth 1993; 71: 25–38

12. Rehberg B, Xiao Y H, Duch D S. Central nervous system sodium channels are significantly suppressed at clinical concentrations of volatile anesthetics. Anesthesiology 1996; 84: 1223–1233

13. Pancrazio J J, Park W K, Lynch III C. Inhalational anesthetic actions on voltage gated ion currents of bovine adrenal chromaffin cells. Mol Pharmacol 1993; 43: 783–794

14. Barann M, Göthert M, Fink K, Bönisch H. Inhibition by anaesthetics of ^{14}C-guanidinium flux through the voltage-gated sodium channel and the cation channel of the 5-HT$_3$ receptor of N1E-115 neuroblastoma cells. Naunyn-Schmiedeberg's Arch Pharmacol 1993; 347: 125–132

15. Ratnakumari L, Hemmings H C. Effects of propofol on sodium channel-dependent sodium influx and glutamate release in rat cerebrocortical synaptosomes. Anesthesiology 1997; 86: 428–439

16. Frenkel C, Duch D S, Urban B W. Effects of i.v. anaesthetics on human brain sodium channels. Br J Anaesth 1993; 71: 15–24

17. Frenkel C, Urban B W. Molecular actions of racemic ketamine on human CNS sodium channels. Br J Anaesth 1992; 69: 292–297

18. Larrabee M G, Posternak J M. Selective action of anesthetics on synapses and axons in mammalian sympathetic ganglia. J Neurophysiol 1952; 15: 91–114

19. Benoit E. Effects of intravenous anaesthetics on nerve axons. Eur J Anaesthesiol 1995; 12: 59–70

20. Jack J B, Noble T, Tiens R W. Electric Current Flow in Excitable Cells. Oxford: Clarendon, 1983; 306–378

21. Butterworth J F, Raymond S A, Roscoe R F. Effect of halothane and enflurane on firing threshold on frog myelinated axons. J Physiol 1989; 411: 493–516

22. Kulkarni R S, Zorn L J, Anatharam V, Bayley H, Treistman S N. Inhibitory effects of ketamine and halothane on recombinant potassium channels from mammalian brain. Anesthesiology 1996; 84: 900–909

23. Bräu M E, Sander F, Vogel W, Hempelmann G. Blocking mechanism of ketamine and its enantiomers in enzymatically demyelinated peripheral nerve as revealed by single channel experiments. Anesthesiology 1997; 86: 394–404

24. Gibbons S J, Núñez Hernandez R, Mazé G, Harrison N L. Inhibition of a fast inwardly rectifying potassium conductance by barbiturates. Anesth Analg 1996; 82: 1242–1246

25. Tas P W L, Kress H G, Koschel K. Volatile anesthetics inhibit the ion flux through Ca^{2+}-activated K^+ channels of rat glioma C6 cells. Biochim Biophys Acta 1989; 983: 264–268

26. Franks N P, Lieb W R. Volatile general anaesthetics activate a novel neuronal K^+ current. Nature 1988; 333: 662–664

27. Kress H G, Tas P W L. Effects of volatile anaesthetics on second messenger Ca^{2+} in neurones and non-muscular cells. Br J Anaesth 1993; 71: 47–58

28. Kress H G. Effects of general anaesthetics on second messenger systems. Eur J Anaesthesiol 1995; 12: 83–97

29. Bertolino M, Llinas R R. The central role of voltage-activated and receptor operated calcium channels in neuronal cells. Annu Rev Pharmacol Toxicol 1992; 32: 399–421

30. O'Regan M H, Kocsis J D, Waxman S G. Depolarization-dependent actions of dihydropyridines on synaptic transmission in the in vitro rat hippocampus. Brain Res 1990; 527: 181–191

31. Fisher T E, Bourque C W. Calcium-channel subtypes in the somata and axon terminals of magnocellular neurosecretory cells. Trends Neurosci 1996; 19: 440–444

32. McDowell T S, Pancrazio J J, Lynch III C. Volatile anesthetics reduce low-voltage activated calcium currents in a thyroid C-cell line. Anesthesiology 1996; 85: 1167–1175

33. Kress H G, Eckhardt-Wallasch H, Tas P W L, Koschel K. Volatile anesthetics depress the depolarization-induced cytoplasmic calcium rise in PC12 cells. FEBS Lett 1987; 221: 28–32

34. Kress H G, Müller J, Eisert A, Gilge U, Tas P W L, Koschel K. Effects of volatile anesthetics on cytoplasmic Ca^{2+} signalling and transmitter release in a neural cell line. Anesthesiology 1991; 74: 309–319

35. Charlesworth P, Pocock G, Richards C D. Calcium channel currents in bovine adrenal chromaffin cells and their modulation by anaesthetic agents. J Physiol 1994; 481: 543–553

36. Bleakman D, Jones M V, Harrison N L. The effect of four general anesthetics on intra-cellular $[Ca^{2+}]$ in cultured rat hippocampal neurons. Neuropharmacology 1995; 34: 541–551

37. Study R E. Isoflurane inhibits multiple voltage-gated calcium currents in hippocampal pyramidal neurons. Anesthesiology 1994; 81: 104–116

38. Hall A C, Lieb W R, Franks N P. Insensitivity of P-type calcium channels to inhalational and intravenous general anesthetics. Anesthesiology 1994; 81: 117–123

39. Salord F, Kaita H, Lecharny J B, Henzel D, Desmonts J M, Mantz J. Halothane and isoflurane differentially affect the regulation of dopamine and gamma-aminobutyric acid release mediated by presynaptic acetylcholine receptors in the rat striatum. Anesthesiology 1997; 86: 632–641

40. Schlame M, Hemmings H C. Inhibition by volatile anesthetics of endogenous glutamate release from synaptosomes by a presynaptic mechanism. Anesthesiology 1995; 82: 1406–1416

41. Perouansky M, Baranov D, Salman M, Yaari Y. Effects of halothane on glutamate receptor-mediated excitatory postsynaptic currents. Anesthesiology 1995; 83: 109–119

42. Larsen M, Hegstad J, Berg-Johnsen B, Langmoen I A. Isoflurane increases the uptake of glutamate in synaptosomes from rat cerebral cortex. Br J Anaesth 1997; 78: 55–59

43. Miyazaki H, Nakamura Y, Arai T, Kataoka K. Increase of glutamate uptake in astrocytes: a possible mechanism of action of volatile anesthetics. Anesthesiology 1997; 86: 1359–1366

44. Casado M, Bendahan A, Zafra F et al. Phosphorylation and modulation of brain glutamate transporters by protein kinase C. J Biol Chem 1993; 268: 27313–27317

45. Hemmings H C, Adamo A I B. Effects of halothane and propofol on purified brain protein kinase C activation. Anesthesiology 1994; 81: 147–155

46. Tas P W L, Kress H G, Koschel K. Volatile Anaesthetika und n-Alkanole hemmen die Aufnahme von Noradrenalin in Phäochromozytom-Zellen. Anaesthesist 1987; 36: 340–344

47. Kress H G, Schömig E. Methoxyfluran und Ethanol hemmen die neuronale Noradrenalin-Aufnahme (Uptake1) nicht an der Desipramin-Bindungsstelle. Anaesthesist 1990; 39: 371–374

48. Griffiths R, Norman I. Effects of anaesthetics on uptake, synthesis and release of transmitters. Br J Anaesth 1993; 71: 96–107

49. Griffiths R, Greiff J M, Boyle E, Rowbotham D J, Norman R I. Volatile anesthetic agents inhibit choline uptake into rat synaptosomes. Anesthesiology 1994; 81: 953–958

50. Unwin N. Neurotransmitter action: opening of ligand-gated ion channels. Cell 1993; 72 (Suppl.): 31–41

51. Flood P, Ramirez Latorre J, Role L. α4β2 neuronal nicotinic acetylcholine receptors in the central nervous system are inhibited by isoflurane and propofol, but α7-type nicotinic acetylcholine receptors are unaffected. Anesthesiology 1997; 86: 859–865

52. Violet J M, Downie D L, Nakisa R C, Lieb W R, Franks N P. Differential sensitivities of mammalian neuronal and muscle nicotinic acetylcholine receptors to general anesthetics. Anesthesiology 1997; 86: 866–874

53. Forman S A, Miller K W, Yellen G. A discrete site for general anesthetics on a postsynaptic receptor. Mol Pharmacol 1995; 48: 574–581

54. Franks N P, Lieb W R. Stereospecific effects of inhalational general anesthetic optical isomers on nerve ion channels. Science 1991; 254: 427–430

55. Johansson J J, Rabanal F, Dutton P L. Binding of the volatile anesthetic halothane to the hydrophobic core of a tetra-α-helix-bundle protein. J Pharmacol Exp Ther 1996; 279: 56–61

56. Eckenhoff R G. An inhalational anesthetic binding domain in the nicotinic acetylcholine receptor. Proc Natl Acad Sci USA 1996; 93: 2807–2810

57. Wachtel R E. Relative potencies of volatile anesthetics in altering the kinetics of ion channels in BC3H1 cells. J Pharmacol Exp Ther 1995; 274: 1355–1361

58. Wachtel R E, Wegrzynowicz E S. Kinetics of nicotinic acetylcholine ion channels in the presence of intravenous anaesthetics and induction agents. Br J Pharmacol 1992; 106: 623–627

59. Dilger J P, Vidal A M, Mody H I, Liu Y. Evidence for direct actions of general anesthetics on an ion channel protein. Anesthesiology 1994; 81: 431–442

60. Pocock G, Richards C D. The action of volatile anaesthetics on stimulus-secretion coupling in bovine adrenal chromaffin cells. Br J Pharmacol 1988; 95: 209–217

61. Sivilotti L, Colquhoun D. Acetylcholine receptors: too many channels, too few functions. Science 1995; 269: 1681–1682

62. Zoli M, Le Novére N, Hill J A, Changeux J P. Developmental regulation of nicotinic ACh receptor subunits in the rat central and peripheral nervous system. J Neurosci 1995; 15: 1912–1939

63. Harris R A, Mihic J S, Dildy Mayfield J E, Machu T K. Actions of anesthetics on ligand-gated ion channels: role of receptor subunit composition. FASEB J 1995; 9: 1454–1462

64. Lin L H, Chen L L, Harris R A. Enflurane inhibits NMDA, AMPA, and kainate-induced currents in *Xenopus* oocytes expressing mouse and human brain mRNA. FASEB J 1993; 7: 479–485

65. Brockmeyer D M, Kendig J J. Selective effects of ketamine on amino-acid mediated pathways in neonatal rat spinal cord. Br J Anaesth 1995; 74: 79–84

66. McFarlane C, Warner D S, Dexter F. Interactions between NMDA and AMPA glutamate receptor antagonists during halothane anesthesia in the rat. Neuropharmacology 1995; 34: 659–663

67. Anis N A, Berry S C, Burton N R, Lodge D. The dissociative anaesthetics, ketamine, and phencyclidine, selectively reduce excitation of central mammalian neurones by N-methyl-D-aspartate. Br J Pharmacol 1983; 79: 565–575

68. Carlá V, Moroni F. General anaesthetics inhibit the responses induced by glutamate receptor agonists in the mouse cortex. Neurosci Lett 1992; 146: 21–24

69. Irifune M, Shimizu T, Nomoto M, Fukuda T. Ketamine-induced anesthesia involves the N-methyl-D-aspartate receptor-channel complex in mice. Brain Res 1992; 596: 1–9

70. Oshima E, Richards C D. An in vitro investigation of the action of ketamine on excitatory synaptic transmission in the hippocampus of the guinea-pig. Eur J Pharmacol 1988; 148: 25–33

71. Kress H G. Wirkmechanismen von Ketamin. Anaesthesist 1997 (Suppl.); 46: S8–S19

72. Orser B A, Pennefather P S, MacDonald J F. Multiple mechanisms of ketamine blockade of N-methyl-D-aspartate receptors. Anesthesiology 1997; 86: 903–917

73. Mori H, Masaki H, Yamakura T, Mishina M. Identification by mutagenesis of a Mg^{2+}-block site of the NMDA receptor channel. Nature 1992; 358: 673–675

74. Bickler P E, Buck L T, Hansen B M. Effects of isoflurane and hypothermia on glutamate receptor-mediated calcium influx in brain slices. Anesthesiology 1994; 81: 1461–1469

75. Yang J, Zorumski C F. Effects of isoflurane on N-methyl-D-aspartate gated ion channels in cultured rat hippocampal neurons. Ann NY Acad Sci 1991; 625: 287–289

76. Huidobro Toro J P, Bleck V, Allen A M, Harris R A. Neurochemical actions of anesthetic drugs on the γ-aminobutyric acid receptor-chloride channel complex. J Pharmacol Exp Ther 1987; 242: 963–969

77. Jones M V, Brooks P A, Harrison N L. Enhancement of γ-aminobutyric acid-activated Cl⁻ currents in cultured rat hippocampal neurons by three volatile anesthetics. J Physiol (Lond) 1992; 449: 279–293

78. Longoni B, Demontis G C, Olsen R W. Enhancement of γ-aminobutyric acid$_A$ receptor function and binding by the volatile anesthetic halothane. J Pharmacol Exp Ther 1993; 266: 153–159

79. Nakahiro M, Yeh J Z, Brunner E, Narahashi T. General anesthetics modulate GABA receptor channel complex in rat dorsal root ganglion neurons. FASEB J 1989; 3: 1850–1854

80. Sieghart W. Structure and pharmacology of γ-aminobutyric acid$_A$ receptor subtypes. Pharmacol Rev 1995; 47: 181–233

81. Lin L H, Chen L L, Zirolli J A, Harris R A. General anesthetics potentiate γ-aminobutyric acid actions on γ-aminobutyric acid$_A$ receptors expressed by *Xenopus* oocytes: lack of involvement of intracellular calcium. J Pharmacol Exp Ther 1992; 263: 569–578

82. Jones M V, Harrison N L. Effects of volatile anesthetics on the kinetics of inhibitory postsynaptic currents in cultured rat hippocampal neurons. J Neurophysiol 1993; 70: 1339–1349

83. Wang T L, Guggino W B, Cutting G R. A novel γ-aminobutyric acid receptor subunit (ρ2) cloned from human retina forms bicuculline-insensitive homo-oligomeric receptors in *Xenopus* oocytes. J Neurosci 1994; 14: 6524–6531

84. Davies P A, Hanna M C, Hales T G, Kirkness E F. Insensitivity to anaesthetic agents conferred by a class of GABA$_A$ receptor subunits. Nature 1997; 385: 820–823

85. Quinlan J J, Gallaher E J, Firestone L L. Halothane's effects on GABA-gated chloride flux in mice selectively bred for sensitivity or resistance on diazepam. Brain Res 1993; 610: 224–228

86. Homanics G E, Ferguson C, Quinlan J J et al. Gene knockout of the α6 subunit of the γ-aminobutyric acid type A receptor: lack of effect on responses to ethanol, pentobarbital, and general anesthetics. Mol Pharmacol 1997; 51: 588–596

87 Hossain M D, Evers A S. Volatile anesthetic-induced efflux of calcium from IP_3-gated stores in clonal (GH_3) pituitary cells. Anesthesiology 1994; 80: 1379–1389

88. Franks J J, Horn J L, Janicki P K, Singli G. Halothane, isoflurane, xenon, and nitrous oxide inhibit calcium ATPase pump activity in rat brain synaptic plasma membranes. Anesthesiology 1995; 82: 108–117

89. Lopez M M, Kosk-Kosicka D. How do volatile anesthetics inhibit Ca^{2+}-ATPase? J Biol Chem 1995; 270: 28239–28245

William C. Bowman

Recent discoveries in neuromuscular transmission

OVERVIEW

Skeletal muscle is innervated by fast-conducting (~100 m.s^{-1}) myelinated A$_\alpha$ nerve fibres that have their cell bodies in the anterior horn cells or in the brain stem. Near its ending, each nerve fibre branches and each branch ends in apposition to a muscle fibre at the neuromuscular junction. A focally-innervated muscle fibre receives only one branch of a nerve fibre at a focus somewhere near its middle. Most mammalian muscles are composed of focally-innervated muscle fibres. A multiply-innervated muscle fibre, common in amphibia and avians and present in a few mammalian muscles (e.g. extra-ocular muscles, some muscles of the oesophagus), receives numerous nerve endings spread over its surface. The nerve fibre, together with the fascicule of muscle fibres that it innervates, is called a motor unit. Physiologically, the motor unit responds as a synchronous unit. Contractions of separate motor units abnormally occurring out of phase with each other are called fasciculations. Fasciculations are indicative of a neuronal origin because the muscle fibres within each unit respond synchronously. Fibrillation occurs when individual fibres contract asynchronously and are indicative of a neuromuscular or muscle fibre abnormality. The number of muscle fibres within a motor unit differs according to the delicacy of movement of which the muscle is capable. For delicate movements (e.g. the muscles of the fingers) the number is small (~15 or so); for crude movements (e.g. the muscles of the back) it is larger (> 100).

The main tenets of the process of neuromuscular transmission have been known for many years. See, for example, a monograph by Katz.[1] Up-to-date information is contained in more recent texts.[2–4] The neurotransmitter,

Professor William C. Bowman PhD DSc FIBiol FRSE FRSA HonFRCA, Department of Physiology and Pharmacology, University of Strathclyde, 204 George Street, Glasgow G1 1XW, UK

acetylcholine, is synthesized in the axoplasm of the nerve endings from choline and acetate under the influence of the enzyme choline acetyltransferase. Choline is transported from the extracellular fluid into the nerve endings by a special choline carrier protein which is capable of being blocked by certain drugs, notably the drugs known as hemicholiniums.[5] About half of the acetylcholine synthesized is loaded into small (~45 nm diameter) vesicles of which there are half a million or more in each nerve ending. The mechanism of loading involves an acetylcholine transporter protein in the vesicular membrane, and this too can be inhibited by drugs, in particular the compound known as vesamicol.[6] Currently, drugs of the hemicholinium and vesamicol types have no therapeutic uses, but this may not always be so.

Acetylcholine is spontaneously released into the junctional gap from the axoplasm by a Ca^{2+}-independent process known as molecular leakage. The concentration in the gap is sufficient to produce a sustained detectable depolarization of the postjunctional membrane but is well below that necessary to initiate the contractile mechanism. Acetylcholine is also released spontaneously from the vesicles (less than 1% of the total spontaneous release) to produce the miniature endplate potentials (MEPPs). Each MEPP is regarded as the effect produced by the acetylcholine contained within one synaptic vesicle. Spontaneous vesicular release is, of course, also far too small to trigger muscle contractions. A nerve impulse leads to the Ca^{2+}-dependent synchronous release of the contents of some hundred or so vesicles which produce the full-sized endplate potential (EPP) that initiates contraction. The contraction evoked by a single nerve impulse is called a twitch. Physiologically, the fine nervous control of muscle is inadequate to permit a single nerve impulse, and hence a twitch, to occur. Instead, bursts of impulses, generally out of phase with each other in separate nerve axons, are conducted to the muscle from the central nervous system. The individual motor units therefore contract at subtetanic frequencies, the contraction of the muscle as a whole being smoothed out because of the asynchrony in the many hundreds of individual motor units.

On traversing the narrow junctional cleft (~60 nm wide at its narrowest), the acetylcholine combines fleetingly with the acetylcholine receptors in the postjunctional membrane of the muscle fibre. At the junctional region, the muscle fibre membrane is thrown into folds. The acetylcholine receptors are located, at a density of around $10\,000/\mu m^2$, on the shoulders of the junctional folds. The rest of the muscle fibre membrane, the sarcolemma, is virtually free from acetylcholine receptors in mature, normally innervated muscle. Henry Dale, in 1914 and subsequent years, observed that some actions of acetylcholine are imitated by the alkaloid muscarine (from a toadstool) and are blocked by atropine, whereas others are imitated by the alkaloid nicotine (from tobacco) and are blocked by tubocurarine. Two main subtypes of acetylcholine receptors are involved and these subsequently came to be called **muscarinic** receptors and **nicotinic** receptors, respectively. The receptors of skeletal muscle belong to the group of nicotinic acetylcholine receptors. Nicotinic receptors belong to the class of transmitter-gated ion channel receptors. Activation of the nicotinic receptors initiates the contractile cycle.

The life time of acetylcholine is fleeting because it is rapidly hydrolysed to inactive choline and acetate by acetylcholinesterase located in the junctional cleft. Most of the acetylcholinesterase is bound to the so-called basement membrane, a collagen-like tangle of material that fills the gap between axon terminal and muscle fibre membrane at the junction. Hence, the acetylcholine, which is released in considerable excess, has to traverse the hurdle of the acetylcholinesterase before reaching the receptors, and some does not reach its goal. Such is the efficiency of the enzyme, that each molecule that does reach a receptor does not survive long enough to make a second receptor interaction.

VESICULAR MEMBRANE PROTEINS AND ACETYLCHOLINE RELEASE

Certain proteins of the vesicular membrane (synaptotagmins, synaptobrevins, synaptophysins, synaptogyrins, rab3A) and of the axoplasmic face of the terminal axon membrane (syntaxin, SNAP-25) play essential roles in the docking, priming, fusion, exocytosis of the contents and reforming of the vesicles, and much research is being devoted to further elucidation of this process which, in its essentials, resembles that of membrane fusions elsewhere.[7-10] SNAP-25 also has a role in axonal growth. Rab3A and associated proteins appear to be responsible for targeting the vesicle to the release site. Synaptotagmin, synaptophysins, and synaptobrevin are some of the integral vesicular membrane proteins involved in the docking of the vesicles at the release sites, in the formation of the fusion pore that allows the escape of the acetylcholine, and possibly in the reforming of the vesicles. The release of vesicular acetylcholine is Ca^{2+}-dependent. The spontaneous vesicular release that gives rise to miniature endplate potentials obtains sufficient Ca^{2+} from internal stores. The much greater release evoked by a nerve impulse is dependent upon extracellular Ca^{2+} which enters the axoplasm mainly through Ca^{2+} channels of the type that are blocked by ω-agatoxin from the American funnel web spider, hence denoting them as P-type calcium channels.[11]

Synaptotagmin and synaptobrevin are Ca^{2+}-binding proteins. When calcium ions enter the terminal axoplasm on the arrival of a nerve impulse, they bind to these proteins and induce a conformational change that allows them, in vesicles already in the immediately available store, to fuse with docking proteins (the syntaxins and SNAP-25) in the active zones of the terminal axonal membrane. Simultaneously with the fusion of the proteins, a pore opens through them and rapidly expands so that the vesicular contents are released into the junctional gap. In the absence of Ca^{2+}, synaptotagmin functions as a 'vesicle clamp', holding the vesicle in a fusion-ready state but blocking release of its contents. Synaptophysin is involved in the formation of the fusion pore. It appears that, under some circumstances, the fusion pore extends with the result that the vesicular membrane temporarily becomes a part of the axon terminal membrane. Vesicular fusion requires a high concentration of Ca^{2+}, yet release of acetylcholine occurs in response to a single nerve impulse. This is possible because the calcium channels responsible for release are located in the active zones so that the local concentration of Ca^{2+} becomes high even after a single nerve impulse. Ca^{2+}-activated K^+ channels are also located close to the calcium channels involved in release.[12] Hence they are strategically located to hyperpolarize the local membrane and switch off transmitter release.

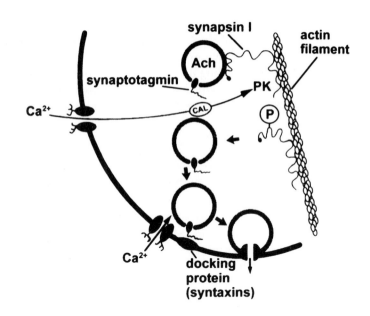

Fig. 2.1 The postulated roles of synapsin I and synaptotagmin in Ca^{2+}-mediated mobilisation and release of vesicular acetylcholine. The membrane calcium channels are opened by the action potential. The channels closely associated with the docking proteins in the active zones provide for a high local concentration of Ca^{2+} which binds to synaptotagmin. This causes synaptotagmin to fuse with the docking proteins. A fusion pore is formed through the combined membranes, enabling the vesicle contents (acetylcholine, ATP, Ca^{2+} and probably a binding protein) to escape into the junctional gap. Synapsin I anchors the reserve vesicles to the cytoskeleton. Ca^{2+} entering the axoplasm combines with calmodulin (CAL) and the combination activates protein kinase II (PK) which in turn phosphorylates synapsin I. This frees the vesicles which are then able to migrate to the active zones. Other proteins (see text) are also important in the targeting and release mechanism.

Synaptotagmin may also be a component of the site in the nerve terminals that acts as an antigen giving rise to the circulating auto-antibody responsible for the Lambert-Eaton myasthenic syndrome.[13]

Synapsin I is a phosphoprotein that forms a cage-like structure around the outside surface of the vesicles. Synapsin I serves to anchor the vesicles in the reserve stores to elements of the cytoskeleton. An additional action of calcium ions on entering the axoplasm, is, after combination with calmodulin, to activate the enzyme calcium/calmodulin-dependent protein kinase II. This enzyme phosphorylates serine residues in the tail region of synapsin I. As a consequence, the binding affinity of synapsin I for the vesicles is greatly reduced, so that they are freed and able to move towards the active zones.[14] Phosphorylation of synapsin I by calcium-activated protein kinases may, therefore, play an important role, not in immediate release or rapid mobilisation of transmitter, but in the slower mobilisation of transmitter necessary to maintain prolonged high outputs during continuous heavy nerve impulse traffic. Since the anchored reserve vesicles are not close to the active zones, opening of additional calcium channels may be necessary to raise the Ca^{2+} concentration of the axoplasm to the level appropriate to activate protein kinase II. Figure 2.1 is a simplified diagram of vesicular exocytosis.

BOTULINUM TOXIN

Botulinum toxin from *Clostridium botulinum* exists in seven polypeptide forms denoted by the letters A to G. These exist in the bacterium in inactive forms in combination with other proteins, but they are released by proteinase enzymes present both in the bacteria and in infected tissues. Each active toxin is a di-chain consisting of a light (50 kDa) and a heavy (100 kDa) component linked together by a disulphide bond. They act to inhibit the release of acetylcholine from peripheral cholinergic nerves and are especially active on somatic motor nerves to skeletal muscle. At the motor nerve endings, 4 steps are necessary for their inhibitory action on acetylcholine release to occur.

1. They bind rapidly and selectively to, as yet, unidentified binding sites on the terminal axon membrane. Probably the different toxins have different binding sites; the C-terminal part of the heavy chain is necessary for binding.

2. The toxin is internalized into an endosome within the axoplasm of the nerve terminal. Here the N-terminal part of the heavy chain plays an essential role.

3. The toxin is translocated into the endosome membrane, an effect which is dependent on acidification of the endosome contents by an ATP driven proton pump in its membrane. Acidification also releases the light chain from the endosome into the axoplasm.

4. The light chains are zinc endopeptidases and they cleave vesicular and active zone proteins necessary for acetylcholine release. Types B, D, F and G cleave synaptobrevin, type C cleaves syntaxin and types A, C and E cleave SNAP-25.

Once internalised, the toxin is protected from antibodies. However, certain 4-aminoquinolines (which happen also to have antimalarial action; e.g. quinacrine) exert some protective action even after internalization, although they are ineffective once the light chain has been released into the axoplasm. They appear to act by preventing acidification of the endosomal contents. As more is learned of the mechanism of action of the toxins, so there is more opportunity to devise drugs to combat their action. For example, the development of selective inhibitors of the zinc endopeptidase enzyme action is an obvious approach.

The late neuromuscular component of the toxicity of tetanus toxin is likewise a consequence of zinc endopeptidase activity destroying synaptobrevin.

Botulinum toxin, as well as being an occasional serious food contaminant, is used clinically to alleviate certain muscle dystonias (strabismus, blepharospasm, torticollis and others, including certain cases of cerebral palsy in children). The actions and uses of botulinum toxin have been reviewed.[15,16]

COTRANSMITTERS

The vesicles, as well as containing acetylcholine, also contain Ca^{2+}, ATP, and possibly a proteoglycan similar to that present in *Torpedo marmorata* vesicles.

All of these are released along with acetylcholine. The Ca^{2+} may simply represent a mechanism for expelling that which enters with the nerve terminal action potential, and the proteoglycan may be an acetylcholine-binding molecule. However, the role of the ATP, which is not only released from nerve but also from contracting muscle, is intriguing.[17] ATP receptors of the P_{2x} subtype, which are coupled to cation channels, are present on both immature and adult muscle cells. Those in the motor endplate membrane are similar to nicotinic acetylcholine receptors, except that the mean open time of their channels is shorter. Those in the extrajunctional membrane may actually be the acetylcholine receptors. Furthermore, ATP potentiates the action of acetylcholine on nicotinic receptors. ATP receptors of the P_2-G protein-coupled type are also present in skeletal muscle. Possibly these are responsible for receptor desensitization through phosphorylation and, on a long term basis, they may play a part in down-regulating the receptors.

ATP is rapidly broken down to adenosine, and adenosine (P_1) receptors of both the inhibitory A_1 and excitatory A_2 subtypes have been detected on motor nerve endings. Under normal circumstances, activation of the inhibitory A_1 subtype is dominant.[17] Ginsborg & Hirst[18] first showed that adenosine inhibits acetylcholine release in the isolated phrenic nerve-diaphragm preparation of the rat, and this has been confirmed repeatedly in isolated nerve-muscle preparations of rodents and amphibia. The inhibitory effect in rodents has been shown to be mediated by an A_1 adenosine receptor and to be abolished by pretreatment with pertussis toxin, indicating the involvement of a G protein.

In mammals (though apparently not in frogs), the inhibitory effect of adenosine on acetylcholine release is a consequence of inhibition of the nerve terminal Ca^{2+} influx that occurs in response to the nerve action potential. Furthermore, the decrease in the Ca^{2+} current and in the endplate potential that occurs on increasing the frequency of nerve stimulation from say 0.1 Hz to 0.5 Hz and 1 Hz is apparently due to endogenous adenosine, since it is prevented by treatment with an adenosine A_1 receptor antagonist. This observation may lead to modification of standard textbooks of physiology.

Drugs that modify adenosine mechanisms are increasingly being developed for therapeutic use in several fields, e.g. cardiovascular and analgesic drugs. The potential for interaction with other drugs that modify neuromuscular transmission should be borne in mind.

In addition to acetylcholine-containing vesicles, motor nerve terminals also contain relatively large dense-cored vesicles which are loaded with the polypeptide, calcitonin gene-related peptide (CGRP). About one hundredth of the vesicles are of the large dense-cored type, which still amounts to a substantial number. The contents of these vesicles are also released by nerve impulses and release is Ca^{2+}-dependent. However, the finer details of the release of CGRP are different from that of acetylcholine, since exocytosis from the larger vesicles requires a higher frequency of nerve impulses and the release is not affected by black widow spider venom. CGRP produces a number of acute effects at the neuromuscular junction including an increase in acetylcholine synthesis, reduction in acetylcholine release, and postjunctional acetylcholine receptor desensitisation. At least some of its actions are probably a consequence of its ability to increase cAMP formation. Changeux and his coworkers[19] have shown that its chronic effect is to stimulate the synthesis of new acetylcholine receptors. It may be therefore that its main physiological role is concerned with the up-regulation of endplate acetylcholine receptors.

PREJUNCTIONAL AND PRETERMINAL RECEPTORS

In addition to CGRP receptors and adenosine (A_1 and A_2) receptors, receptors present on motor nerve endings include both muscarinic (M_1 and M_2) and nicotinic acetylcholine receptors, and both α- and β-adrenoceptors. The acetylcholine, adenosine and CGRP receptors may be regarded as autoreceptors, since all three agonists are released from the motor nerves. This might not be the only source, however, for muscle and Schwann cells also release some acetylcholine, and adenosine may be derived from ATP released from contracting muscle. Japanese workers[20] have elegantly demonstrated the presence in motor nerves and their terminals of nicotinic receptors of the type that contain $\alpha 3$ subunits. The adrenoceptors are clearly heteroreceptors, since there is no evidence of an adrenergic innervation of skeletal muscle. When activated, the α-adrenoceptors enhance acetylcholine release in response to nerve impulses, whereas the β-adrenoceptors enhance acetylcholine synthesis in circumstances in which it is impaired.[21] It is not yet clear whether the nerve terminal adrenoceptors play any physiological or pathological roles in transmission. If they do, they are presumably activated by catecholamines released from the adrenal medullae, or by noradrenaline that spills over from the sympathetic innervation of neighbouring blood vessels.

The familiar tetanic fade and 'train-of-four' (2 Hz for 2 s) fade are commonly produced by drugs of the tubocurarine-type. Not only is the amplitude of contractions reduced by the drug, but, in a tetanus, the tension rapidly wanes to zero despite continued stimulation. With 'train-of-four', the last twitch of the group is a great deal more depressed than the first. The conclusion has been reached that, whereas the depression of amplitude is essentially postjunctional in origin, the fade is the result of the tubocurarine-like drug blocking prejunctional nicotinic receptors that normally act to facilitate mobilization of acetylcholine into the releasable situation, so that output can keep up with the demands of the high frequency stimulation.[22] The inadequate mobilization consequent upon blockade of this process causes the fading tension.

Whatever the prejunctional action of the tubocurarine-like drug is, it is not a consequence of it preventing the entry of Ca^{2+} from the extracellular fluid.[23] Tubocurarine and related drugs reduce the release of radiolabelled acetylcholine and this effect also is independent of extracellular Ca^{2+}.[24] This does not, of course, mean that intracellular Ca^{2+} is not involved. It might be that some of the acetylcholine released from the nerve endings normally acts prejunctionally to release a second messenger that then acts to cause Ca^{2+} release from internal stores, and that this internal Ca^{2+} then enhances mobilisation. The nicotinic antagonist, by blocking this action of acetylcholine, would then prevent the necessary enhanced mobilisation.

There is evidence for a second population of nicotinic receptors near motor nerve endings which may be described as preterminal. Many nicotinic agonists including acetylcholine itself, nicotine, carbachol, dimethylphenylpiperazinium,

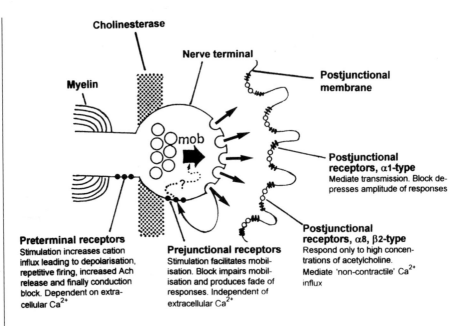

Cholinesterase

Nerve terminal

Myelin

Postjunctional membrane

mob

Postjunctional receptors, α1-type
Mediate transmission. Block depresses amplitude of responses

?

Preterminal receptors
Stimulation increases cation influx leading to depolarisation, repetitive firing, increased Ach release and finally conduction block. Dependent on extracellular Ca^{2+}

Prejunctional receptors
Stimulation facilitates mobilisation. Block impairs mobilisation and produces fade of responses. Independent of extracellular Ca^{2+}

Postjunctional receptors, α8, β2-type
Respond only to high concentrations of acetylcholine. Mediate 'non-contractile' Ca^{2+} influx

Fig. 2.2 The postulated sites and roles of nicotinic receptors at the neuromuscular junction. The preterminal receptors are protected from the neurotransmitter acetylcholine by the junctional acetylcholinesterase which is present, associated with the basement membrane, throughout the junctional gap. The column of cholinesterase depicted in the diagram is not meant to be anatomically accurate but is merely to suggest that it acts as a protective barrier. The question mark indicates that the link between activation of the prejunctional receptors and the process of transmitter mobilisation (mob) is not known. Nicotinic receptors containing α_3 protomers have been detected in the axonal and terminal membranes of motor nerves.

suxamethonium and, in some species, decamethonium, have been shown[22,25,26] to increase the release of acetylcholine measured as tritiated choline. Large concentrations of the same agonists, or even small concentrations left in contact with the preparation, produce a decrease in transmitter release. The enhanced release is entirely dependent upon extracellular Ca^{2+}. The effects are prevented by application of reversible nicotinic antagonists, such as tubocurarine and pancuronium, and high concentrations of hexamethonium, but not by α-bungarotoxin.

The fact that the released transmitter acetylcholine does not itself appear to activate this second population of nerve ending receptors, except after cholinesterase inhibition, suggests that they are normally protected from the transmitter by acetylcholinesterase, and that they are situated more centrally than the prejunctional receptors. They, therefore, have pharmacological relevance, but apparently no physiological role in neuromuscular transmission. They may represent a vestigial remnant of receptors that are present at many nerve endings, including some that are non-cholinergic; for example, those at certain locust nerve endings, at synapses in *Aplysia californica*, and at sensory nerve endings. A similar dual population of nicotinic receptors described as preterminal and presynaptic is proposed to be present at many synapses in the CNS.[27] Figure 2.2 represents the postulated sites and functions of nicotinic receptors at the neuromuscular junction.

Facilitatory (M_1) and inhibitory (M_2) muscarinic receptors are also present on motor nerve endings. Their presence is demonstrable pharmacologically only under unusual physiological conditions and their physiological functions remain unclear. Prejunctional mechanisms involved in neuromuscular transmisssion have recently been reviewed.[22]

POSTJUNCTIONAL ACETYLCHOLINE RECEPTORS

A nicotinic acetylcholine receptor is made up of 5 subunits (a pentamer) joined to form a ring that penetrates through the membrane and projects on each side (Fig. 2.3).[28,29] Each protein subunit is specified by a different gene. The subunits have different molecular weights and different properties, and each general type is denoted by a Greek letter : α (alpha), β (beta), γ (gamma), δ (delta), ε (epsilon). There are 9 different α-type subunits (α1–α9), 4 different β-type subunits (β1–β4) and 1 each of γ, δ and ε. All 16 subunit genes have been cloned from vertebrates. The theoretically possible number of different native nicotinic receptor subtypes is, therefore, huge, a molecular biologist's nightmare, although it is limited to the extent that all nicotinic receptors contain at least two α-type subunits, γ, δ and ε subunits appear to be confined to muscle and are not present in the nervous system, and there are certain restrictions in the abilities of some α-subunits to combine with others.The α-subunits are the ones that bind acetylcholine. The most common subunits present in nicotinic receptors in the brain are α4 and β2 although, with the exception of α1 and β1, all other α and β subunits are present.

The nicotinic receptors responsible for neuromuscular transmission in adult vertebrates have the stoichiometry $(\alpha1)_2\beta1\epsilon\delta$ (Fig. 2.3A). In the fetus, a slightly

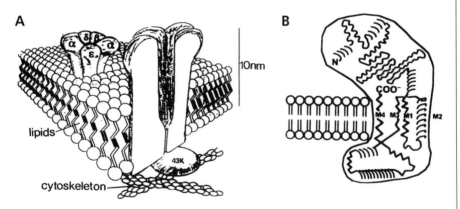

Fig. 2.3 (A) Diagram of a portion of a mammalian postjunctional motor endplate membrane showing two receptor complexes embedded in and spanning the bimolecular lipid layer. The two α–subunits and the β-, δ- and ε-subunits are labelled. These surround a central ion channel. The acetylcholine recognition sites are located on the α-subunits, one on each. The receptors are shown anchored to the actin cytoskeleton via a 43 kDa protein also called rapsyn, but the situation is actually more complicated than this (see also Fig. 2.4). **(B)** The general transmembrane arrangement of the polypeptide chain in a subunit of a nicotinic receptor. M_1–M_4 are the transmembrane domains that span the lipid bilayer. The pore is lined by the five M_2 domains. M_1, M_3 and M_4 are probably β-pleated sheets.

different subunit, denoted γ, is present in place of the ε subunit, but when the nerve grows out to reach the muscle the gene encoding the γ subunit is somehow switched off and that encoding the ε subunit is switched on. When a muscle is chronically denervated, the mechanism that confines the receptors to the neuromuscular junction is destroyed and receptors then re-appear (as in fetal muscle) all over the muscle fibre surface. Such receptors have the fetal-type structure, containing γ instead of ε subunits. The subunits have apparent molecular weights approximately as follow: α, 40 kDa; β, 49 kDa; γ/ε, 60 kDa; and δ, 67 kDa. Each has the general structure illustrated in Figure 2.3B.

Each subunit consists of a chain of amino acids. Most of the evidence is in favour of 4 transmembrane domains (M_1, M_2, M_3 and M_4). A short loop connects M_1 to M_2 and a larger loop connects M_3 to M_4 on the sarcoplasmic side. The M_2 domain of each of the 5 subunits probably lines the ion channel and is in the form of an α-helix. The remaining transmembrane domains (M_1, M_3 and M_4) may be β-pleated sheets. Figure 2.3B illustrates some of these features. The acetylcholine-binding site on the two α-subunits lies 2–3 nm from the membrane surface and involves cysteines 192 and 193, tyrosines 93 and 190 and tryptamine 149.

Although the two α1-subunits of the motor endplate receptor are specified by the same gene and are identical in composition, their binding properties differ because each is surrounded by different subunits which influence the binding. For example, one has a higher binding affinity than the other for tubocurarine. When viewed from the junctional cleft, the subunits are arranged in the clockwise order α1*-γ-α1-δ-β where α1* indicates the subunit with the higher affinity binding site for tubocurarine.[30]

The receptors are located at a density of about $10\,000/\mu m^2$ on the shoulders of the junctional folds, and much is being learned about the various proteins (agrin, rapsyn, laminin, α-dystroglycan, adhalin, utrophin, syntrophin, spectrin, and others) that serve to aggregate the receptors and anchor them appropriately to the cytoskeleton, while maintaining the characteristic junctional folds of the endplate membrane.[31,32] Figure 2.4 is a representation of the possible roles of the various proteins in anchoring the receptors to the cytoskeleton. It seems clear that the high concentration of receptors at the junction is maintained by connections between the receptors and the underlying cytoskeleton via linking proteins. In some congenital myasthenic syndromes, there is an inherited deficiency of nicotinic receptors leading to impaired neuromuscular transmission. It is possible that the basic problem lies in a deficiency or a dysfunction in one or more of the accessory proteins. The extracellular protein agrin is thought to be secreted by the motor nerve and to trigger localized clustering of the receptors in the endplate membrane. Binding of agrin to α-dystroglycan is followed by re-arrangement of the cytoskeleton with localized replacement of dystrophin by utrophin. This effect is unlikely to be concerned with receptor clustering, because most of the utrophin is located in the depths of the junctional folds where there are few acetylcholine receptors. However, utrophin may be concerned with maintaining the integrity of the specialised junctional structures. Rapsyn, also called the 43K protein, which is associated with the inner face of the postjunctional membrane, is able to cluster acetylcholine receptors and link them to the cytoskeleton. Rapsyn may, therefore, be the final link in the chain of events that

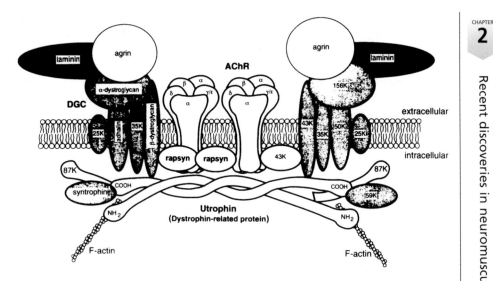

Fig. 2.4 A representation of the molecules proposed to play a role in nicotinic receptor clustering at the neuromuscular junction, arranged with predicted interactions depicted. Apparent molecular weights that originally defined each depicted protein are indicated at the right; on the left, alternative names are shown. It is proposed that rapsyn links the receptor to the dystrophin-glycoprotein complex (DGC), thereby facilitating the association of receptor clusters with the cytoskeleton. It is also proposed that the formation of mature clusters involves the linkage of many receptor–rapsyn small clusters to each dystroglycan molecule. (*Reproduced with permission from* Apel and colleagues,[32] copyright held by *Cell Press*.)

leads to immobilisation of the acetylcholine receptors on the shoulders of the junctional folds. Agrin, released from the nerve may, therefore, serve, via other proteins, to trap the receptor–rapsyn complexes in the appropriate way.

When two molecules of acetylcholine interact with their recognition sites located on the two α-subunits of the receptor, a conformation change in the protein occurs which is transmitted throughout the receptor complex, resulting in the opening of a cation channel and allowing the influx of a current carried mainly by Na^+ ions. Unwin has been able to visualize the activated channel in the open state.[33]

The patch clamp recording electrode system, developed by Neher and Sakmann, enables the activity of a single receptor to be recorded (see, for example, Schuetze[34]). A patch clamp electrode applied to an adult mammalian receptor shows that acetylcholine produces a series of rectangular current pulses of equal amplitude, but different durations, carried by Na^+ through the open channel. The characteristics of the single current pulse (at 37°C and at normal resting membrane potential) are a current amplitude of around 3.5 pA, a conductance of around 60 pS, and a mean duration (i.e. a mean channel open time) of around 6.5 ms. A change in the concentration of acetylcholine produces a corresponding change in the frequency of the channel opening, but amplitude, conductance and mean open time do not change. The isolated patch of endplate membrane adhering to a patch clamp electrode is free from acetylcholinesterase and remains in continuous contact with the same concentration of acetylcholine. Clearly, the acetylcholine molecules repetitively combine with and dissociate from the receptor in order to produce the repeated opening and closing of the receptor channel. The situation in the intact neuromuscular system is different in that acetylcholinesterase is present and highly active. Any one molecule of acetylcholine survives intact long enough to open one receptor ion channel once, at the most. Some molecules are hydrolysed before reaching the receptors. The current of Na^+ flowing across the endplate membrane (the endplate current) in response to acetylcholine released from the nerve is therefore the summed response of the thousands of activated individual channels, each opened only once for a few milliseconds. The endplate current flowing across the endplate membrane lowers the voltage across that membrane (i.e. depolarizes it) to produce the endplate potential (EPP). The resting membrane potential of the whole of the muscle fibre membrane is around 90 mV, inside negative (i.e. conventionally described as –90 mV). Acetylcholine released from the nerve depolarizes the endplate membrane by about 40 mV (i.e. from –90 mV to –50 mV). The depolarized endplate, surrounded by membrane at normal resting potential, acts as a current sink into which local circuit currents flow to initiate a propagating action potential that passes around the muscle fibre membrane to trigger the contractile process. The walls of the junctional folds, though devoid of acetylcholine receptors, are especially richly endowed with voltage gated Na^+ channels which function to amplify the current initiated by the EPP.[35] Neuromuscular transmission is impaired in certain diseases in which the junctional folds are poorly developed.[36] The main events in neuromuscular transmission are summarized in Figure 2.5.

RECEPTOR DESENSITIZATION

Prolonged application of acetylcholine or other agonist to the neuromuscular junction leads to receptor desensitization[37] which may represent a safety mechanism that prevents over-excitation. The mechanisms underlying receptor desensitization are not fully understood, although phosphorylation of certain amino acid residues in the receptor proteins plays a part at least in some instances. Presumably such phosphorylation produces conformational changes in the channel proteins that prevent ion flux. One mechanism that may be involved has recently been proposed by Japanese workers.[38] It was formerly thought that the only acetylcholine receptors present in skeletal muscle membrane were the $(\alpha1)_2\beta1\gamma/\epsilon\delta$ type described above. However, four genes expressing $\alpha4$, $\alpha5$, $\alpha7$ and $\beta4$ receptor subunits are now known to be expressed in developing chick skeletal muscle,[39] and in mammalian muscle, receptors containing $\beta2$ and probably $\alpha8$ subunits have now been shown to be colocalized with the more familiar $(\alpha1)_2\beta1\epsilon\delta$ receptors. The ion channels of the $\beta2/\alpha8$ receptors, when opened by acetylcholine, are highly permeable to Ca^{2+}, but this source of Ca^{2+} is not concerned with the contractile mechanism. Kimura and coworkers[38] describe the $\alpha8/\beta2$ receptor function by the acronym RAMIC (receptor activity modulating intracellular Ca^{2+}). It is initiated only by amounts of acetylcholine in excess of those required for normal neuromuscular transmission, e.g. stimulation in the presence of an anticholinesterase. It has

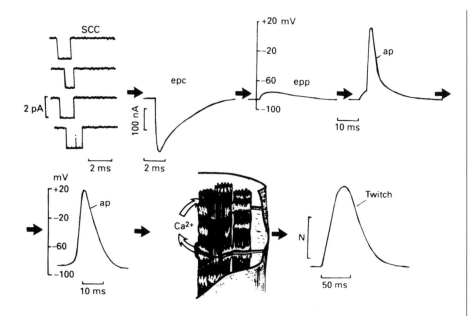

Fig. 2.5 The chain of events in excitation–contraction coupling from the elementary events (the single-channel currents) produced by the interaction of acetylcholine with endplate cholinoceptors, to the muscle fibre twitch. The summation of many single-channel currents (SCC) produces the endplate current (epc) which drives the endplate membrane potential towards zero (i.e. depolarizes it) to produce the endplate potential (epp). When the epp reaches a critical value, it triggers a propagating action potential (ap) which, at the endplate region, is seen superimposed on the epp (top right). The ap passes around the sarcolemma and along the T tubules to cause the release of Ca^{2+} from the sarcoplasmic reticulum. The Ca^{2+} activates the contractile machinery to produce the twitch. The SCC are the type of record obtained with a patch-clamp electrode from a single ion channel. Note the different calibration from that of the epc.

been proposed that the function of RAMIC is to produce desensitization of the $(\alpha 1)_2 \beta \epsilon \delta$ receptors and thereby quell the overexcitation. The influx of Ca^{2+} arising from activation of the $\alpha 8/\beta 2$ receptors causes the translocation of protein kinase C from the sarcoplasm to the endplate membrane, simultaneously activating it. The protein kinase C may then phosphorylate proteins of the $(\alpha 1)_2 \beta 1 \epsilon \gamma$ receptors thereby desensitizing them.

CGRP may also play a part in the desensitizing process by stimulating its receptors in muscle and activating protein kinase A through cAMP production. Protein kinase A enhances the production of RAMIC by acetylcholine. Additionally, ATP, released from nerve and from contracting muscle, may contribute to acetylcholine receptor desensitization by acting on muscle P2-G protein-coupled receptors and thereby increasing the activity of protein kinase C.[17]

NEUROMUSCULAR BLOCK

Although it is only 56 years since Griffith and Johnson,[40] in Montreal, pioneered the use of neuromuscular blocking drugs in anaesthetic practice, physiologists and pharmacologists had been studying their action for almost 100 years before that time. Ever since Claude Bernard in the mid 19th century had demonstrated the site of action of curare in the frog, extensive studies of chemical structure:action relations had been carried out. Curare, and later its purified alkaloid tubocurarine, played an important part in the experiments leading to the elucidation of chemical transmission at the neuromuscular junction. The early history has been reviewed.[41]

Tubocurarine blocks neuromuscular transmission by combining reversibly with the binding sites for acetylcholine on the α1-protomers of the nicotinic acetylcholine receptors in the postjunctional membrane of the motor endplate. What is perhaps not always realized is just how fleeting each combination with the receptor is.[42] Patch clamp recording from a single receptor, with both acetylcholine and tubocurarine together in the pipette, shows that a tubocurarine molecule's interaction with the receptor is on a submillisecond time basis, but interactions are, of course, repetitive. The situation in the patch clamp pipette may be visualized as a mixed cloud of molecules of acetylcholine and tubocurarine in the fluid surrounding the receptor, each type making fleeting but repetitive collisions with the receptor. When two acetylcholine molecules collide with the two binding sites, the receptor channel opens in the normal way, but collision by only one tubocurarine molecule is sufficient transiently to prevent activation by acetylcholine. Hence, tubocurarine does not inactivate the receptor, but rather it reduces the probability that acetylcholine can activate it. Obviously, the more acetylcholine present, the more the dice are loaded in its favour, and vice versa. This is the basis of Gaddum's definition of block by competition, and is the basic reason why neostigmine or other anticholinesterase drug reverses neuromuscular block in the intact neuro-muscular system. By prolonging the life of acetylcholine at the neuromuscular junction, an anticholinesterase gives each molecule a better chance of interacting with a receptor that happens to be free from tubocurarine at the time. It is clear, then, that reversal by neostigmine does not occur because the preserved acetylcholine has in some way cleared the junction of tubocurarine. The tubo-curarine remains present, but the probability of acetylcholine interacting with receptors has been increased. Despite the neostigmine, the tubocurarine disappears from the junction at the normal rate, as determined by redistribution, and excretion. It should be recalled that the situation in the intact junction differs from that in the patch clamp pipette in that, because of the cholinesterase present in the intact junction, each acetylcholine molecule's life is fleeting. Hence, the equilibrium conditions necessary to demonstrate true competitive block of acetylcholine by tubocurarine cannot be met in an intact neuromuscular junction. It is for this reason that some purists object to the terms 'competitive blocking agent' and 'block by competition' to describe tubocurarine and related compounds, and their action in the intact neuromuscular junction.

It is the case that, with very large concentrations of tubocurarine, a second mechanism of action, channel block, comes into play. In this situation, mole-cules of tubocurarine actually plug the open ion channels like so many corks in bottles. However, this type of action is largely experimental. Even with gallamine, which amongst all neuromuscular blocking drugs exhibits channel block to the greatest extent, the concentrations required are probably greatly in excess of any produced in normal clinical practice.

Once the use of tubocurarine had been established as an adjunct to anaesthesia, the difficulty of obtaining it from its natural sources together with some obvious disadvantages in its clinical use, soon led to attempts to find substitutes for it, either by modifying its structure or those of related alkaloids, or by synthesizing new compounds. By the early 1960s, relatively few compounds from the vast number synthesized were available to the anaesthesiologist, the main ones of the nondepolarizing type being tubocurarine and its then so-called dimethyl derivative (metocurine), gallamine, laudexium, benzoquinonium and alcuronium. Generally speaking, as the complexity of surgical procedures increased, anaesthesiologists became dissatisfied with the available neuromuscular blocking drugs because of their side-effects and inappropriate time course of action. The range of unwanted effects that neuromuscular blocking drugs may produce has been reviewed,[43] and the drugs that are currently used in anaesthetic practice have been described in a number of monographs.[2,44–46]

The methonium compounds were synthesized and tested by Paton & Zaimis thereby illustrating an entirely new mechanism of transmission block; that is block by depolarization.[47] Decamethonium, now obsolete, was the clinically available compound that arose from these studies. Because it is stable to the junctional acetylcholinesterase, decamethonium makes repetitive acetylcholine like interactions with the endplate nicotinic receptors, thereby preventing the endplate from repolarizing rapidly. Hence, a zone of depolarization is set up in the middle of the muscle fibre membrane. As a result of this, the local circuit current from the surrounding normally polarized membrane continues to flow into the depolarized endplate. Under normal conditions, the transient endplate depolarization produced by transmitter acetylcholine gives rise to a corresponding transient local circuit current which opens the Na^+ channels in the surrounding membrane thereby triggering the propagating action potential that leads to contraction. It is characteristic of Na^+ channels in excitable membranes, however, that a conformation change in their structure inactivates them soon after the current begins to flow; hence the refractory period of excitable membranes. The prolonged local current consequent upon the prolonged endplate depolarization by decamethonium leads to prolonged inactivation of the surrounding Na^+ channels. Hence, the depolarized endplate is surrounded by a zone of inexcitability so that action potential propapagation, and therefore contraction, cease. In a sense, block by depolarization resembles a prolonged refractory period, and is analogous to cathodal block in nerve.

One of the problems with depolarizing blocking drugs is that their action is not 'pure'; true block by depolarization (the so-called phase 1 block) as described above is complicated by other actions that contribute to the paralysis and that become more pronounced with increase of dose and with time (the so-called phase 2 block). Additional actions include stimulation of preterminal nicotinic receptors on motor nerve endings, postjunctional receptor desensitization, postjunctional receptor channel block leading to penetration of the drug into the muscle sarcoplasm, and a partial agonist action involving a nondepolarizing type of postjunctional receptor block. The stimulation of preterminal nicotinic receptors on nerve initially contributes to the muscle fasciculations produced by depolarizing blocking drugs. Eventually, this effect leads to conduction block at the nerve endings so that a component of reduced transmitter release may contribute to phase 2 block. For fuller discussions of the mechanisms of action of depolarizing drugs a number of longer texts may be consulted.[2,37,45] It remains uncertain as to which of the experimentally demonstrable actions of decamethonium and other depolarizing drugs contribute to the phase 2 block observed in patients. Other depolarizing blocking drugs that for a time entered anaesthetic practice include carbolonium and dioxonium. Like decamethonium, they are now obsolete largely because of the uncertainty surrounding their mechanism of action. The development of decamethonium shortly led to the use of succinylcholine in anaesthesiology, although the compound, as a chemical, had been known since 1906. Succinylcholine is the only depolarizing blocking drug that continues in clinical use. Because of its range of unwanted effects, the use of succinylcholine is now virtually restricted to single dose use, where its rapid onset of action is useful for intubation at the start of an operation.[48] What is required is a nondepolarizing type of muscle relaxant with a time course of action like that of succinylcholine.

The early structure:action studies had shown that for non-depolarizing activity the molecule should be bulky and that it requires two charged centres (preferably nitrogens) around 1.0–1.4 nm apart. All clinically used non-depolarizing blocking drugs, past and present, fulfil these criteria.

About 45 years ago, rudimentary evidence that muscarinic acetylcholine receptors were not a homogeneous group was beginning to accumulate. Perhaps the first indication was the observation by Riker & Wescoe,[49] who showed that gallamine blocked cardiac muscarinic receptors (now called M_2 receptors) without affecting those of the gut or of most other peripheral tissues (now called M_3 receptors). It is now recognised that muscarinic receptors exist in five subtypes. Pancuronium, like gallamine, although to a lesser extent, blocks muscarinic M_2 receptors and, therefore, blocks the cardiac vagus. It also blocks neuronal reuptake of noradrenaline (uptake 1). During surgical operations these effects combined may lead to a mild tachycardia and hypertension which may be undesirable in certain procedures.

The discovery of new neuromuscular blocking drugs necessarily relies more on classical pharmacological and electrophysiological techniques, rather than on molecular biological techniques, because efficacy at the receptor is well understood and can readily be built into a new chemical entity. What is required is freedom from unwanted effects at other sites, together with appropriate pharmacokinetic variables. Though none is perfect, the chloralose-anaesthetized cat gives the best prediction of effective dose and time course of effect in man. Hence, a large number of compounds have been tested in cats for their ability to block a fast-contracting (e.g. tibialis anterior) and a slow-contracting (e.g. soleus) muscle, and to affect the arterial blood pressure,the response to cardiac vagus stimulation, and the contractions of the nictitating membrane to preganglionic stimulation. Effective compounds selected from such a basic screening programme are then subjected to numerous other tests involving electrophysiological analysis, biochemical tests, and metabolism and excretion studies.

After testing a large number of aminosteroidal compounds, it became clear that, in this series, the abilities to block cardiac M_2 receptors and neuronal noradrenaline uptake are associated with the presence of a quaternary nitrogen at the Ring A end of the molecule. Hence, vecuronium which has a tertiary nitrogen instead of a quaternary nitrogen at the ring A end of its molecule is especially notable for its lack of unwanted cardiac effects. For different, and unknown reasons, atracurium also is relatively free from actions on the heart.

The special property of atracurium is its ability to undergo a Hofmann elimination reaction at the pH and temperature of the blood. This means that the molecule will spontaneously disintegrate, becoming ineffective at the neuromuscular junction, even in the absence of kidney or liver function. Amongst other factors, for a Hofmann elimination to occur, the carbonyl group must be nearer to the quaternary nitrogen that is the ether oxygen (i.e. N—CO—O—C—). In contrast, for breakdown by a cholinesterase enzyme (cf acetylcholine, succinylcholine, mivacurium) the compound must be an ester, that is the ether oxygen must be the closer to the quaternary nitrogen (N—O—CO—C—). Atracurium is a mixture of optical isomers. One of these isomers is cis-atracurium. It is 3–4 times more potent than atracurium, and is somewhat slower in onset of action as would be expected because of the inverse relationship between potency and rate of onset as described below. The actions, uses, degradation and pharmacokinetics of cis-atracurium are essentially similar to those of atracurium. Its propensity to cause histamine release is less than that of atracurium.

The chemical structures of mivacurium and doxacurium superficially resemble that of atracurium. However, the ether oxygen and the carbonyl group do not have the relationship that permits Hofmann elimination. Mivacurium is hydrolysed by plasma cholinesterase at around 75% of the rate at which succinylcholine is hydrolysed, and so recovery from mivacurium is rapid. Unfortunately, its onset of action is not rapid. It has been deduced[50] that hydrolysis by cholinesterase is not a mechanism that could lead to rapid onset of action coupled with short duration of a non-depolarizing drug. Doxacurium is relatively stable to cholinesterase for reasons that are not clear. The hydrolysis rate is only about 6% of that of succinylcholine. It is highly potent with a very slow onset of action, a long duration and slow recovery.

A desirable feature in a new nondepolarizing neuromuscular blocking drug is a rapid onset of action that by itself permits intubation without the need for an initial paralysis produced by succinylcholine with its entirely different mechanism of action. Brief duration and rapid recovery (or at least rapid reversibility by another agent) are also desirable properties so that spontaneous breathing quickly recommences in those rare instances when intubation turns out to be impossible.

In studying more than a hundred related aminosteroidal compounds it has become clear that rapid onset of action is generally associated with lack of potency, that is with a high initial plasma concentration. The original observation was made with only 20 compounds.[51] The relationship is illustrated for four of these compounds in Figure 2.6. Numerous further studies have shown the generality of the phenomenon. At one end of the graph relating onset time to effective dose, the curve becomes asymptotic towards the circulation time, because time of onset cannot be shorter than the circulation time. At the other, 'highly potent', end, the curve must become asymptotic towards the number of molecules necessary to block sufficient endplate receptors to prevent muscle activation. Of course rapid onset of block can also be achieved by giving a huge dose of a potent drug, but this occurs only at the expense of what might be called a 'supramaximal' block of very prolonged duration which will last until the plasma concentration falls below the blocking level. For rapid offset coupled with rapid onset, a drug that lacks potency is necessary, unless the potent drug happens to be metabolised or redistributed at an extremely high rate, in which case recovery will be swift. Similar results have been obtained in electrophysiological studies of single motor endplates.[52]

Hence it was observed that rapid onset was usually, although not invariably, associated with brief duration and rapid recovery. This general observation is illustrated for the 4 compounds in Figure 2.6. The relationship is, of course, a general one; there will be exceptions especially in so far as dose is concerned. If, for example, a particular compound has a volume of distribution that is greater than expected, because of some unsuspected pharmacokinetic characteristic, such as excessive binding to plasma proteins or to cartilage, then its concentration in the junctional cleft will be lower than supposed from the dose injected and consequently its speed of onset will be slower.

The results showed that it should be possible to produce a nondepolarizing type of drug with a time course of action resembling that of succinylcholine. Indeed, in animal experiments, especially on anaesthetised cats, compounds with these properties have been found.[51] The problems are that the greater the dose required, the more expensive is the drug to produce and the more likely it is

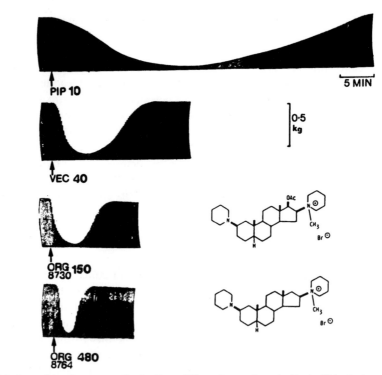

Fig. 2.6 Cats, chloralose anaesthesia. Four different experiments. Typical blocks (approx 90%) are shown for pipecuronium (PIP), vecuronium (VEC), ORG 8730, and ORG 8764. The numbers denote the doses in µg/kg i.v. Generally, highly potent drugs have slower onset and longer duration of action than less potent drugs.

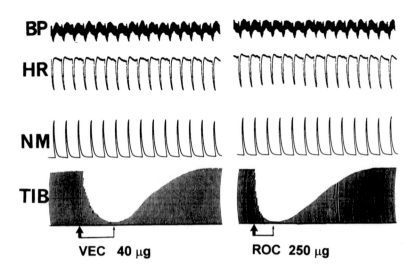

BP

HR

NM

TIB

VEC   40 μg   **ROC   250 μg**

Fig. 2.7 Cat, chloralose anaesthesia; both vagi cut. Records from above downwards; BP, arterial blood pressure; HR, heart rate; the right vagus was stimulated (8 Hz for 5 s every 100 s); NM, contractions of a nictitating membrane evoked by preganglionic stimulation of the cervical sympathetic nerve (10 Hz for 5 s every 100 s); TIB, twitches of a tibialis anterior muscle stimulated through its motor nerve (0.1 Hz). At VEC, 40 μg/kg vecuronium and at ROC, 250 μg/kg rocuronium were injected i.v. Note that, in neuromuscular blocking doses, both drugs are without effect on blood pressure and are free from ganglion blocking action (no effect on nictitating membrane). Rocuronium (but not vecuronium) produces a slight block of cardiac vagus stimulation. The neuromuscular blocks are similar except that rocuronium is about twice as fast in onset as vecuronium.

to produce unwanted side-effects. A compromise is required. Compounds must be acceptable in terms of expense and side-effects and yet fast enough in onset to permit intubation. The compounds rocuronium, and that termed ORG 9487 (rapacuronium), which is presently in clinical trial, are such compromises.

Rocuronium possesses a tertiary nitrogen at the ring A end of the molecule thereby minimising its cardiovascular effects. It does produce a very slight block of the cardiac M_2 receptors because the effective dose is large (about 6 times larger than that of vecuronium). The relatively large dose necessary means that its rate of onset is such as to permit intubation.[53] Figure 2.7 compares the effects of rocuronium and vecuronium. Unusually, its duration of action is little different from that of vecuronium.

It is perhaps easy to see why high potency should result in slow access to the biophase, that is, to the junctional cleft, which is enclosed by its terminal Schwann cells and the nerve terminal. The fewer the molecules in the plasma, the less the concentration gradient driving the drug into the cleft and, therefore, the slower the onset of block. The less potent drug, in its necessarily high concentration, will enter the cleft more rapidly and it has to be assumed that this is the main rate limiting step, overriding the individual differences in the affinity constants for the receptors. Onset, then, is essentially simply mass action-related. The degree of receptor occupancy necessary to cause block is, of course, the same regardless of the potency. Other influences being equal, it appears that the concentration of the less potent drug will more quickly fall below the blocking threshold, so that generally speaking offset of action, as well as onset, will be faster. However, the correlation is less uniform than that with fast onset, because a variety of additional factors may affect rate of recovery. These factors have been thoroughly discussed by several authors.[45,50,54]

Different neuromuscular blocking drugs have relatively different propensities to cause tetanic or train-of-four fade,[55] presumably representing relatively different affinities for pre- and postjunctional receptors. There is evidence that rocuronium has a greater prejunctional component of action than other clinically used neuromuscular blocking drugs.[56] This effect, superimposed upon its more rapidly developing postjunctional action, must contribute to the ease of intubation experienced with the drug.

ORG 9487 is considerably less potent than vecuronium, ranging from 3–20 times in different animal species. It is about 20 times less potent than vecuronium in human patients. Accordingly, its onset of action is rapid and, in accordance with the more usual relationship, its duration of action is short.[57,58] Although its overall time course of action does not quite match that of succinylcholine, it is the closest so far developed, and may represent the limit of what can be economically achieved amongst the traditional type of reversible receptor blocking drugs.

References

1. Katz B. Nerve, Muscle and Synapse. New York: McGraw Hill, 1966
2. Bowman W C. Pharmacology of Neuromuscular Function, 2nd edn. London: Wright,; 1990
3. Vincent A, Wray D. (eds) Neuromuscular Transmission Basic and Applied Aspects. Manchester: Manchester University Press, 1990
4. Salpeter M M. (ed) The Vertebrate Neuromuscular Junction. New York: Alan Liss, 1987
5. Bowman W C, Marshall I G. Inhibitors of acetylcholine synthesis. In: Cheymol J. (ed.) Neuromuscular Blocking and Stimulating Agents. Int Encycl Pharmacol Ther Sect 14, Vol 1, Oxford: Pergamon Press, 1972; 357–390
6. Parsons S M, Prior C, Marshall I G. Acetylcholine transport, storage and release. Int Rev Neurobiol 1993; 35: 279–390
7. Sudhof T C, Jahn R. Proteins of synaptic vesicles involved in exocytosis and membrane recycling. Neuron 1991; 6: 665–677
8. Monck J R, Fernandez J M. The exocytotic fusion pore and neurotransmitter release. Neuron 1994; 12: 707–716
9. Geppert M, Bolshakov V Y, Siegelbaum S A et al. The role of Rab3A in neurotransmitter release. Nature 1994; 369: 493–497
10. Sudhof T C. The synaptic vesicle cycle: a cascade of protein:protein interactions. Nature 1995; 375: 645–653
11. Hong S J, Chang C C. Inhibition of acetylcholine release from mouse motor nerve by a P-type calcium channel blocker. J Physiol 1995; 482: 283–290
12. Robitaille R, Garcia M L, Kaczorowski G J, Charlton M P. Functional colocalization of calcium and calcium-gated potassium channels in control of transmitter release. Neuron 1993; 11: 645–655
13. Leveque C, Hoshino T, David P. The synaptic vesicle protein synaptotagmin associates with calcium channels and is a putative Lambert-Eaton myasthenic syndrome antigen. Proc Natl Acad Sci USA 1992; 89: 3625–3629
14. McGuiness T L, Greengard P. Protein phosphorylation and synaptic transmission. In: Sellin L C, Libelius R, Thesleff S. (eds) Neuromuscular Junction. Amsterdam: Elsevier, 1988; 111–124
15. Montecucco C, Schiavo G, Tugnoli V, de Grandis D. Botulinum neurotoxins: mechanism of action and therapeutic applications. Mol Med Today 1996; 2: 418–423

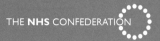

The Pocket Guide to the new NHS

1999/2000

The restructured 2nd edition of the Pocket Guide contains up-to-date information about:

- the role of the NHS
- the history of the NHS
- how the NHS is organised
- the role of NHS boards
- finance, human resources, information and quality strategies

The Pocket Guide is the ideal companion for:

- non-executives
- primary care group board members
- all NHS professionals looking for a useful quick reference guide to the NHS
- local government working with the NHS
- commercial companies working with the NHS
- charities involved in health
- students learning about the NHS

**NEW!
2nd
edition**

The comprehensive A-Z mini-guide to the NHS

I wish to order _____ copies of 'The Pocket Guide to the new NHS' (pub code 509).

Price per copy	
NHS Confederation members	£8.95
Non NHS Confederation members	£10.50
Postage and packaging	£1.50
TOTAL AMOUNT DUE	£ _____

I wish to pay by: (please tick appropriate option)

◯ Cheque: I enclose a cheque made payable to The NHS Confederation Trading Company Ltd
◯ Credit card: Please charge my credit card:

Card type _____   Card number _____

Expiry date _____

◯ Company order/invoice: Please invoice my organisation (order numbers must be supplied if members wish to be invoiced)

NB: Non members of the NHS Confederation must pay in advance by cheque or credit card

Name _____   Job title _____

Organisation _____

Address _____

_____   Tel _____

Address for delivery (if different) _____

_____

Please return this order form to:

The NHS Confederation publications office, Birmingham Research Park, Vincent Drive, Birmingham B15 2SQ. Tel: 0121 471 4444 Fax: 0121 414 1120 Email: lizd@nhsconfed.co.uk

● ● ● Order five or more copies to receive a discount! ● ● ●
Call Elizabeth Dalton on 0121 471 4444
for further information on special bulk buy prices.

16. Tsui J K C. Botulinum toxin as a therapeutic agent. Pharmacol Ther 1996; 72: 13–24

17. Henning R H. Purinoceptors in neuromuscular transmission. Pharmacol Ther 1997; 74: 115–128

18. Ginsborg B L, Hirst G D S. The effect of adenosine on the release of the transmitter from the phrenic nerve of the rat. J Physiol 1972; 224: 629–645

19. Fontaine B, Klarsfeld A, Changeux J-P. Calcitonin gene-related peptide and muscle activity regulate acetylcholine receptor α-subunit mRNA levels by distinct intracellular pathways. J Cell Biol 1987; 105: 1337–1342

20. Tsuneki H, Kimura I, Dezaki K, Kimura M, Sula C, Fumagalli B. Immunohistochemical localization of neuronal nicotinic receptor subtypes at the pre- and post-junctional sites in mouse diaphram muscle. Neurosci Lett 1995; 196: 13–16

21. Bowman W C. Effects on skeletal muscle. Handbook Exp Pharmacol 1980; 54: 47-128

22. Bowman W C. Prejunctional mechanisms in neuromuscular transmission. In: Booij L H D J. (ed.) Neuromuscular Transmission. London: BMJ Publishing, 1996; 1–27

23. Tian L, Prior C, Dempster J, Marshall I G. Nicotinic antagonist-produced frequency-dependent changes in acetylcholine release from rat motor nerve terminals. J Physiol 1994; 476: 517–529

24. Vizi E S, Chaudrey I A, Goldiner P L, Ohta Y, Nagashima H, Foldes F F. The pre- and postjunctional components of the neuromuscular effect of antibiotics. J Anesth 1991; 5: 1–9

25. Wessler I. Acetylcholine at motor nerves: storage, release and presynaptic modulation by autoreceptors and adrenoceptors. Int Rev Neurobiol 1992; 34: 283–384

26. Bowman W C, Gibb A J, Harvey A L, Marshall I G. Prejunctional actions of cholinoceptor agonists and antagonists, and of anticholinesterase drugs. Handbook Exp Pharmacol 1986; 79: 141–170

27. Wonnacott S. Presynaptic nicotinic Ach receptors. Trends Neurosci 1997; 20: 92–98

28. Unwin N. Neurotransmitter action: opening of ligand-gated ion channels. Cell 72/Neuron 10 1993; Suppl: 31–41

29. Sargent P B. The diversity of neuronal nicotinic acetylcholine receptors. Annu Rev Neurosci 1993; 16: 403–443

30. Machold J, Weise C, Utkin Y, Tsetlin V, Hucho F. The handedness of the subunit arrangement of the nicotinic acetylcholine receptor from *Torpedo californica*. Eur J Biochem 1995; 234: 427–430

31. Phillips W D. Acetylcholine receptors and the cytoskeletal connection. Clin Exp Pharmacol Physiol 1995; 22: 961–965

32. Apel E D, Roberds S L, Campbell K P, Merlie J P. Rapsyn may function as a link between the acetylcholine receptor and the agrin-binding dystrophin-associated glycoprotein complex. Neuron 1995; 15: 115–126

33. Unwin N. Acetylcholine receptor channels imaged in the open state. Nature 1995; 373: 37–43

34. Schuetze S. Understanding channel gating: patch clamp recordings from cloned acetylcholine receptors. Trends Neurosci 1986; 9: 140–141

35. Flucher B E, Daniels M P. Distribution of Na^+ channels and ankyrin in neuromuscular junctions is complementary to that of acetylcholine receptors and 43 kd protein. Neuron 1989; 3: 163–175.

36. Fawcett P R W, Slater C R, Baxter P, Young C, Walls T J, Gardner-Medwin D. Congenital myasthenia with reduction of utrophin and acetylcholine receptors at the neuromuscular junction. Electroenceph Clin Neurophysiol 1994; 91: 100P

37. Colquohoun D. On the principles of postsynaptic actions of neuromuscular blocking agents. Handbook Exp Pharmacol 1986; 79: 59–113

38. Kimura I. Calcium-dependent, desensitizing function of the post-synaptic neuronal type nicotinic acetylcholine receptors at the neuromuscular junction. Pharmacol Ther 1998; 77: 183–202

39. Corriveau R A, Romano S J, Conroy W G, Oliva L, Berg D K. Expression of neuronal acetylcholine receptor genes in vertebrate skeletal muscle during development. J Neurosci 1995; 15: 1372–1383

40. Griffith H R, Johnson G E. The use of curare in general anaesthesia. Anesthesiology 1942; 3: 418–420

41. Bowman W C. Peripheral ly acting muscle relaxants. In: Parnham M J, Bruinvels J. (eds) Discoveries in Pharmacology. Amsterdam: Elsevier, 1983; 105–160

42. Sheridan R, Lester H A. Rates and equilibria at the acetylcholine receptor of *Electrophorus* electroplaques. A study of neurally evoked postsynaptic currents and of voltage jump relaxations. J Gen Physiol 1977; 70: 187–219

43. Vizi E S, Lendvai B. Side-effects of nondepolarizing muscle relaxants: relationship to their antinicotinic and antimuscarinic actions. Pharmacol Ther 1997; 73: 75–90

44. Bevan D R, Bevan J C, Donati F. Muscle relaxants in clinical anaesthesia. Chicago: Year Book Medical Publishers, 1988

45. Feldman S. Neuromuscular Block. Oxford: Butterworth-Heinmann, 1996

46. Booij L.H.D.J. (ed.) Neuromuscular Transmission. London: BMJ Publishing, 1996

47. Paton W D M, Zaimis E. The methonium compounds. Pharmacol Rev 1952; 4: 219–253

48. Bevan D R, Donati F. Suxamethonium in clinical practice. In: Booij L H D J. (ed.) Neuromuscular Transmission. London: BMJ Publishing, 1996; 80–90

49. Riker W F, Wescoe W C. The pharmacology of flaxedil with observations on certain analogs. Ann NY Acad Sci 1951; 54: 373–392

50. Midgley J M, Stenlake J B. Neuromuscular blockade: offset anomalies. Are they simply potency-related receptor bonding effects? J Pharm Pharmacol 1997; 49: 416–420

51. Bowman W C, Rodger I W, Houston J, Marshal R J, McIndewar I. Structure:action relationships among some desacetoxy analogues of pancuronium and vecuronium in the anaesthetized cat. Anesthesiology 1988; 69: 57–62

52. Law J C, Bekavac M D, Glavinovic M I, Donati F, Bevan D R. Ionophoretic study of speed of action of various muscle relaxants. Anesthesiology 1992; 77: 351–356

53. Vickers M D. (ed.) Clinical Experiences with Rocuronium Bromide. Eur J Anaesth 1955; Suppl 11: 1–112

54. Bowman W C. The discovery and evolution of aminosteroidal neuromuscular blocking agents. In: Denissen P. (ed.) The Development of Aminosteroidal Neuromuscular Blocking Agents, Turnhout: Interface Symposium, Organon-Teknika, 1992; 3–20

55. Bowman W C, Webb S N. Tetanic fade during partial transmission failure produced by non-depolarizing neuromuscular blocking drugs in the cat. Clin Exp Pharmacol Physiol 1976; 3: 545–555

56. England A J, Richards K M, Feldman S A. The effect of rate of stimulation on force of contraction in a partially paralysed rat phrenic nerve hemidiaphragm preparation. Anesth Analg 1997; 84: 882–885

57. Wierda J M, van den Broek L, Proost JH. Time course of action and endotracheal intubating conditions of ORG 9487, a new short-acting steroidal muscle relaxant: a comparison with succinylcholine. Anesth Analg 1993; 77: 579–584

58. Kahwaji R, Bevan D R, Bikhazi G et al. Dose-ranging study in younger adult and elderly patients of ORG 9487, a new, rapid-onset, short-duration muscle relaxant. Anesth Analg 1997; 84: 1011–1018

Leo L. Bossaert

Ventricular fibrillation and transthoracic defibrillation

VENTRICULAR FIBRILLATION (VF) IS THE LEADING CAUSE OF DEATH

Sudden death, defined as death that occurs naturally, unexpectedly and instantaneously or within the first hour after the onset of premonitory symptoms, is one of the most important challenges of modern medicine. This is due to both the high incidence and the dramatic presentation. Moreover, many of the victims are relatively young and had the prospect of many more years of acceptable quality of life: 'hearts too good to die' and 'brains too good to die'.[1-3] In western Europe, more than 250 000 people die from sudden unexpected death each year. The majority of these deaths are associated with acute myocardial ischaemia. VF is the first recorded arrhythmia in 75–80% of patients who have a sudden cardiovascular collapse. Rarely does sustained ventricular tachycardia (VT) alone cause collapse and unconsciousness. Early application of cardiopulmonary resuscitation (CPR) and rapid defibrillation are essential to ensure survival with satisfactory neurological recovery. Fibrillation of the ventricles of the heart is the result of chaotic electrical activity of the heart chambers, resulting in chaotic mechanical activity and loss of co-ordinated myocardial contraction as a consequence, and causing cessation of blood flow and oxygen supply to the vital organs of the body. Loss of oxygen supply to the brain causes brain damage and eventually brain death after only a few minutes. Restoration of blood flow and oxygen supply to the vital organs of the body can only be achieved by restoration of a co-ordinated electrical activity, which is necessary for a co-ordinated mechanical activity.

In the last 15 years, overall 1 month mortality of acute myocardial infarction (AMI) remains virtually unchanged at about 45%. Death from

Prof. Dr Leo L. Bossaert, Departement Geneeskunde, Universitaire Instelling Antwerpen, Universiteitsplein 1, B-2610 Antwerpen (Wilrijk), Belgium

AMI can arise from electrical instability or from extensive myocardial necrosis. More than 60% of AMI-related early deaths occur within 2 h after onset of symptoms, 10% of deaths occur between day 1 and 2, and 30% die between day 3 and day 28. Early deaths are most frequently related to early VF, unrelated to infarct size. Late deaths are related to the extent of myocardial damage, and are precipitated by cardiac failure, shock and late arrhythmias. Lethal pathways, lethal arrhythmias and lethal loss of functional myocardium, need a different interventional strategy during the first few hours after onset of symptoms. The American College of Cardiology, American Heart Association, European Society for Cardiology and the European Resuscitation Council have prepared recommendations for the early management of patients presenting with acute chest pain.[4,5]

Therapeutic strategies

These aim at the various mechanisms involved.

Early death — Primary prevention, early recognition, defibrillation of lethal arrhythmias, supported by CPR and beta-adrenoceptor blocking drugs.

Subacute death — Limitation of infarct size by early mechanical or pharmacological reperfusion therapy.

Late death — Prevention of re-infarction, cardiac failure and late VF by beta-blockers, aspirin and angiotensin-converting enzyme (ACE) inhibitors; implantable cardioverter-defibrillators and coronary revascularisation.

MECHANISM OF SUDDEN CARDIAC DEATH (SCD) AND VENTRICULAR FIBRILLATION (VF)

The initiation of VF: a vulnerable substrate and a trigger

The mechanism of initiation of VF is the consequence of the simultaneous presence of a vulnerable substrate and a trigger.[6,7]

- The **substrate** is usually an area of ischaemic myocardium or an ischaemic border zone surrounding an infarcted area. Other types of pathological substrate are hypertrophy, dilatation, myopathy and congenital abnormalities. In the minority of cases, no pathological substrate can be found.

- The substrate becomes increasingly **vulnerable** (decreased fibrillation threshold) by elevated levels of circulating catecholamines, sympathetic imbalance, endogenous or exogenous toxic products, metabolic abnormalities, pro-arrhythmogenicity of drugs, hyper- and hypothermia. Sympathetic hyperactivity is arrhythmogenic, an elevated vagal activity has a beneficial effect. Heart rate variability is a non-invasive assessment of cardiac autonomic tone. A reduced circadian heart rate variability after myocardial infarction is associated with an increased risk of arrhythmic death and ventricular tachycardia.

- The **final trigger** is usually an early ventricular premature ectopic beat (VPB). The co-existence of ventricular ectopic beats (increased excitability of the substrate, latent pacemaker activity) and abnormal propagation of the impulse (bradycardia, intraventricular conduction blocks, intramural re-entry phenomena) in the presence of a lowered fibrillation threshold, may generate chaotic electrical activity. Once this chaos is present in a critical mass of ventricular myocardium, fibrillation invades the whole ventricle causing VF.

Holter recordings of patients who died suddenly demonstrate that 80% of cases were due to ventricular tachyarrhythmias (VF 60% and VT or torsades de pointes 20%) and the remaining 20% were due to bradyarrhythmias. In the initiation of VF, a so-called 'R on T' extrasystole is a most important factor. Frequently, a period of VT precedes the degeneration of this rhythm into VF. A late cycle ectopic and idioventricular rhythm initiate VF less frequently.[8]

Epidemiology of VF

Incidence

In 1997, a report was published by the World Health Organization[9] revealing that of the 50.5 million deaths that occur each year world-wide, the leading causes of death were ischaemic heart disease (IHD) with 6.3 million deaths per annum and cerebrovascular accidents with 4.4 million deaths. Road traffic accidents accounted for 1.0 million and lung cancer for 0.9 million deaths. In the next 30 years, world-wide mortality is expected to increase for IHD, traffic accidents, cerebrovascular disease, tobacco-attributable mortality, war injuries and COPD (chronic obstructive pulmonary disease). In Europe, the incidence of SCD (sudden cardiac death) due to VF is about 1 per 1000 inhabitants per year according to the MONICA registry.[10] Death due to ischaemic heart disease is most frequent in Nordic countries (Finland, 390 deaths per 100 000 inhabitants per year) and is lower in southern countries (France, 180 deaths per 100 000 inhabitants per year). This lower incidence of death due to IHD is believed to correlate with a different nutritional and behavioural profile (the 'French paradox').[11] In children, cardiac arrest is primarily of respiratory origin: diphtheria, bronchiolitis, asthma, pneumonia, birth trauma and inhalation of foreign material. Other causes are sepsis and cardiomyopathy. In youngsters and young adults, cardiomyopathy and toxic substances are more important aetiologies.[12]

Circadian distribution

Similar to other symptoms of IHD, the time of onset of VF has a circadian distribution pattern with a relatively high risk during day-time and highest peak in the first 3 h after awakening. This time variation correlates with sympathetic instability and related biochemical variations that increase the likelihood of VF or increase the risk of thrombosis in the morning hours. Also, morning increase in physical and mental activity is likely to act as a trigger of sudden cardiac death.[13] Sympathetic overload could be a possible explanation for cardiac arrest without any overt heart disease.[14]

Survival

In the literature, the reported survival of cardiac arrest (CA) varies from less than 5% to 60% according to the characteristics of the cardiac arrest event (e.g. cardiac aetiology or not, witnessed or not, VF or not) and according to the type and the quality of the intervention.[15–20] CPR results are influenced not only by the resuscitation efforts but also by the pre-CPR conditions. Outcome from CA is a complex interplay of so-called 'fate factors' (e.g. age, underlying disease) and 'programme factors' (e.g. time interval to basic life support and to defibrillation). It is now generally accepted that the time to electrical defibrillation is the single most important determinant of survival from ventricular fibrillation. In countries with a reasonably well-functioning emergency medical service (EMS-system), before introduction of automated external defibrillators operated by ambulance personnel, only some 15% of all prehospital cardiac arrest victims have restoration of spontaneous circulation (ROSC) and reach the hospital alive. Of those, only 50% survived to discharge (5–7%). Considering VF patients only, survival to discharge is about double (15–20%). In areas where early defibrillation by ambulance personnel is implemented, more patients are found in VF, and survival to hospital discharge in VF patients may be as high as 25–28%. About two-thirds of cardiac arrests occur at home, in patients aged > 50 years of age (about 75%), during day-time between 0800–1800 hours (about 75%). In most reports on out-of-hospital cardiac arrest presenting with VF, CA is witnessed in two-thirds of cases. The profile of the cardiac arrest patient is helpful to identify the profile of the potential bystander of a cardiac arrest event and, therefore, the primary target group for teaching citizen-CPR, i.e. the persons being in the neighbourhood of male individuals aged > 50 years, being at home during day-time, i.e. housewives, family members and relatives of cardiac patients.

Aetiology of VF

Primary VF

Primary VF, in the absence of shock or cardiac failure, occurs in the first 5–10 min after the onset of coronary occlusion, and is usually induced by an early R-on-T ventricular premature beat and, less frequently, through degeneration of a ventricular tachycardia. The success rate for resuscitation of patients in the first minute of primary VF is probably 90–95%.

Secondary VF

Secondary VF occurs in the presence of shock or cardiac failure and is caused by several mechanisms including hypertrophy, dilatation, stretching, metabolic disorders, proarrhythmic drugs. Secondary VF has a far lower prognosis for successful resuscitation, with probably less than 30% of patients recovering.[21]

Ischaemic heart disease

Ischaemic heart disease is responsible for more than 80% of cases VF.[22–24] More than 30% of all patients suffering from AMI die from VF within the first 2 h after onset of symptoms. During hospital admission for AMI, about 10% of patients develops VT and another 7–10% develop VF. Myocardial infarction is clearly associated with life threatening arrhythmias, but only 20% of sudden cardiac death victims have actually sustained an AMI. Transient ischaemia and reperfusion rather than infarction have a major role in triggering the arrhythmias leading to sudden cardiac death. Reperfusion arrhythmias and cell damage are also related to oxidative damage incurred during the critical first minute of reperfusion. In ischaemic myocardium, endothelin and free radicals are produced abundantly.[25] Both agents appear in the coronary circulation after spontaneous restoration of coronary flow or after thrombolysis, angioplasty or bypass surgery. Endothelin is a potent vasoconstrictor and is also a pro-arrhythmic agent. It is believed that scavengers of oxygen-derived free radicals protect against reperfusion injury.[26]

Coronary spasm and substance abuse

Coronary spasm and substance abuse can be responsible for VF in patients without significant structural heart disease. Cocaine abuse can provoke lethal cardiac events, including AMI and VF. Cocaine acts as a local anaesthetic (inducing impaired impulse conduction and inhomogeneities in repolarization, which is an ideal substrate for re-entrant arrhythmias) and as a powerful cardiac stimulant that accentuates the actions of the sympathetic nervous system (activating alpha- and beta-adrenergic receptors, which can provoke coronary vasospasm, myocardial ischaemia and cardiac arrhythmias).[27] In youngsters, there is also a steady increase in the number of deaths occurring from volatile substance abuse. Fuel gases and other solvents, such as typewriter correction fluid, dry-cleaning fluids and fire extinguishers, sensitize the heart to circulating catecholamines, such that sudden emotion or exercise may precipitate sudden death.[28]

Ventricular dilatation and congestive heart failure

In patients with dilated cardiomyopathy, ventricular arrhythmias are present in more than 80% of cases. In patients dying from heart failure, 50–70% of deaths are sudden and unexpected before they have deteriorated to NYHA class IV. The substrate for sudden death is myocardial scar tissue, hypertrophy and aberrant conducting pathways; ventricular arrhythmia is a trigger event in the development of fatal arrhythmias; intermittent regional myocardial ischaemia, interaction with inotropes, inodilators, antiarrhythmic drugs, digitalis toxicity, electrolyte or autonomic nervous system imbalance are important additional precipitating factors. Sudden death is most likely to be prevented by interventions that result in improvement of left ventricular function, such as ACE inhibition and probably moderate beta-adrenoceptor blockade.[29–31]

Congenital heart disease: long QT and WPW syndrome

Sudden death due to VF is a well-known, but rare, complication of rapid atrial fibrillation in the Wolff-Parkinson-White (WPW) syndrome. In 1988, the

European Registry on 'sudden death in the WPW syndrome' collected only 26 cases from various centres.[32] Sudden arrhythmic death has also been described in patients with the idiopathic long QT syndrome. The pathogenic mechanism of idiopathic long QT syndrome is probably related to an abnormal myocardial sympathetic innervation.[33]

Hypothermia

Death due to VF or asystole occurs between 28–25°C. Spontaneous reversible VF has been demonstrated in hypothermic experimental animals. In a survey of 234 cases of accidental hypothermia, factors related with survival were rapid cooling rate, presence of VF in cardiac arrest patients and presence of narcotics and/or alcohol during hypothermia. Among the survivors, the coldest patient had a core temperature of 17.5°C and the longest cardiac arrest with a favourable outcome lasted 4.75 h.[34]

The role of anti-arrhythmic drugs

The Cardiac Arrhythmia Suppression Trial (CAST) has demonstrated that certain anti-arrhythmic drugs not only fail to abolish dysrhythmias, but even increase arrhythmic mortality. In patients with IHD and treated with anti-arrhythmic drugs, pro-arrhythmic effects were observed in 8–10%.[35,36] Pro-arrhythmia can be defined as: (i) greater than 4-fold increase in VPBs (premature ventricular beats); (ii) greater than 10-fold increase in repetitive forms; or (iii) new occurrence of ventricular tachycardia or VF (VT/VF). It is most frequently observed in class IC drugs. No arrhythmia-suppressing drug is completely free of this type of reaction. No pro-arrhythmic effect has been observed with calcium antagonists or beta-adrenoceptor blockers. Beta-adrenoceptor blockers remain the only class of agents that, in control trials, have been shown to reduce sudden death. Beta-adrenoceptor blockers appear to act by preventing VF and not by suppressing premature ventricular contractions (VPBs).[37] Therefore, our attention should shift from ectopic-suppressing interventions (class I agents, but also interventional anti-arrhythmic techniques) to agents with antifibrillatory actions by sympathetic antagonism (class II; beta-adrenoceptor blockers) and by lengthening myocardial refractoriness (class III; amiodarone).[38–40]

Electric shock and lightning

Exposure to low voltage alternating current (220–380 V) may reach the heart during the vulnerable phase of the cardiac cycle and may precipitate VF. Lightning acts as a massive unsynchronized DC shock and may produce VF or asystole.[41]

VENTRICULAR DEFIBRILLATION

The rapidly increasing role of transthoracic defibrillation was initiated in the early 1950s, after major contributions by Jude and Knickerbocker (external chest compression), Elam (ventilation), Safar (the ABC concept), Beck, Kouwenhoven, Negovsky, Gurvich and Zoll (defibrillation), Dahl and Pantridge (prehospital defibrillation) and others, and by huge technological improvements.[42,43]

Mechanism of defibrillation

Electrical defibrillation is the only effective method of terminating VF and of restoring a perfusing cardiac rhythm. External defibrillation of the heart works by delivering an adequate electrical current flow through the heart, through electrodes applied to the chest wall, causing simultaneous depolarization of all myocardial cells that are at that moment fully refractory. This current is determined by the applied voltage and the transthoracic impedance. Defibrillators consist of a power source (battery, AC source), a voltage selector, an AC–DC converter, a capacitor and electrodes.[44–46] The output of the defibrillator is usually expressed in terms of energy, where: energy (J) = power (W) × duration (s); power (W) = potential (V) × current (A); and current (A) = potential (V)/resistance or impedance (Ω). Current is responsible for successful defibrillation, but defibrillator output is most commonly measured in units of energy (J).

After defibrillation, myocardial contraction is re-established within moments but, initially, cardiac output may be extremely weak, especially after prolonged VF, and continues to increase over minutes or even hours. This phenomenon was described as the postcountershock pulseless rhythm or postcountershock myocardial depression. Therefore, a short period of CPR is needed after delivery of a successful defibrillation.

Defibrillation waveforms

Defibrillation of the heart is achieved if an electrical current depolarizes the majority of the unsynchronized fibrillating myocardial cells. The applied current or the corresponding voltage described as a function of time is called the waveform.[47,48] The source of voltage is a charged capacitor, the discharge waveform is modified by the inclusion of an inductor in the discharge circuit (damped sine wave) or by direct discharge of a capacitor that is electrically truncated after a given period of time (truncated exponential). The output waveform of most conventional external defibrillators is half sinusoidal (damped Edmark waveform) or truncated exponential with a duration of 4–12 ms.

Inspired by the work of Russian investigators and by the experience of implanted automatic cardioverter-defibrillators (ICD), the use of biphasic waveforms has been introduced. In ICDs, defibrillation threshold is lower when using biphasic waveforms and causes less myocardial dysfunction. Biphasic defibrillation is now the standard of care for ICDs. The step from biphasic ICDs to biphasic external defibrillators was logical. Transthoracic biphasic external defibrillation has now been introduced in clinical practice. Biphasic waveforms have lower defibrillation thresholds than monophasic waveforms of the same duration: the first biphasic defibrillatory shocks with energies as low as 115 J seemed to be equally efficient as conventional first shocks with 200 J. Biphasic waveforms require less energy and, therefore,

Table 3.1 Electrophysiological profile of antiarrhythmic drugs

Drug	Fibrillation threshold	Defibrillation threshold	Pro arrhythmo genicity
Quinidine	++	+++	+
Procainamide	++	0	+
Encainide	++	+++	+
Flecainide	++	+++	+
Lidocaine	++	+	+
Bretylium	++	−	+
Amiodarone	++	−	0/+
Adrenergic agents	−	0	+
Sotalol	+	−	+

+ = increase; − = decrease; 0 = no influence.

capacitors and batteries can be simpler and so this new waveform technology could lead to lighter, simpler and cheaper defibrillators. Also, some reports suggest that less shock-induced myocardial damage is seen after biphasic shocks.[49-52] Further investigation is needed to define the optimum energy level and the optimum shape of the biphasic wave (voltage, slope and duration of positive and of negative wave). It can be expected that, in the near future, most major manufacturers of external defibrillators will include biphasic technology in their programme.

Transthoracic impedance, threshold and energy requirements

The amount of current flowing through the heart depends on the energy of the shock and on the transthoracic impedance. During transthoracic defibrillation in humans, as little as 4% of the delivered transthoracic current traverses the heart because parallel pathways (thoracic cage, lungs) shunt the current around the heart.

Defibrillation threshold

Defibrillation threshold is the minimum shock strength that is able to abolish fibrillation. Defibrillation threshold is influenced by anatomical variations in heart size, ventricular filling, lung volumes, by electrical variables such as defibrillation waveform, metabolic state, and by biochemical and physiological differences in temperature, tissue pH and PO_2, extracellular potassium concentration, ischaemia and drugs. The energy requirement for defibrillation increases with the duration of fibrillation. The success of defibrillation is not only a matter of threshold but also a matter of probability.[53] Electrophysiological studies have documented variable influences of anti-arrhythmic drugs on fibrillation and defibrillation thresholds (Table 3.1).[54,55] The sum of these variables can be responsible for a 5-fold difference in threshold when measuring the threshold at consecutive moments.

Transthoracic impedance

Transthoracic impedance depends on time to defibrillation, electrode size (contact, pressure, distance), previous shocks, and ventilatory phase.[56,57] The transthoracic impedance seems to decrease after the first shock. The average human transthoracic impedance is 70–80 Ω, but can occasionally be as high as 150 Ω and as low as 15 Ω. Attempts at defibrillation (assuming the same energy setting) will thus result in a wide range of delivered currents. It is known that high defibrillation currents produce myocardial damage; conversely, currents which are too low will fail to achieve defibrillation. First shock energy can be predicted and adjusted based on automatic measurement of impedance, and inappropriate low energies can be avoided in high impedance patients. This principle is already implemented in modern equipment.

Energy requirements

Defibrillation at too high energy levels can be pro-arrhythmic and can inflict functional and morphological damage to the myocardium. Shocks below the defibrillation threshold are ineffective and harmful because they may re-initiate VF by stimulating parts of the myocardium during their vulnerable period.[58–62] Clinical investigation has demonstrated that defibrillation success rates and subsequent hospital discharge rates were virtually identical in patients receiving an initial monophasic shock of 175 or 320 J. Therefore, the energy selected for the first shock is a trade-off between probability of success and risk of damage. The following guideline is currently accepted for monophasic waveform defibrillation of an adult presenting with VF: first shock, 200 J; second shock, 200–300 J; subsequent shocks, 360 J. In children, a weight related initial energy of 2 J/kg is recommended, then 2–4 J/kg, then 4J/kg.[63]

Practical considerations[64]

Electrodes

Electrode size, shape and position are important determinants of transthoracic current flow during external countershock.[65] Larger self-adhesive defibrillator pads are associated with a lower transthoracic impedance and improved defibrillation success rates with low energy shocks. The optimum electrode size is about 13 cm diameter in adults. In children, adult electrodes should be used whenever possible, but overlap has to be avoided. If the size of the child is too small, paediatric electrodes have to be used.[66] Unfortunately, there has been no attempt at standardization of the adhesive pads for automated external defibrillators. Paddle position influences current flow through the myocardium. One electrode should be placed below the outer half of the right clavicle and the other just outside the usual position of the cardiac apex (V4-5 position). Anterior-posterior (one paddle over the precordium and the other on the back just behind the heart) electrode placements are recommended in patients with implanted defibrillators or pacemakers. The influence of polarity on the defibrillation threshold is negligible.[67] Disposable coupling pads are as effective as electrode paste and are preferred, as jelly tends to be spread across the chest wall during resuscitative efforts: the delivered shock then arcs across the chest wall, failing to reach the heart in adequate strength.[68]

Safety

Small explosions and burns have occasionally been documented in patients that have been defibrillated while carrying nitro-patches. There is now evidence that it is not the nitroglycerine but the metallic components of transdermal patches that are responsible for the explosions. Therefore all patches should be removed from the chest wall before performing external defibrillation.[69] Airborne defibrillation does not interfere with avionics equipment, so defibrillation can be performed in aircraft and helicopters, provided standard defibrillation cautions are observed.[70]

External defibrillation and pacemakers

Pacemaker malfunction including transient malfunctions of pacing, capture and sensing has been reported after external defibrillation.[71] In the presence of an implanted pacemaker, anterior-posterior electrode placement or a paddle position keeping a distance of 12–15 cm from the pacemaker house is recommended. It is also recommended to check pacing functions in pacemaker patients who have been defibrillated. Pacemaker spikes may interfere with the diagnostic algorithm of automated defibrillators.

Technical problems

In a review of more than 2100 technical reports related to defibrillator problems, some failures were attributable to component malfunctions, but inappropriate operator use and maintenance accounted for the majority of defibrillator failures. In places of high incidence of defibrillator use, such as ambulances, emergency departments, intensive and coronary care units, operating theatres and catheterization labs, it is recommended to assess the operational state of the equipment every day using appropriate checklists. Inadequate training and retraining increase the chances of operator errors at the moment when correct operation is needed most.[72]

The role of time in VF and defibrillation

VF waves have initially a large amplitude of 0.2 mV and a median frequency of about 200 to 300 bpm. Progressively, rate and amplitude decrease and, after some 12–15 min, the fibrillation waves fade out to become a flat iso-electric line. There is a clear association between amplitude of VF and outcome.[73] Median VF frequency can also be used to estimate the time from collapse until assessment.[74,75] Combining amplitude and frequency is helpful to identify patients with a very low probability of survival. The majority of patients presenting with fine and slow VF are highly resistant to resuscitation.[76]

The chances of successful defibrillation decrease rapidly over time, at a speed of more than 5%/min, due to a rapid depletion of left ventricular content in high-energy phosphates.[77,78] After some minutes, the amplitude and the frequency of the VF waveform decreases and after some 15 min the VF degenerates into asystole; therefore, the presence of asystole usually indicates that the time since collapse is long.

The percentage of cardiac arrest patients found in VF is a reflection of the speed of intervention of the EMS. Literature data for incidence of VF in different cities and countries around the world range from 62% to less than 10%. Figures are worse in 'vertical cities' (Chicago, New York) and better in 'horizontal cities' (Seattle, Houston, Miami, many European cities). As could be expected, there is a significant correlation between the incidence of VF as the first presenting rhythm and subsequent survival.

Treatment strategies for VF: the 'chain of survival' concept

People are more likely to survive prehospital cardiac arrest when activation of the EMS-system, basic cardiopulmonary resuscitation (CPR), defibrillation and advanced care occur as rapidly as possible. The concept of the **chain of survival**[86,87] describes the interventions that are needed for optimal survival. This concept illustrates also that the weakness of any of these links condemns EMS to poor results.[79,80]

The first link in the chain of survival, **early access** is essential to bring trained people and appropriate equipment, i.e. the defibrillator, quickly to the patient. This includes recognition of the collapse, decision to call, calling and dispatch, and can be strengthened by public education and availability of an efficient emergency communication system (including a unique simple telephone number for medical emergencies).

The importance of the second link, **early CPR** by the first person witnessing the arrest (lay person or other bystanding health care worker), has been shown abundantly. Bystander CPR is able to keep the heart some 10–12 min longer in VF. Basic CPR is effective at sustaining life until the early arrival of trained and equipped people and is, therefore, a bridge to first defibrillation.

The most crucial link is **early defibrillation**. Initially, prehospital defibrillation was only performed by medical and paramedical personnel, but recently newer and reliable technology has allowed the expansion in the use of a defibrillator to the first-line ambulanceman. First tier ambulances arrive many vital minutes before arrival of the second tier. Primary rescue teams, such as police, security personnel and fire fighters are present at the scene several minutes before the first tier ambulance of the EMS. In remote areas (airplanes, cruise ships, trains), board personnel are the only official personnel who could be in charge of delivering a defibrillatory shock within seconds or minutes. To shorten the time to defibrillation, rescuers in the community other than doctors or paramedics should have access to defibrillation.[81–85] Early defibrillation is of high value as long as the other links in the chain of survival do not fail. In systems where access time is excessively long, only a disappointing limited usefulness of an early defibrillation programme can be expected.

The fourth link, **early advanced life support**, implies early intervention of a well-trained and well-equipped team, working with specially equipped ambulances or rapid intervention vehicles. These teams consist of paramedics (in the USA, UK, Scandinavia) or trained ambulancemen, doctors and/or nurses (in most European countries). It is depressing to observe that more than

Recent Advances in Anaesthesia and Analgesia 20

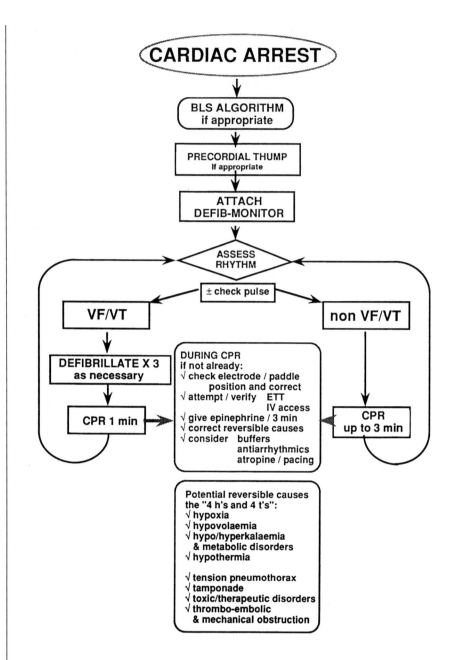

Fig. 3.1 The algorithm for ALS-management of the cardiac arrest patient, according to the International Liaison Committee on Resuscitation (ILCOR).

50% of patients who could initially be resuscitated to restoration of spontaneous circulation (ROSC), do not survive to hospital discharge, and die from the pathology initiating the cardiac arrest, from hypoxic damage of organs including the brain and the heart, and from reperfusion damage. Therapeutic possibilities in this area are still limited.

In optimal conditions with a rapidly responding and highly qualified EMS-system, the initial resuscitation rate for out-of-hospital VF can be as high as 60%, and 25–30% may eventually survive to hospital discharge.

Resuscitation algorithms for VF

In an attempt to produce international guidelines for resuscitation, the major multinational, multidisciplinary guidelines producing resuscitation councils (European Resuscitation Council, American Heart Association, Canadian Heart and Stroke Foundation, Australian Resuscitation Council and Southern African Resuscitation Council) created, in 1992, the International Liaison Committee on Resuscitation (ILCOR). In 1997, ILCOR published advisory statements for basic and advanced life support of newborns, children and adults in the journals *Resuscitation* and *Circulation*.[89]

Based on the available scientific knowledge, a universal algorithm for ALS management of VF patients was proposed.[86–90] After confirmation of cardiac arrest, a precordial thump should be given immediately and the defibrillator pads should be applied. The diagnosis of VF should be followed immediately by 3 electric shocks of 200 J, 200–300 J, 360 J, without interposed CPR. If the initial 3 shocks are unsuccessful, the patient should be intubated, and i.v. access should be achieved – if these manoeuvres have not already been performed. Any intubation attempt should be aborted temporarily if it was unsuccessful after about 30 s. At this stage, 1 mg epinephrine should be given i.v. (2.5 mg when given by tracheal tube), and 10 CPR sequences of 5 chest compressions with 1 ventilation should be given. The next shocks should be given as urgently as possible and the interval between the 3rd and the next (4th) shock should not exceed 2 min: the quicker a co-ordinated rhythm is restored, the better the prospects of long-term success. The 4th shock forms the beginning of a new sequence of 3 shocks. It follows that the doses of 1 mg epinephrine will be given at 2–3 min intervals (Fig. 3.1).

THE AUTOMATED EXTERNAL DEFIBRILLATOR (AED)

Defibrillation was once a medical act which could only be delegated to emergency care providers who are trained in ALS. AEDs eliminate the need for training in rhythm recognition and make early defibrillation by minimally trained personnel practical and achievable.

Technical aspects of AEDs

The term automated defibrillator refers to external defibrillators that incorporate a rhythm analysis system. AEDs are attached to the patient by 2 adhesive pads and connecting cables to analyze the rhythm and to deliver the command to give a shock. The information is given by voice and/or on a visual display and the final delivery of the shock is triggered manually. These systems have great potential for use by basic ambulance men who may not be trained in ECG interpretation. Although specificity for VF is about 100%, sensitivity in the case of coarse VF is about 90–92% and, in the case of fine VF, even lower. Failures of the diagnostic algorithm have been documented when using an AED in patients carrying an implanted pacemaker. The currently available equipment is relatively expensive, and performance is dependent on good maintenance. A new generation of AEDs uses new battery technology and some of them also the new biphasic waveform technology. They are smaller, simpler, reliable and inexpensive. Some of the new devices have the facility for an ECG display, others have not. These new generation AEDs will stimulate widespread availability of defibrillators in ambulances, hospital wards, places of work, public places, airplanes and cruise ships.[91,92]

Early defibrillation by first responding ambulance personnel

Electrical defibrillation is the only effective therapy for VF. The chances of successful defibrillation decrease rapidly over time, with more than 5%/min. Therefore, the time between onset of VF and defibrillation should be as short as possible to increase the chances of survival. Bystander CPR is able to keep the heart longer in VF, for some 10–15 min and is, therefore, a bridge to first defibrillation. In two-tiered EMS-system, the first tier ambulance arrives several minutes before arrival of the second tiered ambulance, which had usually the defibrillator and medically qualified personnel on board. This was illustrated by the Belgian CPCR Registry, where 69% of the studied cardiac arrest patients were initially attended by the first tiered basic ambulance manned by 2 EMTs; the median time interval between collapse and start of BLS resuscitation by the EMTs was 8 min; the median time interval between collapse and defibrillation by the second tiered medical ALS resuscitation team was 16 min. It was concluded that EMTs can be expected to reach a substantial number of VF victims within a few minutes after the collapse and many minutes before arrival of the medical ALS resuscitation team (Fig. 3.2).[93]

Therefore, it is logical to equip first tiered ambulances with defibrillators and to train first line ambulancemen in the use of the AED. The expected result is that EMS, based on early defibrillation by the ambulancemen who respond first, provide significantly shorter times to initial countershock.

A training course of 8–10 h followed by 6-monthly refresher courses is sufficient to instruct a minimally trained ambulanceman in the proper use of an AED according to a standard protocol. The AED training course and the subsequent implementation of an AED programme, should be placed under full medical supervision. Perfect knowledge of basic CPR is a prerequisite for successfully attending an AED course. The course should include background information, knowledge of the equipment and its maintenance, knowledge of the protocol and should be tested by an examination. Refresher courses should include feedback instructions discussing each intervention and formal 6-monthly courses.

Slow implementation of AED in Europe

The first successful defibrillation of VF outside the hospital was achieved by the Belfast Mobile Coronary Care Unit in 1966 and the first automated defibrillators appeared in Brighton and Seattle in the late 1970s.[94–96] After these early experiences with AEDs, the technology was further developed and

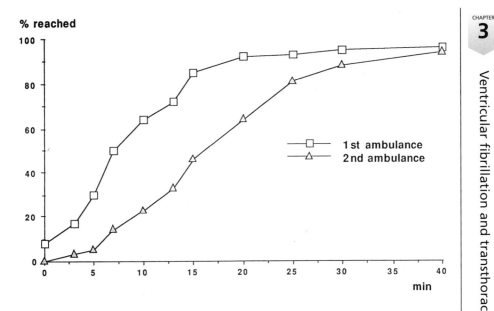

% reached

1st ambulance
2nd ambulance

Fig. 3.2 Cumulative inclusion of 2310 patients presenting with cardiac arrest, treated by the first tiered ambulance (1st ambulance) before arrival of the medical intervention team (2nd ambulance): from Calle et al (1992).[93]

implemented in several centres in the US and Europe. In Europe, the strategy of early defibrillation with AEDs by ambulance personnel is now implemented community-wide in the UK and Scandinavia, and in parts of Germany and Belgium. Pilot experiences are emerging in many European countries. In some European countries, all ambulances are manned with experienced nurses and/or doctors and are equipped with manual defibrillators. As a result of these experiences, it was recognized that an early defibrillation programme has the best chances of success if: (i) the programme is placed under medical control; (ii) the time interval between cardiac arrest and first CPR is usually < 4 min; (iii) the time interval between cardiac arrest and defibrillation is usually < 12 min; (iv) there is a critical number of interventions; (v) there is a programme of training and retraining; and (vi) there is a programme for monitoring performance. AED programmes are only partially implemented in Europe and in the US less than 50% of ambulances are equipped with an AED.[97] The major reasons for slow implementation are awareness, organization and legislation.

Awareness

Public awareness is not only influenced by science but also by the media. Science indicates that more than 45% of mortality in Europe is caused by cardiovascular disease. In a recent survey in a sample of the Belgian adult population, only 8% of respondents answered that cardiovascular disease was their major concern, whereas the answer was 18% for media-prone traffic accidents and 17% for AIDS.

Organization

In all European countries, access to the EMS is available with a specific telephone number. The European Union published in 1991 Recommendation 396: the uniform European emergency telephone number 112 should be available in 1997.[98] This is actually the case in most European countries.

There is a wide variety of systems involved in European EMS: (i) one-tiered systems delivering BLS by an emergency medical technician; (ii) one-tiered systems delivering BLS and defibrillation by an emergency medical technician; (iii) one-tiered systems delivering BLS and ALS by paramedics, doctors and/or nurses; (iv) two-tiered systems delivering BLS followed by ALS; and (v) two-tiered systems delivering BLS and defibrillation, followed by ALS. It was demonstrated that best performance, in terms of survival, is obtained by systems with the highest qualification.[98]

In the majority of European countries, doctors have an active role in prehospital emergency medical care, as part of the first or second tier. In most parts of Scandinavia and in the UK, paramedics serve as members of the second tier. Medical presence in the field could be one of the reasons for slow involvement of ambulance personnel in the act of defibrillation.[99–101] The structure and organization of the EMS in European countries, and the legal background for defibrillation practice, are summarized in Table 3.2.

Legislation

The 'Code Napoléon' influenced law and organization in most European countries. However, due to historical, organizational, political and religious reasons, legislation related to resuscitation and defibrillation is different in European countries. In countries where historically only ambulancemen and paramedics were present in the field, the implementation of early defibrillation by ambulancemen was easy. In countries, however, where medical presence was prominent in the second or even in the first tier, the introduction of defibrillation by ambulancemen who were first to attend was much slower. Data in Table 3.2 indicate that, in at least 11 European countries, law is a major or minor obstacle for nationwide implementation of AED programmes by non-physicians. Fortunately, legal and regulatory aspects of defibrillation are changing very rapidly.

Results of AED programmes: uniform reporting according to the Utstein style

Reported data on survival after cardiac arrest due to VF, using an AED by non-medically qualified personnel, range between 4% and 31%. These differences could be related to differences in the characteristics of the treated population, differences in methodology and quality of registration or real differences in the performance of the AED-programme.[102–108] The **Utstein style** for out-of-hospital and in-hospital cardiac arrest and resuscitation is a glossary of terms and reporting guidelines for the description of cardiac arrest, resuscitation, the EMS and the outcome, and was published by the American Heart Association (AHA), the European Resuscitation Council (ERC), the Heart and Stroke

Table 3.2 Legal and regulatory aspects of EMS in European countries

Country	Ambulance 1st Tier	Ambulance 2nd Tier	Emergency phone	Allowed to start CPR	Allowed to stop CPR	Allowed to defibrillate
Austria	emt	md	144	anyone trained	md	md, rn, emt (md present)
Belgium	emt-(d)	md	100	anyone	md	md, rn, emt-d
Bulgaria	md	md	150	anyone trained	emt	md, rn, emt-d
Croatia	md	–	94	no law	md	md
Czech Rep	emt	md	155	anyone	md (evidence)	md,pm
Denmark	emt-(d)	(pm)	112	anyone	md	md, rn, emt-d
Finland	emt-(d)	md	112	anyone	md (evidence)	anyone trained
France	emt	md	15	anyone	md (no law)	md, rn, emt-d
Germany	emt-(d)+pm	md	112	anyone trained	md	md, pm
Greece	emt	–	166	anyone trained	md	md
Hungary	emt-(d)	rn/md	104	anyone	md (no law)	md, pm, emt-d
Iceland	emt-(d)	md	0112	anyone trained	md	md, emt (md present)
Ireland	emt	md	999	no law	md, pm	md, rn, pm
Italy	emt	(md)	118	anyone	md	md, rn
Netherlands	rn	–	06-11	anyone	no law	md, rn
Norway	emt-d	md/pm	113	anyone	no law	md, emt
Poland	md	md	999	no law	md	md, emt (md present)
Portugal	md	.	115	anyone	md	md, emt (md present)
Romania	rn/md	md	06	anyone trained	md (no law)	md, rn
Russia	md	–	03	anyone trained	md	md, rn, emt-d
Slovakia	md/pm/rn	md	155	anyone trained	md	md, rn, emt-d, pm
Slovenia	md	–	94	anyone	md	md, rn, emt-d
Spain	emt/rn/md	–	061	anyone trained	no law	md, rn (no law)
Sweden	emt-d	pm	112	anyone	md	md, rn, emt-d
Switzerland	emt	(md)	114	anyone trained	md	md, rn, pm
Turkey	md	–	118	anyone trained	md	md
UK	emt-(d)	(pm)	999	no law	no law	no law
Yugoslavia (former)	md	md	94	anyone	md	md, rn, emt

Figures for 1st and 2nd tier between parentheses indicate local variations in the country. md = medical doctor; rn = nurse; pm = paramedic; emt = emergency medical technician; emt-d = emergency medical technician qualified for use of AED.

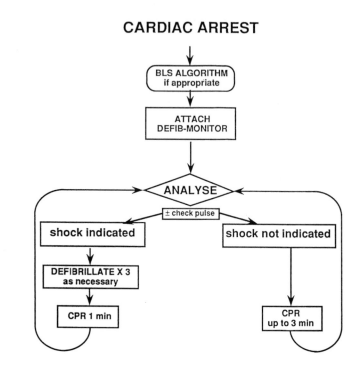

CARDIAC ARREST

Fig. 3.3 The algorithm for the use of automated external defibrillators in the management of VF patients, according to the International Liaison Committee on Resuscitation (ILCOR).

Foundation of Canada and the Southern African and Australian Resuscitation Councils.[109,110]

The ILCOR advisory statements for automated external defibrillation

Based on the available scientific knowledge, a universal algorithm for the use of automated external defibrillators in the management of VF patients was proposed by ILCOR (Fig. 3.3).[111,112] To achieve the earliest possible defibrillation, in many settings, non-medical individuals must be allowed and encouraged to use defibrillators. ILCOR recommends that all resuscitation personnel be authorized, trained, equipped and directed to operate a defibrillator, if their professional responsibilities require them to respond to persons in cardiac arrest. This recommendation includes all first-response emergency personnel, in both the hospital and out-of-hospital setting, whether physicians, nurses, or non-medical ambulance personnel. The widespread availability of automated external defibrillators now provides the technological capacity to provide early defibrillation by ambulance crews and by lay responders.

Early defibrillation by first-response ambulance personnel

ILCOR urges the medical profession to increase the awareness of the public, and of the people who are responsible for emergency medical services, of the importance of early defibrillation by ambulance personnel. In some locations, the medical profession will need to encourage medical and regulatory authorities to initiate changes in regulations and legislation. EMS leaders may need to overcome obstacles that include: non-enabling legislation, economic priorities, unsuitable EMS structure, lack of awareness, inadequate motivation and tradition. ILCOR recommends the following actions:

- to promulgate explicit written policies and guidelines similar to those already developed by the ERC and the AHA.
- to establish a training and quality maintenance programme that ensures a high level of supervision.
- to place the programme under the direction and responsibility of a physician.
- to use only AEDs that contain internal recording facilities to permit documentation and review of all clinical interventions.

All resuscitation efforts should be accurately recorded and reviewed using the out-of-hospital Utstein style.

Early defibrillation by first responders in the hospital

ILCOR encourages the following steps:

- to develop early defibrillation programmes for first responders in the hospital.
- to regularly train all hospital staff in basic life support.
- to establish and encourage AED training as a basic skill for health care providers working in settings where advanced life support professionals are not available immediately.
- to extend training and authorization to use conventional and automated defibrillators to all appropriate non-physician staff, including nurses, respiratory therapists, and physician assistants.
- to make defibrillators available in strategic areas throughout the hospital.

All resuscitation efforts should be accurately recorded and reviewed using the in-hospital Utstein style. An interdisciplinary committee should be established, with expertise in CPR, to assess the quality and efficacy of the resuscitation efforts.

Early defibrillation by first responders in the community

As considerable time may elapse between the onset of VF and the arrival of the EMS, immediate defibrillation by first-response trained bystanders may be the long-term realization of the concept of early defibrillation. The term 'first responder' is defined as a trained individual acting independently in a medically controlled system. Immediate defibrillation by first responders in the community offers a promising direction for the future evolution of early defibrillation. First responders may include the police, security officers, life guards, airline cabin attendants, railroad station officers, voluntary aiders and those assigned to provide first aid at their workplace or in the community, and are trained in how to use AEDs. Research has not yet demonstrated that the widespread dissemination of defibrillators into public places, accessible by random witnesses to an arrest, can increase overall community survival rates. Programmes should be developed to test the principle that first responders assigned to the management of cardiac arrest in the community should be trained and permitted to defibrillate. Every programme designed to implement first responder defibrillation should be co-ordinated by a physician and be critically evaluated to confirm that first responder defibrillation increases survival.

Early defibrillation and the chain of survival concept

Early defibrillation answers just part of the problem of sudden cardiac death. Early defibrillation initiatives will succeed only when implemented as part of the chain of survival concept. The links in the chain of survival include early recognition of cardiopulmonary arrest, early activation of trained responders, early CPR, early defibrillation when indicated, and early initiation of advanced life support. Establishment of early defibrillation within a strong chain of survival will ensure the highest possible survival for both out-of-hospital and in-hospital events.

CONCLUSIONS

Cardiorespiratory arrest due to sudden arrhythmias as a consequence of myocardial ischaemia or infarction will continue to be a leading cause of unexpected death in the community. Expanded public education of the recognition of the early symptoms and signs of a heart attack is likely to achieve a significant reduction in the present mortality and morbidity from of out-of-hospital heart attack. Electrical defibrillation is the single most important therapy for the treatment of VF. The time interval between the onset of VF and the delivery of the first defibrillation shock is clearly the main determinant of survival. To achieve the goal of early defibrillation, it is mandatory to allow for individuals other than doctors to defibrillate. Overwhelming scientific and clinical evidence re-inforces early defibrillation as the standard of medical practice. At present, however, early defibrillation by ambulance personnel using automated external defibrillation (AED), is not yet widely implemented.

References

1. Beck C, Leighninger D. Death after a clean bill of health. JAMA 1960; 174: 133–135
2. Brugada P, Andries E W, Mont L, Gursoy S, Willems H, Kaissar S. Mechanisms of sudden cardiac death. Drugs 1991; 41 Suppl 2: 16–23
3. Myerburg R, Kessler K M, Castellanos A. Sudden cardiac death: epidemiology, transient risk, and intervention assessment. Ann Intern Med 1993; 119: 1187–1197
4. Chamberlain D, Arntz R, Bossaert L et al. The prehospital management of acute heart attacks. Recommendations of a task force of the European Society for Cardiology and the European Resuscitation Council. Resuscitation 1998: 37: (In press)

Key points for clinical practice

- The medical profession is urged to increase awareness of the public, of those responsible for emergency medical services and of those with regulatory powers, to permit changes in practice and legislation where necessary.

- It is essential to integrate the concept of early defibrillation into an effective emergency cardiac care system. This is best characterized by the 'chain of survival' concept, which includes early access to the emergency medical services, early cardiopulmonary resuscitation when needed, early defibrillation when indicated, and early advanced cardiac care.

- All emergency personnel should be trained and permitted to operate an appropriately maintained defibrillator if their professional activities require that they respond to persons experiencing cardiac arrest. This includes all first-response emergency personnel working in an organized emergency medical service, both hospital and non-hospital.

- All emergency ambulances and other emergency vehicles that respond to or transport cardiac patients should be equipped with a defibrillator.

- Defibrillation should be a core competence of all health care professionals, including nurses, and defibrillators should be widely available on general hospital wards.

- All defibrillator programmes must operate within medical control by qualified and experienced physicians. They should ensure that every link in the chain of survival is in place and should have access to all information required to permit system audit.

- To monitor the programme, there must be appropriate registration of the interventions according to the Utstein style.

5. ACC/AHA Guidelines for the management of patients with acute myocardial infarction. A report of the ACC/AHA task force on practice guidelines (committee on management of acute myocardial infarction). J Am Coll Cardiol 1996; 28: 1328–1428

6. Willich S N, Maclure M, Mittleman M, Arntz H R, Muller J E. Sudden cardiac death. Support for a role of triggering in causation. Circulation 1993; 87: 1442–1450

7. Davies M J. Anatomic features in victims of sudden coronary death: coronary artery pathology. Circulation 1992; 85: I-19–I-24

8. Bayes de Luna A, Coumel P, Leclercq J F. Ambulatory sudden death: mechanism of production of fatal arrhythmias on the basis of data from 157 cases. Am Heart J 1989; 117: 151–159

9. Murray C J, Lopez A D. Mortality by cause for eight regions of the world: Global Burden of Disease Study. Lancet 1997; 349: 1269–1276, 1498–1504

10. Chambless L, Keil U, Dobson A et al. Population versus clinical view of case fatality from acute coronary heart disease: results from the WHO MONICA Project 1985–1990. Multinational MONItoring of trends and determinants in CArdiovascular disease. Circulation 1997; 96(11): 3849–3859

11. Renaud S, De Lorgeril M. Wine, alcohol and platelets, and the French paradox for coronary heart disease. Lancet 1992; 339: 1523–1526

12. Mogayzel C, Quan L, Graves J R, Tiedeman D, Fahrenbruch C, Herndon P. Out-of-hospital ventricular fibrillation in children and adolescents: causes and outcomes. Ann Emerg Med 1995; 25: 484–491

13. d'Avila A, Wellens F, Andries E, Brugada P. At what time are implantable defibrillator shocks delivered? Evidence for individual circadian variance in sudden cardiac death. Eur Heart J 1995; 16: 1231–1233

14. Wellens H J, Lemery R, Smeets J L et al. Sudden arrhythmic death without overt heart disease. Circulation 1992; 85: 192–197

15. Eisenberg M, Horwood B, Cummins R, Reynolds-Haertle R, Hearne T. Cardiac arrest and resuscitation: a tale of 29 cities. Ann Emerg Med 1990; 19: 238–243

16. Mullie A, Lewi P, Van Hoeyweghen R. Pre-CPR conditions and the final outcome of CPR. The Cerebral Resuscitation Study Group. Resuscitation 1989; 17 Suppl: S11–S21

17 Becker L, Ostrander M, Barret J, Kondos G. Outcome of CPR in a large metropolitan area: where are the survivors? Ann Emerg Med 1991; 20: 355–361

18. Lombardi G, Gallager J, Gennis P. Outcome of out-of-hospital cardiac arrest in New York City: the Pre-Hospital Arrest Survival Evaluation (PHASE) Study. JAMA 1994; 271: 678–683

19. Tunstall-Pedoe H, Bailey L, Chamberlain D, Marsden A, Ward M, Zideman D. Survey of 3765 cardiopulmonary resuscitations in British hospitals (the BRESUS study). BMJ 1992; 304 :1347–1351

20. Herlitz J, Ekstrom L, Wennerblom B, Axelsson A, Bang A, Holmberg S. Hospital mortality after out-of-hospital cardiac arrest among patients found in ventricular fibrillation. Resuscitation 1995; 29: 11–21

21. Jensen G V, Torp Pedersen C, Kober L et al. Prognosis of late versus early ventricular fibrillation in acute myocardial infarction. Am J Cardiol 1990; 66: 10–15

22. Bayes de Luna A, Guindo J. Sudden death in ischemic heart disease. Rev Port Cardiol 1990; 9: 473–479

23. Schomig A, Haass M, Richardt G. Catecholamine release and arrhythmias in acute myocardial ischaemia. Eur Heart J 1991; 12 Suppl F: 38–47

24. Farb A, Tang A L, Burke A P et al. Sudden coronary death: frequency of active coronary lesions, inactive coronary lesions, and myocardial infarction. Circulation 1995; 92: 1701–1709

25. Gelvan D, Saltman P, Powell S R. Cardiac reperfusion damage prevented by a nitric oxide free radical. Proc Natl Acad Sci USA 1991; 88: 4680–4684

26. Salvati P, Chierchia S, Dho L et al. Proarrhythmic activity of intracoronary endothelin in dogs: relation to the site of administration and to changes in regional flow. J Cardiovasc Pharmacol 1991; 17: 1007–1014

27. Billman G E. Cocaine: a review of its toxic actions on cardiac function. Crit Rev Toxicol 1995; 25: 113–132

28. Adgey A A, Johnston P W, McMechan S. Sudden cardiac death and substance abuse. Resuscitation 1995; 29: 219–221

29. Oakley C. Genesis of arrhythmias in the failing heart and therapeutic implications. Am J Cardiol 1991; 67: 26–28

30. Kjekshus J. Arrhythmias and mortality in congestive heart failure. Am J Cardiol 1990; 65: 421–481

31. Podrid P J. Potassium and ventricular arrhythmias. Am J Cardiol 1990; 65: 33E–44E

32. Montoya P T, Brugada P, Smeets J et al. Ventricular fibrillation in the Wolff-Parkinson-White syndrome. Eur Heart J 1991; 12: 144–150

33. Gohl K, Feistel H, Weikl A, Bachmann K, Wolf F. Congenital myocardial sympathetic dysinnervation: a structural defect of idiopathic long QT syndrome. Pacing Clin Electrophysiol 1991; 14: 1544–1553

34. Locher T, Walpoth B, Pfluger D, Althaus U. Akzidentelle Hypothermie in der Schweiz (1980–1987) – Kasuistik und prognostische Faktoren. Schweiz Med Wochenschr 1991; 121: 1020–1028

35. The Cardiac Arrhythmia Suppression Trial (CAST) Investigators. Preliminary report: effect of encainide and flecainide on mortality in a randomized trial of arrhythmia suppression after myocardial infarction. N Engl J Med 1989; 321: 406–412

36. Singh B N . Do antiarrhythmic drugs work? Some reflections on the implications of the Cardiac Arrhythmia Suppression Trial. Clin Cardiol 1990; 13: 725–728

37. Olsson G, Ryden L. Prevention of sudden death using beta-blockers. Review of possible contributory actions. Circulation 1991; 84: 133–137

38. Camm A, Julian D, Janse M et al on behalf of the European Myocardial Infarction Amiodarone Trial Investigators. The European Myocardial Infarction Amiodarone Trial (EMIAT). Am J Cardiol 1993; 72: 95F–98F

39. Cairns J, Connolly S, Roberts S, Gent M for the Canadian Amiodarone Myocardial Infarction Arrhythmia Trial Investigators. Randomized trial of outcome after myocardial infarction in patients with frequent or repetitive premature depolarisations: CAMIAT. Lancet 1997; 349: 675–682

40. Domanski M, Zipes D, Schron E. Treatment of sudden cardiac death. Current understandings from randomized trials and future research directions. Circulation 1997; 95: 2694–2699.

41. Cooper M. Emergency care of lightning and electrical injuries. Semin Neurol 1995; 15: 268–278

42. Zoll P, Linenthal A, Gibson W, Paul M, Norman L. Termination of ventricular fibrillation in man by externally applied electric countershock. N Engl J Med 1956; 254: 727

43. Safar P. On the history of modern resuscitation. Crit Care Med 1996; 24 (Suppl 2): S3–S11

44. Walcott G P, Walcott K T, Ideker R E. Mechanisms of defibrillation. Critical points and the upper limit of vulnerability. J Electrocardiol 1995; 28 Suppl: 1–6

45. Dalzell G, Adgey A. Determinants of successful transthoracic defibrillation and outcome in ventricular defibrillation. Br Heart J 1991; 65: 311–316

46. Lerman B B, Deale O C. Relation between transcardiac and transthoracic current during defibrillation in humans. Circ Res 1990; 67: 1420–1426

47. Gurvich N L, Makarychev V A. Defibrillation of the heart with biphasic electrical impulses. Kardiologiya 1967; 7: 109–112

48. Behr J, Hartley L L, York D K, Brown D D, Kerber R E. Truncated exponential versus damped sinusoidal waveforms for transthoracic defibrillation. Am J Cardiol 1996; 78: 1242–1245

49. Bardy G H, Gliner B E, Kudenchuk P J et al. Truncated biphasic pulses for transthoracic defibrillation. Circulation 1995; 91: 1768–1774

50. Greene H L, DiMarco J P, Kudenchuk P J et al. Comparison of monophasic and biphasic defibrillating pulse waveforms for transthoracic cardioversion. Biphasic Waveform Defibrillation Investigators. Am J Cardiol 1995; 75: 1135–1139

51. Walcott G P, Walker R G, Cates A W, Krassowska W, Smith W M, Ideker R E. Choosing the optimal monophasic and biphasic waveforms for ventricular defibrillation. J Cardiovasc Electrophysiol 1995 ; 6: 737–750

52. Tomassoni G, Newby K, Deshpande S et al. Defibrillation efficacy of commercially available biphasic impulses in humans. Circulation 1997; 95: 1822–1826

53. Jones D L, Irish W D, Klein G J. Defibrillation efficacy. Comparison of defibrillation threshold versus dose-response curve determination. Circ Res 1991; 69: 45–51

54. Babbs C. Effect of drugs on defibrillation threshold. In: Tacker W. (Ed) Defibrillation of the Heart. St Louis: Mosby Year Book 1994;. 223–258

55. Ujhelyi M R, Schur M, Frede T, Gabel M, Markel M L. Differential effects of lidocaine on defibrillation threshold with monophasic versus biphasic shock waveforms. Circulation 1995; 92: 1644–1650

56. KenKnight B H, Eyuboglu B M, Ideker R E. Impedance to defibrillation countershock: does an optimal impedance exist? Pacing Clin Electrophysiol 1995; 18: 2068–2087

57. Charbonnier F M. Selection of optimum defibrillation level. Energy-based, current-based, or impedance-based defibrillation. J Electrocardiol 1990; 23: 29

58. Trouton T G, Allen J D, Yong L K, Rooney J J, Adgey A A. Metabolic changes and mitochondrial dysfunction early following transthoracic countershock in dogs. Pace 1989; 12: 1827–1834

59. Sweeney R J, Gill R M, Reid P R. Characteristics of multiple-shock defibrillation. J Cardiovasc Electrophysiol 1995; 6: 89–102

60. Kerber R E. Energy requirements for defibrillation. Circulation 1986; 74 (Suppl IV): 117–119

61. Jakobsson J, Rehnqvist N, Nyquist O. Energy requirement for early defibrillation. Eur Heart J 1989; 10: 551–554

62. Weaver W, Cobb L, Copass M, Hallstrom A. Ventricular defibrillation: a comparative trial using 175-j and 320-j shocks. N Engl J Med 1982; 307: 1101–1106

63. Gutgesell H, Tacker W, Geddes L, Davis J, Lie J, McNamara D. Energy dose for ventricular defibrillation of children. Pediatrics 1976; 58: 898–901

64. Bossaert L, Koster R. Defibrillation: methods and strategies. Resuscitation 1992; 24: 211–225

65. Dalzell G, Cunningham S, Anderson J, Adgey A. Electrode pad size, transthoracic impedance and success of external ventricular defibrillation. Am J Cardiol 1989; 64: 741–744

66. Atkins D L, Kerber R E. Pediatric defibrillation: current flow is improved by using 'adult' electrode paddles. Pediatrics 1994; 94: 90–93

67. Weaver W D, Martin J S, Wirkus M J et al. Influence of external defibrillator electrode polarity on cardiac resuscitation. Pacing Clin Electrophysiol 1993; 16: 285–290

68. Aylward P E, Kieso R, Hite P, Charbonnier F, Kerber R E. Defibrillator electrode-chest wall coupling agents: influence on transthoracic impedance and shock success. J Am Coll Cardiol 1985; 6: 682–686

69. Panacek E A, Munger M A, Rutherford W F, Gardner S F. Report of nitropatch explosions complicating defibrillation. Am J Emerg Med 1992; 10: 128–129

70. Dedrick D K, Darga A, Landis D, Burney R E. Defibrillation safety in emergency helicopter transport. Ann Emerg Med 1989; 18: 69–71

71. Monsieurs K G, Conraads V M, Goethals M P, Snoeck J P, Bossaert L L. Semi-automatic external defibrillation and implanted cardiac pacemakers: understanding the interactions during resuscitation. Resuscitation 1995; 30: 127–131

72. Cummins R, Chesemore K, White R. Defibrillator failures, causes of problems and recommendations for improvement. JAMA 1990; 264: 1019–1025

73. Weaver W D, Cobb L A, Dennis D, Ray R, Hallstrom A P, Copass M K. Amplitude of ventricular fibrillation waveform and outcome after cardiac arrest. Ann Intern Med 1985; 102: 53–55

74. Brown C G, Griffith R F, Van Ligten P et al. Median frequency – a new parameter for predicting defibrillation success rate. Ann Emerg Med 1991: 20; 787–789

75. Strohmenger H-U, Lindner K H, Lurie K G, Welz A, Georgieff M. Frequency of ventricular fibrillation as a predictor of defibrillation success during cardiac surgery. Anesth Analg 1994; 79: 434–438

76. Monsieurs K, De Cauwer H, Wuyts F, Bossaert L. A rule for early outcome classification of out-of-hospital cardiac arrest patients presenting with ventricular fibrillation. Resuscitation 1998; 36: 37–44

77. Kern K B, Garewal H S, Sanders A B et al. Depletion of myocardial adenosine triphosphate during prolonged untreated ventricular fibrillation: effect on defibrillation success. Resuscitation 1990; 20: 221–229

78. Lerman B B, Engelstein E D. Metabolic determinants of defibrillation. Role of adenosine. Circulation 1995; 91: 838–844

79. Ahnefeld F W. Die Wiederbelebung bei Kreislaufstillstand. Verh Dtsch Ges Inn Med 1968; 74: 279–287

80. Cummins R O, Ornato J P, Thies W H, Pepe P E. Improving survival from sudden cardiac arrest: the 'chain of survival' concept. Circulation 1991; 83: 1832–1847

81. Kaye W, Mancini M E, Richards N. Organizing and implementing a hospital-wide first-responder automated external defibrillation program: strengthening the in-hospital chain of survival. Resuscitation 1995; 30: 151–156

82. O'Rourke M F, Donaldson E. An airline cardiac arrest programme. Circulation 1994; 90 (Suppl): 1548

83. Macdonald J W, Brewster M F, Isles C G. Defibrillation by general practitioners: an audit of resuscitation in a Scottish rural practice. Scot Med J 1993; 38: 79–80

84. Schneider T, Mauer D, Diehl P et al. Early defibrillation by emergency physicians or emergency medical technicians? A controlled prospective multicentric study. Resuscitation 1994; 27: 197–206

85. White R D, Asplin B R, Bugliosi T F, Hankins D G. High discharge survival rate after out-of-hospital ventricular fibrillation with rapid defibrillation by police and paramedics. Ann Emerg Med 1996; 28: 480–485

86. European Resuscitation Council. The 1998 European Resuscitation Council Guidelines for Adult Simgle Rescuer Basic Life Support. Resuscitation 1998; 3(2): 67–80

87. European Resuscitation Council. (1) The 1998 European Resuscitation Council Guidelines for Adult Advanced Life Support. (2) Guidelines for the use of Automated External defibrillators by EMS providers and first responders. Resusitation 1998; 37(2): 81–89 and 91–94

88. Emergency Cardiac Care Committee, American Heart Association. Guidelines for CPR and emergency cardiac care. JAMA 1992; 268: 2171–2302

89. Chamberlain D, Cummins R. Advisory statements of the International Liaison Committee on Resuscitation. Circulation 1997; 95: 2172–2173 and Resuscitation 1997; 34: 99–100. (2) Zideman D A et al. Recommendations on resuscitation of babies at birth. Resuscitation 1998; 37(2): 103–110

90. Chamberlain D, Cummins R, Albarran Sotelo A et al. International emergency cardiac care: support, science and universal guidelines. Ann Emerg Med 1993; 22: 508–511

91. Niskanen R. Automated external defibrillators. Experiences with their use and options for their further development. New Horizons 1997; 5: 137–144

92. Kroll M, Brewer J. Automated external defibrillators: design considerations. New Horizons 1997; 5: 128–136

93. Calle P, Van Acker P, Buylaert W et al. Should semi-automatic defibrillators be used by emergency medical technicians in Belgium ? Acta Clin Belg 1992; 47: 6–14

94. Pantridge J, Geddes J. A mobile intensive care unit in the management of myocardial infarction. Lancet 1967; ii: 271–273

95. Eisenberg M, Copass M, Hallstrom A et al. Treatment of out-of-hospital cardiac arrests with rapid defibrillation by emergency medical technicians. N Engl J Med 1980; 302: 1379–1383

96. Jaggerao N, Heber M, Grainger R, Vincent R, Chamberlain D. Use of an automated external defibrillator-pacemaker by ambulance staff. Lancet 1982; ii: 73-75

97. Cummins R O, White R D, Pepe P E. Ventricular fibrillation, automatic external defibrillators, and the United States Food and Drug Administration: confrontation without comprehension. Ann Emerg Med 1995; 26: 621–631

98. Van den Broeck G. Council decision of 29 July 1991 on the introduction of a single European emergency call number. Official Journal of the European Council. 1991/396/EEC

99. Bossaert L L. The complexity of comparing different EMS-systems: a survey of EMS-systems in Europe. Ann Emerg Med 1993; 22: 99–102

100. WHO Regional Office for Europe. Monitoring of the strategy for health for all by the year 2000. Eur/RC38/11. Copenhagen: WHO, 1989

101. Conseil de l'Europe. Etude comparative sur l'organisation et le fonctionnement des services d'aide médicale urgente. Comparative study of the organisation and functioning of emergency medical assistance services. Strasbourg: Conseil de l'Europe, 1990

102. Auble T E, Menegazzi J J, Paris P M. Effect of out-of-hospital defibrillation by basic life support providers on cardiac arrest mortality: a meta analysis. Ann Emerg Med 1995; 25: 642–648

103. Cummins R. From concept to standard-of-care? Review of the clinical experience with automated external defibrillators. Ann Emerg Med 1989; 18: 1269–1276

104. Arntz H R, Oeff M, Willich S N, Storch W H, Schroder R. Establishment and results of an EMT-D program in a two-tiered physician-escorted rescue system. The experience in Berlin, Germany. Resuscitation 1993; 26: 39–46

105. Sedgwick M L, Dalziel K, Watson J, Carrington D J, Cobbe S M. Performance of an established system of first responder out-of-hospital defibrillation. The results of the second year of the Heartstart Scotland Project in the 'Utstein style'. Resuscitation 1993; 26: 75–88

106. Mauer D, Schneider T, Diehl P et al. Erstdefibrillation durch Notèrzte oder durch Rettungsassistenten? Eine prospektive, vergleichende Multicenterstudie bei ausserklinisch aufgetretenem Kammerflimmern. Anaesthesist 1994; 43: 36–49

107. Mols P, Beaucarne E, Bruyninx J et al. Early defibrillation by EMTs: the Brussels experience. Resuscitation 1994; 27: 129–136

108. Ekstrom L, Herlitz J, Wennerblom B, Axelsson A, Bang A, Holmberg S. Survival after cardiac arrest outside hospital over a 12-year period in Gothenburg. Resuscitation 1994; 27: 181–187

109. Cummins R, Chamberlain D, Abramson N et al Special Report. Recommended guidelines for uniform reporting of data from out-of-hospital cardiac arrest: the Utstein style. Resuscitation 1991; 22: 1–26 and Circulation 1991; 84: 960–975

110. Cummins R, Chamberlain D, Hazinski M F et al. Recommended guidelines for reviewing, reporting and conducting research on in-hospital resuscitation, the 'in-hospital Utstein style'. Resuscitation 1997; 34: 151–185 and Circulation 1997; 95: 2213–2239

111. Weisfeldt M L, Kerber R E, McGoldrick R P et al. Public access defibrillation: a statement for healthcare professionals from the American Heart Association Task Force on Automatic External Defibrillation. Circulation 1995; 92: 2763

112. Bossaert L, Cummins R, Callanan V. Early defibrillation. An advisory statement from the advanced life support working group of the international liaison committee on resuscitation. Resuscitation 1997; 34: 101–102 and Circulation 1997; 95: 2183–2184

D. A. J. Walker

Anaesthetic management of the brain-injured patient presenting for non-neurosurgical procedures

The problems associated with anaesthesia and surgery for non-neurosurgical procedures in patients who have suffered a recent head injury are two-fold. Firstly, interrupting the clinical and/or physiological monitoring of the neurological condition of the patient, with consequent delay both in detecting significant changes and in instituting an appropriate response, i.e. further investigation, possible transfer or specific medical or neurosurgical management of the intracranial pathology. Secondly, there is the risk or fear of exacerbating the effects of the head injury because of the anaesthetic technique or the surgery itself.

It has been recognised for some time that the consequences of a head injury can usefully be considered in terms of a primary injury – the direct damage to intracranial contents both neural and vascular, occurring at the time of the injury – and a secondary injury, which begins at the time of the initial trauma and can continue for hours or days subsequently. The prolonged course of the secondary injury has two consequences: first, its extent is not immediately apparent; and second, it is open both to limitation and exacerbation by subsequent events. Factors which are known to worsen the secondary injury directly or indirectly include tissue hypoxia and acidosis, hypercapnia, elevated intracranial pressure (ICP), release of excitatory amino acids and free radical formation.

Of those patients who have who have suffered head trauma, 80% have an injury which is classified as mild on the Glasgow Coma Scale at initial assessment, (GCS 13–15), 10% as moderate (GCS 8–12) and 10% severe (GCS 3–7). While the vast majority of patients with a mild head injury will make a full and uneventful recovery, a small proportion will deteriorate due to the development of potentially lethal intracranial bleeding and/or brain swelling,

Dr D A J Walker MA DPhil BM BCh FRCA, Consultant Neuroanaesthetist, Department of Neuroanaesthesia, Institute of Neurological Sciences, Southern General Hospital, 1345 Govan Road, Glasgow G51 4TF, UK

diagnosis and management of which may be delayed by anaesthesia and surgery for incidental procedures. In addition, a larger proportion may be at risk for at least temporary worsening of their neurological condition through use of injudicious anaesthetic techniques. It is clear, therefore, that only urgent surgery should be undertaken at this time. The questions are: (i) which surgery is urgent?; (ii) which anaesthetic techniques should be used?; and (iii) for how long is the patient at risk?

For patients with more serious head injuries, the problems are those of establishing priorities for a number of procedures which should seemingly all be carried out immediately but frequently, for practical reasons, have to be carried out sequentially, in different departments or even in different hospitals. For these patients, what are the priorities? How should the patient be managed during and between the procedures?

PATIENTS WITH A SEVERE HEAD INJURY

Resuscitation

The involvement of the anaesthetist with patients with a moderate or severe head injury is likely to start with the patient's resuscitation. This may already have started at the scene of the injury, where simple actions may prove life-saving: in a series of 49 patients with head injuries, 45% had airway obstruction at the scene of the accident.[1]

The indications for intubation and ventilation of the head-injured patient in hospital are well established: inadequate gas exchange, inability to protect the airway, irregular or abnormal respiration and neurological deterioration.[2] However, while both hypoxia and hypotension are associated with poor outcome after head injury, the latter is frequently more difficult to manage and probably contributes more to exacerbation of the secondary injury.[3] In a series of 74 patients with a head injury in whom ICP was measured, episodes of reduced cerebral perfusion pressure (CPP) during the first 24 h were caused more often by a reduction in arterial pressure than by an increased ICP, and low CPP due to reduced blood pressure was in turn correlated with the Injury Severity Score, suggesting that correction of hypovolaemia was inadequate in these patients.[4] Many studies have confirmed the deleterious effect of hypotension: for example, analysis of data from more than 700 patients with severe head injury in the Traumatic Coma Data Bank (TCDB) study revealed a 150% increase in mortality in those patients who were hypotensive (systolic pressure < 90 mmHg) at some point.[5] Similarly, in children, hypotension with or without hypoxia, increases mortality.[6]

A substantial proportion of patients with a severe head injury have associated life-threatening multiple trauma. The first priority is correction of hypoxia and hypotension and control of bleeding before diagnostic procedures, such as CT scanning, are performed. The anaesthetist's duty is continuing resuscitation of the patient during this time when a variety of different surgeons may each be involved, with competing claims for priority.

It is essential, following the securing of the airway and initial fluid resuscitation of the hypovolaemic patient, to establish the source of blood loss.

In adults, lacerations are unlikely to lead to sufficient blood loss to cause hypotension unless there is major vascular damage as well, and this should be evident on examination. This is not the case in children, in whom scalp lacerations alone may be sufficient to cause hypotension.

Multiple fractures are less easy to assess as a source of haemorrhage. Although fractures of the pelvis and femur may result in substantial blood loss, this is likely to occur over a period of several hours and a patient with multiple fractures who is hypotensive soon after the injury should be assumed to have another source of blood loss until there is proof to the contrary.

Expeditious diagnosis of abdominal injuries in unconscious patients and appropriate surgical intervention can be difficult. Diagnostic peritoneal lavage (DPL) is the procedure of choice and is indicated in patients with an abnormal or equivocal physical examination, hypotension, low haematocrit, a history of blunt or penetrating abdominal injury and an altered conscious level, and those with a severe head injury who have already been sedated and ventilated. The incidence of false positive and false negative results with selective DPL are both about 2%.[7] Abdominal ultrasonography has also been used as a rapid screening procedure to identify those multiple trauma patients requiring urgent laparotomy before a head CT scan but, compared with DPL, the accuracy of the technique is more dependent on the experience of the operator.[7,8] Sequential head and abdominal CT scanning has been advocated for investigating children with moderate or severe head injury and suspected abdominal injuries.[9] Surgically remediable abdominal injury is much more common than surgically remediable head injury: of more than 700 hypotensive trauma patients, while 21% required urgent laparotomy and 26% had an abnormal head CT scan, only 2.5% required an emergency craniotomy for evacuation of a haematoma.[10] Patients who require both an emergency laparotomy and craniotomy are fortunately rare: only 3 were found in a review of 800 trauma patients who had clinical evidence of both head and abdominal injuries.[11] In this situation, DPL should be done first followed by head CT scanning if the DPL is negative.

Anaesthesia for emergency surgery to control bleeding

Pre-operative management

The patient with a severe head injury will already have been intubated, following established guidelines.[2] The emphasis at this stage should be on maintaining adequate cerebral oxygenation by treating hypoxia appropriately and restoring circulating volume promptly. Pre-operative investigations should include at a minimum, a chest X-ray and blood taken for haematology, coagulation, biochemistry and cross-matching, as well as arterial blood gases. Routine monitoring – ECG, pulse oximetry, capnography and temperature – are assumed. Adequate venous access should be secured (at least two large bore cannulae), together with an arterial cannula and urinary catheter. A central venous catheter is desirable for monitoring fluid status and delivering inotropic drugs if required, but its placement is not without hazard: it may delay life-saving surgery, both the subclavian or internal routes are often facilitated by putting the patient in a head-down position which may compromise CPP and both may result in a pneumothorax. Use of the antecubital or femoral route will avoid the latter problems but may give an inaccurate value of central venous pressure if the catheter tip is not intrathoracic. Ideally a second anaesthetist should monitor and manage the blood pressure and fluid therapy during the placement of a central line.

Induction

The procedure for induction will depend on the assessment of the patient's airway and haemodynamic state. If the airway is potentially difficult, the ability to ventilate the lungs must be established before any hypnotic or muscle relaxant is given. If there is time, a fibreoptic intubation may be performed or, alternatively, a cricothyroidotomy or tracheostomy may be appropriate. If the airway appears normal, intubation should proceed following induction with the head maintained in a neutral position by an assistant if there is any doubt about the cervical spine. Because the head-injured patient is at a high risk of regurgitation and aspiration and because subsequent hypoxia is likely to worsen the secondary injury, a rapid sequence induction with cricoid pressure is mandatory. Choice and dose of induction and ancillary agents should be based on assessment of the patient's haemodynamic state, the aim being to maintain an adequate cerebral perfusion pressure without the surge in ICP which may follow laryngoscopy and intubation. Thiopentone or propofol can be used if the patient is haemodynamically stable but etomidate may be preferred if there is a possibility of hypovolaemia. Lignocaine, esmolol or rapidly-acting opioids, such as alfentanil or remifentanil, may be used to obtund the hypertensive response to intubation provided hypotension is avoided: a fall in CPP in a hypovolaemic patient may be more harmful than the transient rise in ICP caused by intubation.

The use of suxamethonium is still the subject of debate and high-dose rocuronium has been advocated as an alternative.[12] However, in adequately anaesthetised patients with a head injury, the adverse effects of suxamethonium on ICP appear to be minimal[13] and the relaxant of choice in this situation is the one with which the anaesthetist is most familiar.

Maintenance

The ideal technique is one which has the least effect on cerebral autoregulation, maintains cardiovascular stability (see below) and has a potentially beneficial effect on ICP without compromising cerebral perfusion. The volatile agents all reduce cerebral autoregulation in a dose-dependent manner; halothane is the most potent vasodilator and potentiates the arrhythmogenic effects of catecholamines. Enflurane is also a vasodilator and can provoke seizure-like activity in the hyperventilated patient. Autoregulation is relatively well preserved with 1 MAC isoflurane anaesthesia, but is lost when the concentration is increased to 2 MAC.[14] Of the newer inhalational anaesthetics, desflurane has been found to increase cerebrospinal fluid (CSF) pressure more than isoflurane in equipotent concentrations in patients with supratentorial mass lesions, but not to differ from isoflurane in its effect on cerebral blood flow or CO_2 reactivity.[15,16] Sevoflurane did not affect CSF pressure in dogs in circumstances in which both halothane and enflurane did cause an increase but, unfortunately, isoflurane was not compared in the same study.[17] Nitrous oxide is a cerebral vasodilator and increases cerebral blood flow both when used alone and together with propofol or isoflurane anaesthesia.[18-20] Although there may be theoretical reasons for preferring an i.v. technique, evidence that choice of agent actually influences outcome is lacking. However, an infusion technique will ensure a more stable anaesthetic if the patient is to be transferred to another department or hospital. Full muscle relaxation should be maintained and analgesia provided. Of more importance than choice of specific agents is the overall conduct of the anaesthetic and again avoidance of hypotension is crucial. In a study of 53 patients with severe head injury, who were initially normotensive and required surgery within 3 days of injury, the mortality in those patients who became hypotensive (systolic pressure < 90 mmHg) during surgery was 82%, but was only 25% in those who remained normotensive.[21] Such findings emphasise that the assumption that general anaesthesia may offer some degree of 'cerebral protection' against the effect of hypotension is unwarranted.

Ventilation

The ventilatory management of the patient with a severe head injury has changed over the last decade as a result of increased understanding of cerebral haemodynamics in the injured brain. Immediately following a head injury many patients have a cerebral blood flow less than half that of normal with areas of both hyperaemia and oligaemia.[22] In a study of regional cerebral blood flow in 27 ventilated head injured patients, hyperventilation ($PaCO_2$ reduced from 4.8 to 3.5 kPa, 36 to 26 mmHg) dramatically increased both the number of oligaemic regions and its severity.[23] Continuous monitoring of jugular venous bulb oxygen saturation ($SjvO_2$) is an increasingly widespread means of assessing cerebral oxygenation[24] and has revealed the dangers of a previously widespread therapeutic intervention. Hyperventilation to a $PaCO_2$ of 3.6 kPa produced a fall in $SjvO_2$ in a heterogeneous group of patients with intracranial pathology.[25] Episodes of jugular venous desaturation are more common in patients with a reduced cerebral blood flow and correlate strongly with outcome: in one study, 55% of patients with no episodes of desaturation had a poor outcome, rising to 74% of those with one episode and 90% of those with multiple episodes of jugular venous desaturation.[26] Prophylactic hyperventilation has been shown to result in a worse outcome in a prospective trial[27] and its routine use is not recommended for head-injured patients. Instead it should be reserved for those situations where there is appropriate monitoring (ICP and $SjvO_2$) with evidence of hyperaemia, or in an acutely deteriorating patient prior to emergency craniotomy.

Fluid therapy

Reference has already been made to the vital importance of adequate and continuing treatment of hypovolaemia in a head-injured patient. The requirements are for restoration of an adequate blood pressure, maintenance of normal plasma electrolytes and osmolality and avoidance of hyperglycaemia.

Although oncotic pressure is not a factor in the development of cerebral oedema, smaller volumes of colloid than crystalloid are required to restore circulating volume and, hence, resuscitation may be achieved more rapidly with the former. Administration of more than 500 ml hetastarch has been associated with increased bleeding in neurosurgical patients and should be avoided;[28,29] gelatin and plasma protein solutions do not have this effect.

Because the blood-brain barrier is impermeable to ions, plasma osmolality determines water flux into and out of brain tissue. Ringer's lactate solution is hypotonic (about 274 mOsm/kg) and volumes in excess of 1–2 l should be avoided; normal saline (osmolality about 300 mOsm/kg) is a preferable crystalloid solution.[30,31] The dangers of even moderately elevated blood glucose after cerebral damage are now well recognised and glucose-containing solutions should be avoided.[32]

There has been considerable interest in the US, where gelatin solutions are not available in the use of hypertonic (7.5%) saline as a resuscitation fluid, since it achieves more rapid volume replacement than equal volumes of isotonic solutions and at the same time reduces cerebral oedema.[33] Such hypertonic solutions are not currently available in the UK.

Positioning of the patient

The patient should be placed in a slight head-up position with the head in a neutral position. Care should be taken that tape securing the endotracheal tube does not obstruct venous return.

Temperature

Head-injured patients undergoing surgery of any kind should have their core temperature monitored. Whereas pyrexia has been shown to be a significant predictor of mortality,[3] induced mild hypothermia to 32–34°C in ventilated patients has been shown to be effective in lowering elevated ICP[34,35] and improving outcome.[36] A head injury patient's temperature should not be allowed to fall below 32°C, however, and even mild hypothermia should be corrected prior to reversal of muscle relaxation to prevent shivering.

Monitoring

In addition to recording the usual cardiovascular and respiratory parameters, it is important to continue to observe and record pupil size regularly in a head injured patient following intubation and sedation or while undergoing surgery. Neither the Cushing reflex to an elevated ICP (a rising blood pressure and bradycardia) nor pupillary dilatation resulting from uncal herniation will be masked by general anaesthetic agents. If one or both pupils dilate during the course of emergency surgery, the surgeon should be informed and requested to complete the surgery as rapidly as possible while any obvious causes such as hypoxia, hypotension, hypo- or hypercarbia or obstructed venous return are corrected. The development of asymmetric pupils is not a reliable guide to either the presence or the location of an intracranial haematoma: analysis of data from the TCDB showed that, even in patients with marked (> 3 mm) pupil asymmetry, fewer than one-half had a haematoma and, of these, the haematoma was ipsilateral to the larger pupil in only two-thirds of the cases:[37] there is, therefore, little justification for 'blind' burr holes. Evidence of uncal herniation should be treated promptly with mannitol 0.25 g/kg and hyperventilation, which may 'buy time' to allow investigation and possible transfer for neurosurgical intervention. While not good, the prognosis for these patients is not hopeless: 25% of patients with fixed dilated pupils undergoing craniotomy for evacuation of a traumatic haematoma had a good outcome or only moderate disability.[38] Factors associated with a better outcome included the presence of an extradural rather than a subdural clot, younger age and less than a 3 h interval between loss of pupillary reactivity and craniotomy.

The extent and duration of emergency surgery in the presence of a severe head injury should be kept to an absolute minimum, i.e. to repair major vascular damage. Surgery to stop major bleeding should take precedence over CT scanning, even if there is evidence of neurological deterioration: pupillary dilatation in the presence of severe hypotension does not indicate a cerebral cause.[39] The only exception to this could be in a situation where the patient was haemodynamically stable, CT scanning was immediately available, there was clinical evidence for an intracranial haematoma and the facilities for performing emergency craniotomy and laparotomy simultaneously if necessary. Needless to say, this is a rare scenario.

The vast majority of orthopaedic injuries do not require emergency surgery and the suggestion that such surgery could be carried out under the same anaesthetic, either simultaneously with or following an emergency laparotomy or thoracotomy should be resisted. Anything other than a manipulation under anaesthetic and splinting is likely to add significantly to operating time.

Following the end of an emergency laparotomy or thoracotomy with the patient more stable, CT scanning and further management of the head injury can be carried out. Sedation, ventilation and monitoring should, of course, continue during this time and during subsequent transfer to a neurosurgical unit if required.[2]

PATIENTS WITH A MILD OR MODERATE HEAD INJURY

Far more common than patients with a severe head injury are those with a mild or moderate head injury. If requiring life-saving surgery for haemorrhage, anaesthetic management will be similar to that already described. More commonly, however, will be the requirement for surgery – for example, ortho-paedic, maxillofacial or plastic – which would normally be carried out in the first day or so after injury. Are these patients at added risk if submitted to anaesthesia and surgery during this time? Are there hazards from particular techniques?

The natural history of mild or moderate head injury

The vast majority of patients with a mild or moderate head injury at initial assessment make a good recovery. Notoriously, a few do not but go on to develop life-threatening intracranial bleeding and/or brain swelling. A review of 183 such patients who deteriorated showed that, while most had one or more factors which might indicate the presence of a significant intracranial injury (such as a history of altered consciousness, headache or vomiting, a focal neurological deficit or skull fracture), some did not.[40] Early CT scanning is the investigation of choice to detect intracranial abnormalities: of more than 1500 patients with a mild head injury (GCS 13–15) and no neurological deficit who underwent routine early CT scanning, more than 80% had a normal scan and none of these subsequently deteriorated.[41] In a smaller series, all patients with a mild head injury, no focal deficit and a normal CT scan were discharged home from the emergency department with no adverse sequelae.[42] Thus, the risk of a patient with a mild head injury who has a normal CT scan deteriorating coincidentally while undergoing surgery seems minimal. However, the question remains whether particular anaesthetic techniques put patients with a mild or moderate head injury at risk.

It is becoming increasingly clear that it is not only patients with a severe head injury who are endangered by the consequences of hypotension.[43] More than a quarter of patients with a mild head injury were found to have poor or absent cerebral autoregulation when tested within 48 h of their injury, i.e. cerebral blood flow became pressure-dependent at all levels of arterial blood pressure.[44] The consequences of this may be serious: the effects of transient hypotension on outcome are more evident in patients with mild or moderate head injuries than those with severe injuries in whom the severity of the primary injury will contribute more to overall outcome.[45] The ideal anaesthetic is, therefore, the 'copybook' example of a smooth anaesthetic avoiding hypo- and hypertension, hypo- and hypercarbia and hypoxia.

General anaesthesia

Choice of technique

A spontaneously breathing technique is contraindicated for two reasons. First, a potential full stomach should be suspected even if the patient has been fasted for more than 6 h. Patients with a moderate head injury may have impaired lower oesophageal sphincter function and delayed gastric emptying initially and an abnormal pattern of emptying may persist for more than 2 weeks.[46–48] Second, the combination of the vasodilatation and respiratory depression characteristic of anaesthetic agents is likely to lead to a rise in ICP in a patient who may have compromised intracranial elastance, starting some way along the classical intracranial pressure–volume curve or who has localised dysfunction in a damaged area.[49] While such adverse effects might be reversible at the end of the anaesthetic it is clearly prudent to minimise their likelihood.

A rapid sequence induction and intubation are indicated (see above). High concentrations of inhalational agents should be avoided, both to prevent excessive cerebral vasodilatation and to reduce the magnitude and duration of postoperative respiratory depression. The potentially adverse effect of nitrous oxide as a cerebral vasodilator has been noted previously.[18–20] Hypertension should be avoided because of the risk of exacerbating any pre-existing intracranial haematoma[50] and hypotension because of the vulnerability of the damaged brain with impaired autoregulation. Short-acting opioids, such as alfentanil or remifentanil, may be valuable in providing potent analgesia without the fear of prolonged respiratory depression. Even so, a general anaesthetic in the presence of increased intracranial elastance may prove fatal.[51]

Postoperatively, the patient should be nursed in a recovery or high dependency area with frequent monitoring of cardiovascular, respiratory and neurological function. For a discussion of postoperative analgesia, see below.

Regional techniques

With the potential hazards of a general anaesthetic, a regional technique may be thought preferable in a patient with a recent head injury. However, these techniques have their own disadvantages.

Epidural anaesthesia

Standard epidural injections of 5 or 10 ml of anaesthetic solutions (or 0.9% saline) produced a substantial rise in ICP in two patients who had suffered a head injury more than a week previously, explicable as the effect of compression of the dural sac shifting CSF back into the intracranial compartment.[52] The authors concluded that epidural anaesthesia should be used with extreme caution in patients with increased intracranial elastance. The dramatic effect of epidural injection on ICP in the presence of an intracranial mass lesion has also been demonstrated in an animal model.[53] If an epidural is used, injections should be of small volume and made very slowly.[52]

Spinal anaesthesia

Despite the standard teaching that spinal anaesthesia is contra-indicated following head injury because of the perceived risk of precipitating tentorial herniation, there are several circumstances where lumbar puncture (LP) has been widely used in patients with raised intracranial elastance without apparent adverse effect: to diagnose subarachnoid haemorrhage and intracranial infections,[54] and in the management of both benign intracranial hypertension and refractory raised ICP in severely head injured children.[55] A patient who has suffered a mild head injury who has no neurological signs and who has a normal CT scan is unlikely to be at risk from a spinal anaesthetic, but this conclusion cannot be made in the absence of a CT scan.

Intravenous regional anaesthesia (IVRA, Bier's block) and orthopaedic tourniquets

There are several case reports of the effects on intracranial pressure in head-injured patients of deflating arterial tourniquets applied to the lower limbs to improve operating conditions.[56–58] In each case, tourniquet release was followed by a rise in ICP which, together with the normal and expected fall in blood pressure which occurs at this time, resulted in a substantial fall in CPP. As ICP was being monitored in each case, immediate measures could be taken to correct the situation and none of the patients apparently suffered any sequelae. The effect of releasing an arm tourniquet is, of course, likely to be smaller. Another potential danger from the use of tourniquets is the possibility of sudden severe bleeding when the tourniquet is released and this, in conjunction with the rise in ICP, could have a significant effect on outcome.

The timing of orthopaedic procedures in patients with head injuries has been subject to several reviews of orthopaedic outcome with no firm evidence to support either early or delayed fixation.[59–62] In the absence of data suggesting that orthopaedic outcome or complications are worsened by delaying fixation, it is prudent to make the management of the head injury the first priority and minimize the number of potential physiological insults which might exacerbate the secondary brain injury.

In contrast to the potential problems with epidural, spinal or IVRA techniques, local nerve blocks would seem to be a good choice for providing anaesthesia in patients with head injury. An additional problem which is common to all regional techniques, however, is the question of sedation. Patients with a recent head injury may be uncooperative, but their response to sedation may be unpredictable and, if respiratory depression or airway obstruction occur, the result could be hazardous.

Analgesia and the head-injured patient

The question of postoperative analgesia was referred to above; in addition, the head-injured patient may require analgesia because of other injuries sustained.

Systemic analgesics

Opioids are effective, but there is the likelihood of respiratory depression if given in excess. The i.v. route is preferable to intermittent i.m. injections, but a drowsy or uncooperative patient may be unable to use a PCA device effectively. Any head-injured patient receiving parenteral opioids should be appropriately monitored. Non-steroidal analgesics inhibit platelet function which could result in the expansion of an intracranial haematoma and also increase cerebral blood flow and, hence, potentially raise ICP.

Epidural analgesia

This has been discussed above.

Local nerve blocks

These may be useful for surgical procedures but the requirement for repeated injections limits their value for prolonged analgesia unless a catheter can be inserted (e.g. continuous brachial plexus block).

The head-injured patient with multiple rib fractures presents a particular problem: pain restricting breathing can result in hypoxia, hypercarbia, sputum retention, atelectasis and pneumonia. Ventilation with ICP monitoring is a possibility but is likely to be required for several days and may necessitate transfer to a neurosurgical centre. Such patients have been managed successfully with a thoracic epidural or intermittent injections via either a paravertebral or intercostal catheter.[63,64] Clearly, each patient has to be assessed individually having regard to the availability of local resources.

TIME COURSE: FOR HOW LONG IS THE HEAD-INJURED PATIENT AT RISK?

Data from case reports suggest that the head-injured patient is vulnerable for a surprisingly long time even after apparently complete neurological recovery.

A child suffered a temporary focal neurological deficit induced by anaesthesia more than 2 weeks after the initial injury and 12 days after neurological recovery.[49] The pathological rises in ICP produced by epidural injections reported by Hilt and colleagues[52] were observed in the second and fifth weeks after injury in their two patients, one being without neurological deficit at this time. In addition, a patient undergoing spinal surgery 10 days after a mild head injury was observed to have an abnormal flow pattern on transcranial Doppler monitoring of the middle cerebral artery, indicating persisting altered intracranial haemodynamics.[65] The available evidence, therefore, suggests that, following even a mild head injury or after complete recovery from a moderate or severe head injury, the brain is abnormal and potentially vulnerable for several weeks at least and anaesthetic management during this time should take account of this.

Key points for clinical practice

- Hypotension and hypoxia are the major treatable causes of secondary brain injury.

- The control of bleeding is the first priority after intubation and ventilation in a patient with a severe head injury and takes priority over other investigations. Non life-saving surgery should be deferred.

- Mannitol and hyperventilation should not be used routinely in a patient with a head injury but only if there is progressive neurological deterioration.

- A patient with a mild or moderate head injury is still at risk of complications from anaesthesia and surgery: there may be adverse consequences from the use a spontaneously breathing technique, spinal and epidural anaesthesia, IVRA and orthopaedic tourniquets.

- A patient may be at increased risk of complications for several weeks even after a mild head injury.

ACKNOWLEDGEMENTS

I am very grateful to Dr M Soutar and Dr T Park for their comments.

References

1. Stocchetti N, Furlan A, Volta F. Hypoxemia and hypotension at the accident scene in head injury. J Trauma 1996; 40: 764–767
2. Recommendations for the transfer of patients with acute head injuries to neurosurgical units. The Neuroanaesthesia Society of Great Britain and Ireland and the Association of Anaesthetists of Great Britain and Ireland. London, 1996
3. Jones P A, Andrews P J, Midgley S et al. Measuring the burden of secondary insults in head-injured patients during intensive care. J Neurosurg Anesth 1994; 6: 4–14
4. Cortbus F, Jones P A, Miller J D, Piper I R, Tocher J L. Cause, distribution and significance of episodes of reduced cerebral perfusion pressure following head injury. Acta Neurochir (Wien) 1994; 130: 117–124

5. Chesnut R M, Marshall L F, Klauber M R et al. The role of secondary brain injury in determining outcome from severe head injury. J Trauma 1993; 34: 216–222

6. Pigula F A, Wald S L, Shackford S R, Vane D W. The effect of hypotension and hypoxia on children with severe head injuries. J Pediatr Surg 1993; 28: 310–314

7. Robertson C, Redmond A D. The management of major trauma, 2nd edn. Oxford: Oxford University Press, 1994: 85–87

8. Huang M S, Shih H C, Wu J K et al. Urgent laparotomy versus emergency craniotomy for multiple trauma with head injury patients. J Trauma 1995; 38: 154–157

9. Beaver B L, Colombani P M, Fal A et al. The efficacy of computed tomography in evaluating abdominal injuries in children with major head trauma. J Pediatr Surg 1987; 22: 1117–1122

10. Thomason M, Messick J, Rutledge R et al. Head CT scanning versus urgent exploration in the hypotensive blunt trauma patient. J Trauma 1993; 34: 40–44

11. Wisner D H, Victor B S, Holcroft J W. Priorities in the management of multiple trauma: intracranial versus intra-abdominal injury. J Trauma 1993; 35: 271–276

12. Schramm W M, Strasser K, Bartunek A, Gilly H, Spiss, C K. Effects of rocuronium and vecuronium on intracranial pressure, mean arterial pressure and heart rate in neurosurgical patients. Br J Anaesth 1996; 77: 607–611

13. Brown M M, Parr M J A, Manara A R. The effects of suxamethonium on intracranial pressure and cerebral perfusion pressure in patients with severe head injuries following blunt trauma. Eur J Anaesth 1996; 13: 474–477

14. Olsen K S, Henriksen A, Owen-Falkenberg A, Dige-Petersen H, Rosenorn J, Chraemmer-Jorgenson B. Effect of 1 or 2 MAC isoflurane with or without ketanserin on cerebral blood flow autoregulation in man. Br J Anaesth 1994; 72: 66–71

15. Muzzi D A, Losasso T J, Dietz N M, Faust R J, Cucchiara R F, Milde L N. The effect of desflurane and isoflurane on cerebrospinal fluid pressure in humans with supratentorial mass lesions. Anesthesiology 1992; 76: 720–724

16. Ornstein E, Young W L, Fleischer L H, Ostapkovich N. Desflurane and isoflurane have similar effects on cerebral blood flow in patients with intracranial mass lesions. Anesthesiology 1993; 79: 498–502

17. Takahashi H, Murata K, Ikeda K. Sevoflurane does not increase intracranial pressure in dogs. Br J Anaesth 1993; 71: 551–555

18. Field L M, Dorrance D E, Krzeminska E K, Barsoum L Z. Effect of nitrous oxide on cerebral blood flow in normal humans. Br J Anaesth 1993; 70: 154–159

19. Matta B F, Lam A M. Nitrous oxide increases cerebral blood flow velocity during pharmacologically induced EEG silence in humans. J Neurosurg Anesth 1995; 7: 89–93

20. Reinstrup P, Ryding E, Algotsson L, Berntman L, Uski T. Regional cerebral blood flow (SPECT) during anaesthesia with isoflurane and nitrous oxide in humans. Br J Anaesth 1997; 78: 407–411

21. Pietropaoli J A, Rogers F B, Shackford S R, Wald S L, Schmoker J D, Zhuang J. The deleterious effects of intraoperative hypotension on outcome in patients with severe head injuries. J Trauma 1992; 33: 403–407

22. Bouma G J, Muizelaar J P. Cerebral blood flow, cerebral blood volume and cerebrovascular reactivity after severe head injury. J Neurotrauma 1992; 9 (Suppl 1): S333–S348

23. Cold G E. Does acute hyperventilation provoke cerebral oligaemia in comatose patients after head injury? Acta Neurochir (Wien) 1989; 96: 100–106

24. Andrews P J D, Dearden N M, Miller J D. Jugular bulb cannulation: description of a cannulation technique and validation of a new continuous monitor. Br J Anaesth 1991; 67: 553–558

25. von Helden A, Schneider G H, Unterberg A, Lanksch W R. Monitoring of jugular venous oxygen saturation in comatose patients with subarachnoid haemorrhage and intracerebral haematomas. Acta Neurochir Suppl (Wien) 1993; 59: 102–106

26. Gopinath S P, Robertson C S, Contant C F et al. Jugular venous desaturation and outcome after head injury. J Neurol Neurosurg Psychiatry 1994; 57: 717–723

27. Muizelaar J P, Marmarou A, Ward J D et al. Adverse effects of prolonged hyperventilation in patients with severe head injury: a randomized clinical trial. J Neurosurg 1991; 75: 731–739

28. Cully M D, Larson C P, Silverberg G D. Hetastarch coagulopathy in the neurosurgical patient. Anesthesiology 1987; 66: 706–711

29. Trumble E R, Muizelaar J P, Myseros J S, Choi S C, Warren B B. Coagulopathy with the use of hetastarch in the treatment of vasospasm. J Neurosurg 1995; 82: 44–47

30. Poole G V, Prough D S, Johnson J C et al. Effects of resuscitation from hemorrhage shock on cerebral hemodynamics in the presence of an intracranial mass. J Trauma 1987; 27: 18–22

31. Tommasino C, Moore S, Todd M M. Cerebral effects of isovolemic hemodilution with crystalloid or colloid solutions in normal rabbits. Crit Care Med 1988; 16: 862–868

32. Lam A M, Winn H R, Cullen B F et al. Hyperglycemia and neurologic outcome in patients with head injury. J Neurosurg 1991; 75: 545–550

33. Vassar M J, Fischer R P, O'Brien P E et al. A multicenter trial for resuscitation of injured patients with 7.5% sodium chloride. The effect of added dextran 70. Arch Surg 1993; 128: 1003–1011

34. Clifton G L, Allen S, Barrodale P et al. A phase II study of moderate hypothermia in severe brain injury. J Neurotrauma 1993; 10: 263–271

35. Marion D W, Obrist W D, Carlier P M, Penrod L E, Darby J M. The use of moderate therapeutic hypothermia for patients with severe head injuries: a preliminary report. J Neurosurg 1993; 79: 354–362

36. Shiozaki T, Sugimoto H, Taneda M et al. Effect of mild hypothermia on uncontrolled intracranial hypertension after severe head injury. J Neurosurg 1993; 79: 363–368

37. Chesnut R M, Gautille T, Blunt B A, Klauber M R, Marshall L E. The localising value of asymmetry in pupillary size in severe head injury: relation to lesion type and location. Neurosurgery 1994; 34: 840–845

38. Sakas D E, Bullock M R, Teasdale G M. One-year outcome following craniotomy for traumatic hematoma in patients with fixed dilated pupils. J Neurosurg 1995; 82: 961–965

39. Andrews B T, Levy M L, Pitts L H. Implications of systemic hypotension for the neurological examination in patients with severe head injury. Surg Neurol 1987; 28: 419–424

40. Miller J D, Murray L S, Teasdale G M. Development of a traumatic intracranial hematoma after a "minor" head injury. J Neurosurg 1990; 27: 669–673

41. Stein S C, Ross S E. Mild head injury: a plea for early CT scanning. J Trauma 1992; 33: 11–13

42. Livingston D H, Loder P A, Koziol J, Hunt C D. The use of CT scanning to triage patients requiring admission following minimal head injury. J Trauma 1991; 31: 483–487

43. Strebel S, Lam A M, Matta B F, Newell D W. Impaired cerebral autoregulation after mild brain injury. Surg Neurol 1997; 47: 128–131

44. Junger E C, Newell D W, Grant G A et al. Cerebral autoregulation after minor head injury. J Neurosurg 1997; 86: 425–432

45. Winchell R J, Simons R K, Hoyt D B. Transient hypotension. A serious problem in the management of head injury. Arch Surg 1996; 131: 533–539

46. Saxe J M, Ledgerwood A M, Lucas C E, Lucas W F. Lower esophageal sphincter dysfunction precludes safe gastric feeding after head injury. J Trauma 1994; 37: 581–584

47. Ott L, Young B, Phillips R et al. Altered gastric emptying in the head-injured patient: relationship to feeding intolerance. J Neurosurg 1991; 74: 738–742

48. Power I, Easton J C, Todd J G, Nimmo W S. Gastric emptying after head injury. Anaesthesia 1989; 44: 563–566

49. Sconzo J M, Lawson D, Lambert P. Extending the indications for cerebral protection. Anesth Analg 1990; 71: 434–439

50. Lee S T, Lui T N. Delayed intracranial haemorrhage in patients with multiple trauma and shock-related hypotension. Acta Neurochir (Wien) 1991; 113: 121–124

51. Vender J R, Black P, Natter H M, Katsetos C D. Post-anesthesia uncal herniation secondary to a previously unsuspected temporal glioma. J Forensic Sci 1995; 40: 900–902

52. Hilt H, Gramm H-J, Link J. Changes in intracranial pressure associated with extradural anaesthesia. Br J Anaesth 1986; 58: 676–680

53. Grocott H P, Mutch W A. Epidural anaesthesia and acutely raised intracranial pressure. Lumbar epidural space hydrodynamics in a porcine model. Anesthesiology 1996; 85: 1086–1091

54. Archer B D. Computed tomography before lumbar puncture in acute meningitis: a review of the risks and benefits. Can Med Assoc J 1993; 148: 961–965

55. Levy D I, Rekate H L, Cherny W B, Manwaring K, Moss S D, Baldwin H Z. Controlled lumbar drainage in pediatric head injury. J Neurosurg 1995; 83: 453–460

56. Eldridge P R, Williams S. Effect of limb tourniquet on cerebral perfusion pressure in a head-injured patient. Anaesthesia 1989; 44: 973–974

57. Conaty K R, Klemm M S. Severe increase of intracranial pressure after deflation of a pneumatic tourniquet. Anesthesiology 1989; 71: 294–295

58. Sparling R J, Murray A W, Choksey M. Raised intracranial pressure associated with hypercarbia after tourniquet release. Br J Neurosurg 1993; 7: 75–78

59. Poole G V, Miller J D, Agnew S G, Griswold J A. Lower extremity fracture fixation in head-injured patients. J Trauma 1992; 32: 654–659

60. Malisano L P, Stevens D, Hunter G A. The management of long bone fractures in the head-injured polytrauma patient. J Orthop Trauma 1994; 8: 1–5.

61. Reynolds M A, Richardson J D, Spain D A, Seligson D, Wilson M A, Miller F B. Is the timing of fracture fixation important for the patient with multiple trauma? Ann Surg 1995; 222: 470–478

62. Schmeling G J, Schwab J P. Polytrauma care. The effect of head injuries and timing of skeletal fixation. Clin Orthop 1995; 318: 106–116.

63. Williamson S, Kumar C M. Paravertebral block in head injured patient with chest trauma. Anaesthesia 1997; 52: 276–290

64. Graziotti P J, Smith G B. Multiple rib fractures and head injury – an indication for intercostal catheterisation and infusion of local anaesthetics. Anaesthesia 1988; 43: 964–966

65. Lam A M. Changes in cerebral blood flow velocity pattern during induced hypotension: a non-invasive indicator of increased intracranial pressure. Br J Anaesth 1992; 68: 424–428

Michael Wang

Learning, memory and awareness during anaesthesia

Why should clinical anaesthetists be interested in the apparently arcane subject of learning and memory during general anaesthesia? Two principal responses to this question deserve careful and critical examination: firstly, because it is claimed that intra-operative information and stimulation may have important effects on postoperative outcome; and secondly, because the intra-operative learning literature, perhaps rather unexpectedly, turns out to bear directly on our understanding of the very nature of general anaesthesia and, in particular, the quantification of anaesthetic depth.

Recent interest in the topic can be traced back to the publication of a provocative study by Levinson (1965).[1] Levinson had trained on an anaesthetic rotation in London in the 1950s. He was disturbed by comments made by surgical staff during operations about the patient on the table. By the early 1960s, Levinson had entered psychiatry, but remained convinced that such intra-anaesthetic remarks were processed at some level, and that these would have subsequent detrimental effects. In order to demonstrate this, he conducted an experiment with 10 patients undergoing dental surgery with ether general anaesthesia. Shortly after induction, the anaesthetist called to the surgeon 'stop the operation, I don't like the patient's colour. His/her lips are turning too blue. I'm going to give a little oxygen' at which point the surgeon did indeed stop. After a few moments, the anaesthetist indicated that all was now well, and the surgery could continue. One month later, Levinson probed for evidence of assimilation of this manufactured intra-operative crisis by inducing hypnosis, regressing the patient back to the time of the operation, and checking for evidence of knowledge of the experimental event. Of the 10 patients, four were able to quote verbatim the words spoken by the anaesthetist in the operation, and a further four showed evidence, in the form of appropriate emotional distress, of having registered the occurrence of a worrying intra-operative event.

Dr Michael Wang BSc MSc PhD CPsychol AFBPsS, Clinical Director, Department of Clinical Psychology, School of Medicine, University of Hull, Hull HU6 7RX, UK

Table 5.1 Effects of positive suggestions presented during general anaesthesia

Author (date)	n	Maintenance anaesthesia (premed./induction)	Significant outcome variables	Outcome variables with no effect
Moix (1996)[5]	27	(Diazepam, fentanyl, propofol) N_2O, isoflurane 0.1–0.5%, fentanyl	Awakening time	Postop. hospital stay, analgesic utilisation, pain, vomiting, perception of recovery, periods of raised temp., body function
Van Leeuwen (1996)[6]	60	(Fentanyl, propofol) N_2O, isoflurane $\geq$1.0 MAC, fentanyl	–	Morphine utilisation (PCA-system[a]), pain, nausea, anxiety
De Houwer (1996)[7]	40	(Lorazepam, etomidate, sufentanil) N_2O, sufentanil, midazolam	–	Postop. hospital stay, recovery rating, days in ICU, anxiety, time to extubation
Oddby-Muhrbeck E (1995)[8]	35	(Midazolam, thiopentone) N_2O, isoflurane, fentanyl	Subject recall of vomiting and nausea (less)	Analgesic and antiemetic utilisation, nausea, vomiting
Caseley-Rondi (1994)[9]	96 (74)	(Diazepam, droperidol, sufentanil, thiopentone) N_2O, isoflurane 0.5%, sufentanil	Analgesic utilisation (PCA-system)	Postop. hospital stay, nausea, mood, anxiety, nurse/subject recovery-rating
Williams (1994)[10]	51	(Hyoscine, thiopentone) N_2O, isoflurane 1.0%	Incidence and severity of nausea and vomiting (requirement of metochlopramide)	Blood loss (intraop.)
Bethune (1993)[11]	49	N_2O and trichlorethylene 0.5%, or fentanyl and midazolam, and enflurane or propofol	Postop. hospital stay	Pain, nausea, recovery (day 2), time in ICU, anxiety, mood
Liu (1993)[12]	143 (> 55 y)	Volatile agent (not known)	–	Postop. hospital stay, analgesic and anti-emetic utilisation, pain, mobility (ADL[b]), mental confusion (MMSE[c]), trail making test
Furlong (1993)[13]	108	(Various benzodiazepines) various volatile and i.v. agents	Incidences of sore throat, anxiety (STAI)	Postop. hospital stay, complications (nausea, vomiting)

Table 5.1 (continued) Effects of positive suggestions presented during general anaesthesia

Author (date)	n	Maintenance anaesthesia (premed./induction)	Significant outcome variables	Outcome variables with no effect
Jelicic (1993)[14]	82	(Thiopentone, droperidol, and sufentanil or fentanyl) N$_2$O, sufentanil, fentanyl	Postop. hospital stay (only if both, affective and non-affective sugg.)	Postop. hospital stay (if either affective, or non-affective sugg.), subject well-being
Couture (1993)[15]	26	(Thiopentone) isoflurane	Only for specific sugg: wellbeing (PANAS[d]), [pain and discomfort, both $P < 0.10$]	For general sugg.: well-being, pain, discomfort, nausea; for specific sugg.: nausea
Rondi (1993)[16]	64	(Diazepam, droperidol, sufentanil, sodium thiopentone) N$_2$O, isoflurane ≥0.5%, sufentanil	–	Pain, nausea, vomiting, anxiety (STAI), subject/nurse recovery-rating, first flatus
Steinberg (1993)[17]	60	N$_2$O, isoflurane 0.6–1.4%, fentanyl	Analgesic utilisation (8–16 h postop., PCA-system)	Postop. hospital stay, analg. utilisation (0–8, 16–24 h postop.), pain, nausea, vomiting
Korunka (1992)[18]	163, 140	(Flunitrazepam, or lormetazepam, thiopentone) N$_2$O 70%, fentanyl, and halothane or isoflurane 0.2–0.5 MAC	First time of analgesic utilisation, pain rating (MSS[e])	Postop. hospital stay, pain (overall score on visual analogue scale), anxiety (STAI)
Block (1991)[19]	209 (< 55 y)	(Morphine, thiopentone) N$_2$O, isoflurane 1.0–1.5 MAC, or fentanyl, sufentanil, alfentanil	–	Postop. hospital stay, analgesic utilisation, pain, fever incidences, recovery rating, anxiety
McLintock (1990)[20]	60	(Thiopentone, morphine) N$_2$O, enflurane 0.8–1.2%	Analgesic utilisation (24 h postop., PCA-system)	Pain
Furlong (1990)[21]	19	(Various benzodiazepines or antidepressants), N$_2$O, or various volatile agents, or opioids	Analgesic utilisation (day 1)	Postop. hospital stay, complications (nausea, vomiting, etc.), mood
Münch (1990)[22]	36	N$_2$O, fentanyl, dihydrobenzperidol, midazolam, fentanyl, enflurane 0.5–1.0% if required	Well-being	Pain, nausea

Table 5.1 (Continued) Effects of positive suggestions presented during general anaesthesia

Author (date)	n	Maintenance anaesthesia (premed./induction)	Significant outcome variables	Outcome variables with no effect
Boeke (1988)[23]	106	(Fentanyl-droperidol, or lorazepam, thiopentone) N_2O, enflurane, fentanyl	–	Postop. hospital stay, analgesic utilisation, pain, fluid loss, vomiting, well-being
Evans (1988)[24]	39	Halothane or enflurane	Postop. hospital stay, pyrexia, bowel difficulties, nurse-rating of recovery	Analgesic utilisation, pain/distress (day 5), mobilisation rating, vomiting, nausea, flatulence, urinary difficulties
Woo (1987)[25]	31	(Morphine, merepedine, thiopentone) N_2O, enflurane 0.8–1.9%	–	Postop. hospital stay, analgesic utilisation, time to beginning oral intake, volume of wound drainage
Bonke (1986)[26]	91	(Thiopentone sodium), N_2O, fentanyl, and/or dehydrobenzperidol	Protection of prolonged hospital stay for => 55-year-olds	Postop. hospital stay for < 55-year-olds
Abramson (1966)[27]	45	Not known	–	Postop. hospital stay, sedative, tranquilizer, analgesic utilisation, number of catheterisations
Pearson (1961)[4]	81	Not known	Postop. hospital stay	Number of doses of narcotics, rating of postop. course

[a]Patient controlled analgesia system; [b]activities of daily living; [c]mini-mental state examination; [d]positive and negative affect scale; [e]multi-dimensional pain scale (Mehrdimensionale Schmerzskala).

Despite the obvious methodological flaws, such as absence of a control group, non-random selection of subjects, absence of double blind study design, the possibility of the investigator asking leading questions under hypnosis and the subjective nature of the interpretation of responses, not to mention important ethical considerations, Levinson's study prompted much serious thought about the potential effects of intra-operative auditory information.

POSITIVE SUGGESTION STUDIES

Previously, several authors[2–4] had begun experimenting with the corollary of the Levinson study: if negative intra-operative information can be assimilated and perhaps produce negative postoperative effects, could positive intra-operative information produce positive postoperative effects? Like the Levinson study, the earliest reports were of uncontrolled case series.[2,3] Pearson[4] in 1961 described the first double blind controlled study in which intra-operative suggestions for relaxation and postoperative coping were given. The outcome variables included the surgeon's ratings of recovery, dose of narcotic required, and days to discharge. A statistically significant difference between the groups on this latter variable was obtained.

In the typical design of these studies, two audiotapes for intra-operative presentation are prepared: one contains positive suggestions such as 'the operation is going extremely well, you are doing fine, you are going to recover unusually quickly, etc.'; the other contains a story which bears no relationship to the operative situation, or alternatively, white masking noise. The tapes are coded so that theatre staff and the investigators cannot tell which is which. A randomisation code is then used to allocate a tape to each successive patient entered into the trial. Closed headphones are used so that theatre staff and investigators cannot tell which tape is being played. Relevant postoperative outcome variables are carefully monitored by recovery ward staff who again do not know which tape the patient has received. Patients are checked for any evidence of conscious knowledge of the taped material. In this way blinding is assured.

Table 5.1 summarises the double blind controlled trials published thus far, in terms of those obtaining a statistically significant difference between experimental and control groups versus those that found no such difference. A great variety of outcome variables have been monitored in these studies, e.g. postoperative narcotic dose, days till discharge, ratings of pain, postoperative pyrexia and other complications, etc. One immediate methodological difficulty here is that the use of a large number of outcome variables in the same study increases the probability of obtaining a significant result, and statistical adjustment to take account of this problem is rarely employed.

It can be seen from Table 5.1, that the ratio of studies obtaining a significant difference compared with those which did not is about 2:1. A particular feature of this literature is the invariable failure to replicate an originally significant study, even when it involves the same author(s). Moreover, Millar has eloquently identified the numerous and often serious methodological difficulties associated with these studies.[28] One salutary example concerns the first study of this type to be conducted in the UK. Evans & Richardson appeared to demonstrate a significant difference between experimental and control groups in terms of time to discharge.[24] A subsequent attempt to replicate these findings not only failed to show a significant difference between the groups, but demonstrated that the control group had been kept in hospital following surgery for an unusually lengthy period and, thus, it was the abnormality of the control group that accounted for the difference in the original report.[29] A further difficulty is that for those few, methodologically sound studies obtaining statistically significant results, it is usually the case that extremely small actual differences in variables give rise to statistical significance: there may be little or no *clinical significance* attaching to such differences.

Merikle & Daneman conducted a meta-analysis of memory for events during anaesthesia, which considered all positive suggestion and implicit verbal learning studies published up to 1995.[30] Forty-four studies satisfied the inclusion criteria, involving a cumulative total of 2179 patients. Merikle & Daneman calculated effect sizes for individual outcome variables, and demonstrated that only amount of morphine delivered by PCA reached unequivocal significance. Duration of hospital stay in the total of 5 studies up to 1989 was associated with a highly significant effect size ($P < 0.0003$), but no effect was associated with the 9 studies published between 1989 and 1995 ($P < 0.488$). The authors deliberately omitted studies involving cardiac surgery from the main meta-analysis, arguing that the nature of the anaesthetic and surgery was quite different from that associated with the bulk of the studies. However, they did perform a separate analysis on these cardiac studies, and found a considerably larger effect size for duration of hospital stay than that for the other studies, leading them to conclude that cardiac patients may be more likely to benefit from intra-operative positive suggestion.

The recent literature is characterised by a preponderance of negative results, and it may be no coincidence that this period has also been associated with the more widespread use of volatile agents in general anaesthesia. Various studies have demonstrated that the use of volatile agents even at subanaesthetic concentrations (0.2–0.4 MAC) abolishes intra-operative assimilation and learning, whether implicit or explicit.[31,32] This is certainly not the case for similar MACs of nitrous oxide[33] and, indeed, nitrous oxide administered in combination with a volatile agent such as isoflurane tends to antagonise this effect.[34] Thus, in studies involving nitrous oxide/narcotic/muscle relaxant, many of the patients were probably wakeful during surgery, hearing suggestions in a conscious state, but with postoperative amnesia due to the effects of narcotic and other drugs (see below).

SUGGESTIONS FOR POSTOPERATIVE BEHAVIOUR CHANGE

Smoking cessation

Most studies investigate the effects of intra-operative suggestion on aspects of postoperative recovery. Some studies have attempted to modify postoperative behaviour. Hughes and colleagues presented intra-operative suggestions to

Table 5.2 Effects of ideo-motor suggestions presented during general anaesthesia

Author (date)	n	Maintenance anaesthesia (premed./induction)	Time of measurement	Significant effect
Gonsowski (1995)[39]	12 (vol.)	(Propofol), desflurane 0.6–1.7 MAC, or isoflurane 0.6–1.7 MAC	< 12 h	−
Chortkoff (1995)[30]	21 (vol.)	Desflurane 3.5–6.6%, or propofol 1.5–2.0 MAC-awake	12–36 h	−
Bethune (1993)[11]	49	N_2O and trichlorethylene 0.5%, or fentanyl, and midazolam, and enflurane or propofol	> 36 h	−
Chortkoff (1993)[32]	10 (vol.)	Isoflurane 0.4 MAC	< 12 h	−
Chortkoff (1993)[34]	24 (vol.)	N_2O/isoflurane (0.68 MAC-comb.)	< 12h	−
Dwyer (1992)[41]	39	Isoflurane => 0.6 MAC	12–36 h	−
Bethune (1992)[42]	43	(Midazolam, fentanyl, droperidol) methohexital or propofol	≥ 36 h	−
Dwyer (1992)[31]	17 (vol.)	Isoflurane 0.4 MAC or N_2O	12–36 h	−
Block (1991)[43]	48	(Morphine and/or glycopyrrolate/thiopentone) N_2O and isoflurane 0.5–0.8%, or fentanyl, alfentanil	< 12 h, > 12 h	+, −
Jansen (1991)[44]	80	(Lorazepam or midazolam, thiopentone, fentanyl) N_2O, enflurane 0.2–0.4 MAC, fentanyl if required	12–36 h, > 36 h	−
Goldmann (1987)[45]	30	(Hyoscine and/or lorazepam) N_2O, fentanyl, and/or halothane	> 36 h	(+)[a]
Bennett (1985)[37]	32	(Thiopentone) N_2O and enflurane 0.5–3% or halothane 0.2–0.6%	> 36 h	+

[a]A re-analysis by Merikle & Rondi (1993) suggested the group difference not to be significant; vol. = volunteer study.

reduce or stop smoking postoperatively, in a double blind randomised controlled study.[35] They found a significant difference between the groups at one month follow-up in the expected direction, but this difference had disappeared by the 6 month point (Sanders, personal communication). An attempt to replicate the finding using a more substantial sample failed to demonstrate a significant effect.[36]

Ideomotor studies

A number of studies have sought to demonstrate that intra-operative suggestions to touch a particular part of the body, such as the ear or nose, have resulted in a significant increase in such behaviour during postoperative interview, as compared with a control group which did not receive such suggestions.

In one of the first of this type of study, Bennett and colleagues presented surgical patients with intra-operative suggestions to touch their ear at postoperative interview, in a randomised, double blind design involving 33 subjects.[37] The authors reported that patients in the experimental group did indeed touch their ears more frequently, despite having no conscious knowledge of the intra-operative suggestion. The study was subsequently criticised by Millar on the grounds of there having been no pre-operative baseline assessment of ear-touching frequency, and the small size of the experimental group.[38] The statistically significant group difference was accounted for by only two members of the latter.

There is a clear preponderance of negative results in these studies. Of the 13 studies listed in Table 5.2, only 3 yielded significant results. None of the 8 studies since 1991 have found evidence of ideomotor learning.

Intra-operative music

A further group of studies has investigated the effects of the intra-operative presentation of music. Some of these studies have attempted to demonstrate postoperative therapeutic effects, whilst others have tested patients to see if they have any form of implicit memory for the particular music presented. Once again, there is a preponderance of negative results. Of the 4 studies listed in Table 5.3, only one obtained evidence of an effect of intra-operative music on postoperative outcome.

UNDERLYING ASSUMPTIONS

Studies which attempt to demonstrate the effects of intra-operative suggestion on postoperative recovery or behaviour have at their heart two basic assumptions: (i) that general anaesthesia is a consistent, unitary state characterised by unconsciousness (subjective oblivion); (ii) that general anaesthesia is associated with a special cognitive state, in which verbal suggestions have much more powerful effects (psychological and even physiological) than when the same suggestions are presented in the normal, conscious, waking state.

Table 5.3 Effects of music presented during general anaesthesia

Author (date)	n	Maintenance anaesthesia (premed./induct.)	Significant outcome variables	Outcome variables with no effect
Caseley-Rondi (1994)[9]	96	(Diazepam, droperidol, sufentanil, sodium thiopental) N_2O, isoflurane 0.5%, sufentanil if required	–	Preference judgement, forced-choice recognition (> 36 h)
Rondi (1993)[16]	64	(Diazepam, droperidol, sufentanil, sodium thiopentone) N_2O, isoflurane (≥0.5%, sufentanil	–	Preference judgement, forced-choice recognition (> 36 h)
Winograd (1991)[46]	20 (vol.)	Isoflurane, fentanyl	–	Preference judgement (> 36 h)
Korunka (1992)[18]	163	(Flunitrazepam or lormetazepam, thiopenthone) N_2O, fentanyl and halothane or isoflurane 0.2–0.5 MAC	Analgesic utilisation (at first day and total), postop. hospital stay, pain (MSS)[a]	Pain (visual analogue scale), anxiety (STAI)

[a]MMS = multi-dimensional pain scale (Mehrdimensionale Schmerzskala); vol. = volunteer study.

Clearly these assumptions are open to question. Surprisingly, the second assumption is not addressed in the literature, in that studies do not compare the effects of intra-operative suggestion with those of *extra*-anaesthetic suggestion, i.e. the same suggestions presented in the unanaesthetised waking state. We cannot know whether the same kind of remarks made with authority to the patient by the surgeon or anaesthetist prior to surgery might not have similar or even more potent effects on outcome.

There is now good evidence to the effect that, not only is there typically large variation in levels of consciousness in the patient during surgery under a general anaesthetic, but that anaesthetists are remarkably poor at detecting such variation. In particular, the introduction of muscle relaxants in the early 1950s has greatly complicated the problem. Careful and systematic monitoring of intra-operative state is seldom a feature of these studies. Thus the possibility that, in some cases, the intra-operative stimuli or suggestions are being presented to the patient in a wakeful or conscious state cannot be ruled out. In clinical practice, there is a widespread belief that light anaesthesia and even full consciousness can be detected by the presence of so-called clinical signs, such as tear production, increased sweating, and increases in haemodynamic variables. In a recent study,[47] experienced anaesthetists were unable to distinguish clear cases of anaesthetic awareness (with full postoperative recall) when their anaesthetic records were mixed with matched control cases in which such problems did not occur. Moreover, in a number of studies using the isolated forearm technique (IFT), intra-operative episodes of coherent, conditional and complex motor response to command and question, were not associated with significant changes in clinical signs.[48,49] The isolated forearm technique has been criticised on the grounds that only a small proportion of patients making positive intra-operative responses have postoperative recall. It is often erroneously assumed that absence of postoperative recall is synonymous with intra-operative oblivion and, therefore it is argued that either the IFT is unreliable giving misleading results, or, at the very least, the significance of isolated forearm responding is questioned. In fact, IFT studies clearly indicate intra-operative consciousness when, for example, a patient is asked to squeeze their fingers twice if they are comfortable, and does so. Yet commonly there is no postoperative recall or elevated intra-operative 'clinical signs'.

What are we to make of this circumstance in which there is intra-operative evidence of high levels of consciousness, but with apparent postoperative amnesia? Some[50] have argued that these are 'ideal circumstances for surgery', whilst others have been concerned about the ethics of this state of affairs, particularly if there is intra-operative distress.[51,52] Readers who are in any doubt about the potential for this state should consider the rather dramatic results obtained by Russell in an investigation of midazolam-alfentanil 'anaesthesia' using the IFT.[53] He found it necessary to discontinue the trial after 20 out of 33 patients clearly indicated they were in pain during surgery. None of the patients had postoperative recall.

Reports of psychopathology following intra-operative wakefulness without explicit recall

In 1961, Meyer & Blacher described a postoperative 'traumatic neurosis' in a series of patients who appeared to have awakened during heart surgery whilst paralysed.[54] The main features of this were: anxiety and irritability, repetitive nightmares, a pre-occupation with death, and a reluctance to discuss the symptoms lest they be thought insane. These symptoms correspond closely with those associated with the contemporary psychiatric diagnosis of post-traumatic stress disorder. Most significantly, according to Meyer & Blacher's account, these patients were uncertain of the cause of their difficulties, and had no clear recollection of intra-operative wakefulness.

Tunstall reported a case in which a woman requiring a second caesarian section described distressing, recurrent nightmares since the previous operation.[55] The nightmare was of floating in black space, being alone, and being unable to hold on to anything or any person. It recurred with greater frequency at the approach of the second caesarian section. Tunstall gave the patient a general anaesthetic with muscle relaxant, but used the IFT to communicate with her when the anaesthetic lightened after 16 min. The patient was asked to indicate whether this was the condition she found herself in during the previous operation. She indicated with her hand that this indeed was the case. Tunstall then proceeded to provide verbal reassurance whilst holding her hand. Postoperatively, the patient had no conscious recall but was left with an inner confidence that the nightmares had gone. This turned out to be the case, and no further nightmares had occurred at an 18-month follow-up.

Howard[56] describes two further case examples in which apparent intra-operative perception without conscious recall gave rise to psychological problems: firstly, a case of chronic insomnia, which persisted for 3 years, and secondly, relapse and return of an eating disorder. In both cases, Howard obtained evidence of episodes of intra-operative wakefulness by means of regression under hypnosis. Tinnin reported a case in which a patient with an inexplicable phobia of surgery was regressed back to a previous operation in which she described 'a transient frightening pain which she experienced in a state of paralysis'.[57]

Clearly these are anecdotal accounts and do not carry the authority of a systematic trial. What is needed is a prospective double blind study involving a large cohort of surgical patients, with careful monitoring of intra-operative state using either the IFT or auditory evoked potentials, to determine the incidence of wakefulness. Patients would then be screened over a number of months postoperatively for evidence of psychological abnormality. To date, no such study has been reported. However, given the anecdotal evidence, *it is unsafe to assume that the occurrence of intra-operative episodes of wakefulness with subsequent amnesia are of no consequence.* Furthermore, the absence of pain during an episode of intra-operative wakefulness is not, in itself, a safeguard against the development of postoperative psychological disorder: it is clear from the foregoing accounts and the literature documenting the experience of intra-operative awareness with full recall that it is often the unexpected paralysis which is the most traumatic aspect for the patient.

INTRA-OPERATIVE VERBAL LEARNING

Psychologists have attempted a more detailed analysis of the cognitive processes occurring during general anaesthesia, making use of sophisticated memory tests which were initially developed in the context of the study of neurological patients with organic amnesia. There is now a burgeoning literature in which various types of word learning are attempted. To understand this work, a brief review of some basic concepts in the psychology of memory is necessary.

Contemporary model of human memory

Human memory has been characterised as comprising two distinct functional stages: short term storage (more recently described as *working memory*) and long term storage (see Fig. 5.1). Working memory is associated with attention and concentration, and has limited capacity.[58] It includes at least two sub systems which are under the control of the central executive (awareness): the *phonological loop* can extend the existence of verbal material through repetition by an inner voice; the *visuo-spatial sketch pad* likewise extends the existence of visual material. If no such rehearsal takes place, information is only maintained within the short term storage phase for about 20 s. If information has not been transferred to the long term memory store by the end of this period, it will be lost. It is important to note that many psychotropic and anaesthetic drugs, such as the benzodiazepines, opioids, and barbiturates interfere with this transfer or *encoding* process, without necessarily greatly disturbing the operation of working memory itself.[59] What this means in practice is that these drugs can easily produce a state in which the subject has

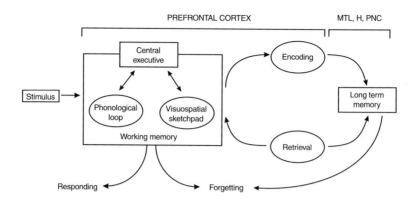

Fig. 5.1 A model of working and long term memory identifying the processes and their anatomical locations. MTL, medial temporal lobe; H, hippocampus; PNC, posterior neocortex. Reprinted from Bailey A R, Jones J G. *Anaethesia* 1997; 52: 460–476 with permission from Blackwell Science Ltd.

a relatively clear and alert sensorium, and yet is not laying down their moment-to-moment experience in the long term memory store. Thus, perhaps just 10 min or more later, they will have no explicit recollection of earlier events or information, even though they may have appeared to be perfectly conscious at the time they occurred.

Implicit memory

A distinction is made between two types of learning: *explicit* versus *implicit* learning. Briefly, *explicit recall* of an event or stimulus is said to be present when the subject provides evidence of memory of both the *content* and *context* of the learning episode. So, for example, in the specific situation of intra-operative learning, the patient having postoperative memory that they heard the word 'gooseberry' (content) spoken by a man's voice at some point in the operation (context), would be classed as explicit recall.

Implicit recall is said to be present when, although there is no recollection of a learning episode or its context, changes in response showing that learning has taken place can be demonstrated. This is the case when although the patient has no postoperative recall of any intra-operative events or stimuli, nevertheless responds 'gooseberry' (rather than the more common responses of 'apple' or 'orange') following the instruction to think of the first fruit that comes into their mind (the word 'gooseberry' having been presented intra-operatively). A more mundane example of implicit recall is that of riding a bicycle without any specific recollection of the period when the skill of bike-riding was first acquired.

The assumption in all intra-operative learning studies is that *explicit* recall indicates absence of, or inadequate, general anaesthesia: studies invariably attempt to demonstrate evidence of *implicit* learning in the context of assumed adequate general anaesthesia.

A range of implicit memory tasks have been employed in the context of general anaesthesia. The 'gooseberry' example given above is known as *category association*, where one or two slightly unusual examples of a category of words (in this case fruit) are presented intra-operatively. The investigator would normally have first established the natural frequency of fruit names in the local population for comparison, in order to select the most appropriate word(s) for presentation.

Word stem completion involves presenting a two-syllable word such as 'carton' intra-operatively, and then asking the patient to complete the word stem 'car...' following the operation. Again, the natural frequency of responses to this task in the general population needs to be ascertained beforehand, but in this case, the response of 'carpet' is common, whereas the response of 'carton' would be extremely unusual. *Word association* simply involves presenting unusual word-pair combinations such as 'sharp–apple' intra-operatively, and then asking for the first word that comes to mind in response to 'sharp' postoperatively. *Unfamiliar knowledge* tasks involve the intra-operative presentation of uncommonly known or trivial facts, such as the blood pressure of an octopus. Patients are then asked to guess the answers to these questions at postoperative interview.

Table 5.4 lists the studies of implicit verbal learning. Whilst 15 studies demonstrated intra-operative learning, 30 others found no such evidence. In the meta-analysis mentioned previously, Merikle & Daneman[30] show how when considering both explicit and implicit memory for intra-operative information combined, significant evidence of recall is obtained if the postoperative test takes place *less than 12 h after intra-operative presentation*. Their analysis shows there is no evidence of persistence of memory, either implicit or explicit, beyond 36 h. Furthermore, when examining implicit versus explicit recall separately, Merikle & Daneman found rather similar effect sizes for each, undermining the notion that implicit memory effects are more potent and persistent than those for explicit memory.

Intra-operative wakefulness and implicit memory

Over the last decade, it has become increasingly difficult to demonstrate evidence of implicit learning during general anaesthesia. There has been a preponderance of negative outcome studies, including many attempts to replicate studies which were previously successful at demonstrating this phenomenon. It has already been noted that this same period has been associated with an increase in the use of volatile agents. A number of studies demonstrate that the use of volatile agents, even at sub anaesthetic concentrations, preclude implicit and explicit learning.[31,32]

To understand this further, it is necessary to look at a basic model of the progressive cognitive effects of general anaesthetic agents. Jones & Konieczko[92] have proposed the following: (i) conscious awareness without amnesia (with explicit recall); (ii) conscious awareness with amnesia (with possible implicit recall) [*wakefulness*]; (iii) subconscious awareness with amnesia (with possible implicit recall); and (iv) no awareness.

It is usually assumed in implicit memory studies that patients are consistently in level (iii). However, there is good reason to suspect that in the majority of studies demonstrating implicit memory, information was assimilated intra-operatively whilst patients were actually in level (ii). The reasons for believing

Table 5.4 Learning of verbal material presented during general anaesthesia

Author (date)	n	Maintenance anaesthesia (premed./induction)	Significant outcome variables	Outcome variables with no effect
Russell (1997)[60]	68 (48)	(Temazepam, thiopentone) N_2O, halothane 0.5%	–	Category generation, word association, (with/without hypnosis) (< 12 h, > 36 h)
Bonebakker (1996)[61]	80, 80	(Sufentanil, thiopentone) N_2O, isoflurane 0.25–0.5%, and sufentanil if required	Word-stem completion, forced-choice recognition (< 12, 12–36 h)	–
Cork (1996)[62]	31	(Propofol, fentanyl) propofol	Word-pair association (< 12 h)	(Cued) recognition (< 12 h)
van Leeuwen (1996)[6]	60	(Fentanyl, propofol) N_2O, isoflurane $\geq$1 MAC, fentanyl	Word association (Peter Pan narrative) (< 12, 12–36 h)	Word association (Robinson Crusoe narrative) (< 12, 12–36 h)
Alkire (1996)[63]	10 (vol.)	Propofol	Familiarity rating (12–36 h)	–
Millar (1996)[64]	75	(Propofol) N_2O, enflurane 0.3–1.1%	–	Category association (< 12 h)
Donker (1996)[65]	63	Propofol and sufentanil	–	Fame-rating, familiar/unfamiliar names, fact learning (< 12 h)
Hughdal (1996)[66]	37	(Oxazepam, thiopentone, fentanyl, dihydrobenzperidol) N_2O, isoflurane 0.6–1.0 MAC, fentanyl if required	–	Category association (12–36 h)
De Houwer (1996)[7]	40	(Lorazepam, etomidate, sufentanil) N_2O, sufentanil, midazolam	–	Preference judgement, recognition (non-words) (> 36 h)
Kalff (1995)[67]	30 (ch.)	(Propofol or halothane) N_2O and halothane or isoflurane	–	Colour/object-word preference judgement (< 12 h)
Chortkoff (1995)[40]	21 (vol.)	Desflurane 3.5–6.6% or propofol 1.5–2 times MAC-awake	–	(Keyword) recall under hypnosis (emotionally charged words), identification certainty, fact learning (12–36 h)
De Roode (1995)[68]	83	(Midazolam) N_2O, alfentanil	–	Fact learning, fame rating (names)

Table 5.4 (continued) Learning of verbal material presented during general anaesthesia

Author (date)	n	Maintenance anaesthesia (premed./induction)	Significant outcome variables	Outcome variables with no effect
Van Hooff (1995)[69]	9	(Morphine) propofol, alfentanil, cephalozin	–	Category association (12–36 h)
Gonsowski (1995)[39]	12 (vol.)	(Propofol) desflurane 0.6–1.7 MAC or isoflurane 0.6–1.7 MAC	–	Fact learning, category association
Schwender (1994)[70]	45	(Fentanyl or etomidate and flunitrazepam) fentanyl or flunitrazepam or isoflurane 0.6–1.2%, or propofol	Word association (Robinson Crusoe narrative) (> 36 h)	–
Andrade (1994)[71]	7 (vol.)	Isoflurane 0.8%	–	Category generation, forced choice recognition (< 12 h)
Parker (1994)[72]	48	(Thiopentone, midazolam) N_2O, fentanyl	–	Category association, within-list recognition
Villemure (1993)[73]	10	(Propofol and fentanyl) N_2O, isoflurane 0.4%, fentanyl if required	Category generation (< 12 h, 12–36 h)	–
Jelicic (1993)[74]	43, 50	(Thiopentone and droperidol) N_2O and sufentanil or fentanyl, if required	Category generation, fact learning, fame rating (names), (< 12 h)	–
Schwender (1994)[75]	45	(Flunitrazepam/fentanyl) fentanyl, flunitrazepam	Word association (Robinson Crusoe narrative) (> 36 h)	–
Schwender (1994)[75]	45	(Etomidate) fentanyl and isoflurane 0.6–1.2% or propofol	–	Word association (Robinson Crusoe narrative) (> 36 h)
Cork (1993)[76]	25	(Thiopentone) isoflurane,	Free association (< 12, > 36 h)	Cued recall (< 12 h, > 36 h)
Cork (1993)[76]	25	(Thiopentone) N_2O, sufentanil	–	Free association, cued recall, word-pair recognition (< 12 h, > 36 h)
Bonebakker (1993)[77]	81	(Diazepam, temazepam, oxazepam if required; thiopentone) sufentanil, N_2O, isoflurane 0.25–0.5%	–	Category generation (< 12 h)
Westmoreland (1993)[78]	48	(Ranitidine, metochlorpramide, midazolam, propofol and fentanyl) N_2O, isoflurane 1.0 MAC	–	Category generation, free association, homophone association, and spelling (< 12 h, > 36 h)

Table 5.4 (continued) Learning of verbal material presented during general anaesthesia

Author (date)	n	Maintenance anaesthesia (premed./induction)	Significant outcome variables	Outcome variables with no effect
Charlton (1993)[79]	44	(Propofol) N$_2$O and isoflurane 0.5%	–	Category association, word preference judgement, and recognition (< 12 h)
Jelicic (1993)[80]	41	(Morphine, cyclicine, thiopentone) enflurane 1.1%	–	Fact learning, fame rating (12–36 h)
Couture (1993)[15]	26	Isoflurane	–	Probability-rating of word encounter (12–36 h)
Chortkoff (1993)[34]	24 (vol.)	N$_2$O/isoflurane 0.68 MAC-combined	–	Category association (< 12 h)
Bonke (1993)[81]	80 (ch.)	(A)mimazine/thiopentone), N$_2$O, halothane 1–3.5%	–	Object/colour preference judgement (12–36 h)
Bethune (1993)[11]	49	N$_2$O and trichlorethylene 0.5%, or fentanyl and midazolam and enflurane or propofol	–	Free word-association (> 36 h)
Bethune (1992)[42]	43	(Midazolam, fentanyl, droperidol) methohexitone or	–	Sentence-cued word association (≥ 36 h)
Bethune (1992)[42]	43	Propofol	Sentence-cued word association (≥ 36 h)	–
Brown (1992)[82]	10	(thiopentone, fentanyl) N$_2$O, isoflurane 0.5–1.0%, fentanyl	–	Homophone, pair-association, signal suppression of three times presented words (> 36 h)
Cork (1992)[83]	25	(Thiopentone) N$_2$O, sufentanil	–	Pair-association, within-list recognition (< 12 h, > 36 h)
Dwyer (1992)[41]	45	Isoflurane ≥0.6 MAC	–	Fact learning
Block (1991)[43]	24, 48	(Morphine and/or glycopyrrolate, thiopentone) N$_2$O and isoflurane 1.0/1.3/1.5 MAC, or fentanyl, alfentanil	Preference judgement, forced-choice within-list recognition of (nonsense) words, word-stem completion (12–36 h)	Category generation, within-list recognition (names), for $n = 24$, isofl. 1.0–1.5 MAC nonsense-word recognition (12–36 h)
Roorda-Hrdlickova (1990)[84]	81	(Thalamonal/propofol, sufentanil) N$_2$O, isoflurane 0.5–1.0%, sufentanil if required	Category generation (< 12 h)	–

Table 5.4 (continued) Learning of verbal material presented during general anaesthesia

Author (date)	n	Maintenance anaesthesia (premed./induction)	Significant outcome variables	Outcome variables with no effect
Kihlstrom (1990)[85]	25	(Thiopentone) isoflurane 1.0%	Pair-association (< 12 h, > 36 h)	Within-list recognition (< 12 h, > 36 h)
Goldmann (1987)[45]	30	Fentanyl and/or halothane	–	Sentence recognition (> 36 h)
Standen (1987)[86]	41 (ch.)	(Diazepam or trimeprazine, droperidol, thiopentone) halothane 0.5–1.0%	–	Category association (< 12 h, 12–36 h)
Stolzy (1986)[87]	22 (vol.)	(Diazepam, glycopyrrolate, thiopentone) N$_2$O, isoflurane 2.1 ± 1.0 MAC	Within-list familiarity judgement	–
Eich (1985)[88]	48	(Thiopentone or sodium hexobarbital, blutopharnol, diazepam, glycopyrrolate) N$_2$O, various volatile agents (enflurane, halothane,isoflurane, meperidine) or fentanyl	–	Homophone spelling, recognition (> 36 h)
Millar (1983)[89]	53	(Scopolamine and omnopon, and/or fentazin, or pethidine and phenergan, or lorazepam, or diazepam/thiopentone or althesin) N$_2$O, halothane 0.25–1.0%	d' in within-list word recognition (12–36 h)	Within-list word recognition (12–36 h)
Dubovsky (1976)[90]	36, 12	Halothane 1.3 MAC, or enflurane 1.3 MAC	–	Letter-word pair within-list recognition (12–36 h)
Terrell (1969)[91]	37	(Morphine and scopolamine, or a barbiturate) halothane, or methoxyflurane, or compound 347, or ethyl ether, d-tubocurarine, N$_2$O	–	Recall of words (non-meaningful, meaningful, stressful) under hypnosis (ideomotor finger-signaling) (> 36 h)

vol. = volunteer study; ch. = child study.

this to be the case, in addition to the increasing level of study failure in recent times associated with the wider use of volatile agents, are as follows:

1. A very large study of nitrous oxide anaesthesia without muscle relaxation demonstrated that, with a concentration of 75% nitrous oxide in oxygen, 50% of subjects were in fact in level (ii) and not level (iii) or (iv).[93] Given the safe upper limit of 70% nitrous oxide, many would suggest that an agent that gives rise to this proportion of patients in a wakeful but amnesic state is technically not a general anaesthetic.

2. In the search for the Holy Grail of an electronic 'consciousness monitor', of greatest promise is auditory evoked potentials, in which a repetitive series of audible clicks is presented to the patient at a rate of about 10 per second. The EEG is averaged over a number of clicks, and the averaged EEG pattern evoked by the clicks delineated. In the wakeful state, a typical evoked three-peak waveform occurs between 10 and 100 ms after the click stimulus, and is known as the mid-latency auditory evoked potential (MLAEP). A number of studies have demonstrated that these MLAEP peaks are suppressed in a dose-dependent manner during general anaesthesia. Nitrous oxide, opioids, and benzodiazepines have little effect on MLAEPs, whereas volatile agents, such as desflurane and isoflurane, markedly reduced peak amplitudes of the waveform.[94] Other studies have demonstrated that the unsuppressed MLAEP wave form is associated with response to command and, therefore, equated with wakefulness.[95]

What we can conclude from this, is that anaesthetic techniques which employ nitrous oxide, opioids and benzodiazepines, either singularly or in combination, will not guarantee the absence of wakefulness in a large proportion of patients, whereas the reverse is true for volatile inhalational agents at MAC 0.4 or greater. It is highly likely, therefore, that in the majority of studies which hitherto have demonstrated implicit learning, patients have been in Jones & Konieczko's level (ii) rather than level (iii).

The Robinson Crusoe study

In an unusual and innovative study in patients undergoing cardiothoracic surgery, Schwender and colleagues monitored cognitive state around the time of the presentation of an audiotape stimulus, using MLAEPs.[75] For the experimental patients, the tape comprised a 10 min synopsis of the story of *Robinson Crusoe*. One reason for choosing this particular story was that it was thought that it might serve as an allegory of the experience of undergoing surgery and might, therefore, have more meaning for the wakeful and possibly distressed surgical patient than a series of subjectively irrelevant word stimuli. The control group received no audiotaped stimulus. In the postoperative interview, all patients were asked to say what came into their mind in response to the word 'Friday'. Seven out of 30 patients had some association with *Robinson Crusoe*, whereas none of the controls had any such association. Even more significantly, those exhibiting such evidence of implicit memory were found to have relatively unsuppressed MLAEPs at the time of tape presentation, suggesting wakefulness, in comparison with other experimental subjects who showed no implicit memory. None of the patients in the study had any conscious recollections of intra-operative events, and those experimental patients who mentioned the *Robinson Crusoe* story denied that this had anything to do with their operation or anaesthetic.

Absence of wakefulness and response to word stimuli

Of particular relevance here are two studies which made certain that intra-operative word stimuli were presented in the *absence* of wakefulness.

In contrast with the majority of studies, Charlton and colleagues chose to investigate patients undergoing elective gynaecological procedures *not* involving muscle relaxants in a double-blind design.[79] Care was taken to make sure that there was no evidence of patient movement at the time of stimulus presentation. In order to enhance the possibility of obtaining evidence of implicit memory, the study included four different probes or tests of implicit recall for the same stimulus words (category association, graded detection through progressive white noise masks, cued recognition, and guessing on the basis of familiarity). Despite this deliberate bias in favour of obtaining a significant result, no such evidence was found.

Russell & Wang used the isolated forearm technique to determine absence of wakefulness at the time of intra-operative stimulus presentation in 68 women having major gynaecological surgery.[60] Again, several different implicit memory probes were used postoperatively in this controlled study attempting to obtain evidence of intra-operative priming. Once more, no such evidence was obtained.

Taken in combination with Dutton and colleagues' work which demonstrated the relationship between memory formation and response to command,[96] these studies provide good circumstantial evidence to the effect that many previous studies which found significant intra-operative implicit memory involved patients who were wakeful [Jones & Konieczko level (ii)] at the time of stimulus presentation.

CONCLUSION

A rather similar pattern emerges for the various types of intra-operative learning studies, from positive suggestion to implicit word learning: initial reports are predominantly encouraging, indicating clear effects, but there are methodological shortcomings; later studies employing more rigorous study design and volatile anaesthetic agents predominantly fail to replicate these effects. Circumstantial evidence indicates that, in many studies obtaining significant results, subjects have been wakeful intra-operatively, with subsequent explicit amnesia. This leads to the question as to whether 'general anaesthesia' which allows for substantial numbers of patients being wakeful but unable to indicate their predicament because of the presence of muscle relaxants and subsequently amnesia, is acceptable. As the use of volatile agents increases, so evidence of implicit memory and learning declines. It might be said that this is a vindication of Dubovsky & Trustman's conclusion in 1976 that an adequate anaesthetic precludes learning of any kind whether implicit or explicit.[90] If adequate general anaesthesia is defined as intra-operative subjective oblivion, then the problem is

Key points for clinical practice

- Empirical evidence for the therapeutic effects of intra-operative suggestion is, at best, equivocal, with numerous failures to replicate. Early positive outcome studies were associated with variable and unsystematic anaesthetic regimens which omitted volatile agents. Over the last decade, the more widespread use of volatile agents has been associated with increasing failure to demonstrate intra-operative learning.

- Evidence of intra-operative learning is associated with lengthy surgery using muscle relaxants, and an absence of systematic intra-operative monitoring of anaesthetic depth.

- Rigorous intra-operative consciousness monitoring and maintenance of sufficient depth to abolish motor response to command obliterates any form of learning, implicit or explicit.

- Volatile agents used at MAC 0.4 or greater abolish all learning, explicit and implicit.

- Absence of postoperative recall is not synonymous with intra-operative oblivion: high states of consciousness may occur intra-operatively only to be forgotten due to the amnesic effects of anaesthetic agents.

- It is probable that implicit learning only occurs during episodes of intra-operative wakefulness undetected by the anaesthetist, and without explicit postoperative recall.

- The postoperative psychological and emotional effects of an episode of intra-operative wakefulness (without explicit recall) are unknown: at the present time it is not safe to assume they are inconsequential.

- Irrespective of whether postoperative recall is present, there are serious ethical issues associated with complacency about episodes of wakefulness, particularly when involving distress.

that in many studies, less than adequate anaesthesia has been provided, giving rise to significant periods of level (ii), when patients were able to process auditory stimuli in a wakeful state.

As a final footnote, in a recent study which included Levinson as a co-author, an attempt was made to replicate his original findings, but this time using a randomised, double-blind design with 22 volunteer subjects.[40] Anaesthesia was maintained using desflurane (rather than ether). Subjects were exposed to either a neutral (control) drama or a mock crisis in which the oxygen delivery system had failed. Postoperative interviews, which included hypnotic debriefing by Levinson, took place one day after anaesthesia. No evidence of memory for the intra-operative crisis, either implicit or explicit, was obtained.

ACKNOWLEDGEMENTS

The author is grateful to Thilo Womelsdorf and Dr Ian F. Russell for their assistance in the preparation of this chapter.

References

1. Levinson B. States of awareness under general anaesthesia. Br J Anaesth 1965; 37: 544–546
2. Wolfe L S, Millett J B. Control of post-operative pain by suggestion under general anaesthesia. Am J Clin Hypn 1961; 3: 109–112
3. Hutchings D D. The value of suggestion given under anaesthesia: a report and evaluation of 200 consecutive cases. Am J Clin Hypn 1961; 4: 26–29
4. Pearson R P. Response to suggestions given under general anesthesia. Am J Clin Hypn 1961; 4: 106–114
5. Moix J, Bayes R, Burrel L M, Casas J M, Nieto E. Effects of intraoperative suggestions on intra- and postoperative variables: preliminary report. In: Bonke B, Bovill J G, Moerman N. (eds) Memory and Awareness in Anaesthesia. Assen: Van Gorcum, 1996; 227–234
6. Van Leeuwen B L, van der Laan W H, Sebel P S, Winograd E, Baumann P, Bonke B. Therapeutic suggestion has no effect on postoperative morphine requirement. In: Bonke B, Bovill J G, Moerman N. (eds) Memory and Awareness in Anaesthesia. Assen: Van Gorcum, 1996; 235–244
7. De Houwer J, Demeyere R, Verhamme B, Eelen P. Intra- and postoperative effects of information presented during CABG-surgery with sufentanil anaesthesia. In: Bonke B, Bovill J G, Moerman N. (eds) Memory and Awareness in Anaesthesia. Assen: Van Gorcum, 1996; 244–253
8. Oddby-Muhrbeck E, Jakobsson J, Enquist B. Implicit processing and therapeutic suggestion during balanced anaesthesia. Acta Anaesthesiol Scand 1995; 39: 333–337
9. Caseley-Rondi G, Merikle P M, Bowers K S. Unconscious cognition in the context of general anesthesia. Consc Cog 1994; 3: 166–195
10. Williams A R, Hind M, Sweeney B P. The incidence and severity of postoperative nausea and vomiting in patients exposed to positive intra-operative suggestions. Anaesthesia 1994; 49: 340–342
11. Bethune D W, Ghosh S, Walker I A, Carter A, Kerr L, Sharples L. Intraoperative positive suggestions improve immediate postoperative recovery following cardiac surgery. In: Sebel P S, Bonke B, Winograd E. (eds) Memory and Awareness in Anaesthesia. Englewood Cliffs, NJ: Prentice Hall, 1993; 154–161
12. Liu D H, Standen P J, Aitkenhead A R. The influence of intratherapeutic suggestions on postoperative recovery after surgical repair of fractured neck of femur. In: Sebel P S, Bonke B, Winograd E. (eds) Memory and Awareness in Anaesthesia. Englewood Cliffs, NJ: Prentice Hall, 1993; 162–165
13. Furlong M, Read C. Therapeutic suggestions during general anesthesia. In: Sebel P S, Bonke B, Winograd E. (eds) Memory and Awareness in Anaesthesia. Englewood Cliffs, NJ: Prentice Hall, 1993; 166–175
14. Jelicic M, Bonke B, Millar K. Different intra-anesthetic suggestions and their effect on postoperative course. In: Sebel P S, Bonke B, Winograd E (eds) Memory and Awareness in Anaesthesia. Englewood Cliffs, NJ: Prentice Hall, 1993; 176–181
15. Couture L J, Kihlstrom J F, Cork R C, Behr S E, Hughes S. Therapeutic suggestions presented during isoflurane anesthesia: preliminary report. In: Sebel P S, Bonke B, Winograd E. (eds) Memory and Awareness in Anaesthesia. Englewood Cliffs, NJ: Prentice Hall, 1993; 182–186
16. Rondi G J, Bowers K S, Buckley D N, Merikle P M, Dunn G L, Rondi P M. Postoperative impact of information presented during general anesthesia. In: Sebel P S, Bonke B, Winograd E. (eds) Memory and Awareness in Anaesthesia. Englewood Cliffs, NJ: Prentice Hall, 1993; 187–195
17. Steinberg M E, Hord A H, Reed, B, Sebel P S. Study of the effect of intraoperative suggestion on postoperative analgesia and well-being. In: Sebel P S, Bonke B, Winograd E. (eds) Memory and Awareness in Anaesthesia. Englewood Cliffs, NJ: Prentice Hall, 1993; 205–208
18. Korunka C, Guttmann G, Schleinitz D, Hilpert M, Haas R, Fitzal S. Die Auswirkungen von Suggestionen und Musik waehrend Vollnarkose auf postoperative Befindlichkeit

[The effects of suggestions and music presented during general anaesthesia on postoperative well-being]. Z Klin Psychol Psychopathol Psychother 1991; 21: 272–285

19. Block R I, Gonheim M M, Sum Ping S T, Ali M A. Efficacy of therapeutic suggestions for improved recovery presented during general anesthesia. Anesthesiology 1991; 75: 746–755

20. McLintock T T C, Aitken H, Downie C F A, Kenny G N C. Postoperative analgesic requirement in patients exposed to positive intraoperative suggestions. BMJ 1990; 301: 788–790

21. Furlong M. Positive suggestions presented during anaesthesia. In: Bonke B, Fitch W, Millar K. (eds) Memory and Awareness in Anaesthesia. Amsterdam: Swets & Zeitlinger, 1990; 170–175

22. Münch F, Zug HD. Do intraoperative suggestions prevent nausea and vomiting in thyroidectomy-patients? An experimental study. In: Bonke B, Fitch W, Millar K, eds. Memory and Awareness in Anaesthesia. Amsterdam: Swets & Zeitlinger, 1990: 185–188.

23. Boeke S, Bonke B, Bouwhuis-Hoogerwerf M L, Bovill J G, Zwaveling A. Effects of sounds presented during general anaesthesia on postoperative course. Br J Anaesth 1988; 60: 679–702

24. Evans C, Richardson P H. Improved recovery and reduced postoperative stay after therapeutic suggestions during general anaesthesia. Lancet 1988; 2: 491–492

25. Woo R, Seltzer J R, Marr A. The lack of response to suggestions under controlled surgical anaesthesia. Acta Anaesthesiol Scand 1987; 31: 567–571

26. Bonke B, Schmitz P I M, Verhage F, Zwaveling A. Clinical study of so-called unconscious perception during general anaesthesia. Br J Anaesth 1986; 56: 957–964

27. Abramson M, Greenfield R, Herron W T. Response to or perception of auditory stimuli under deep surgical anesthesia. Am J Obstet Gynecol 1966; 96: 584–585

28. Millar K. The neglected factor of individual variation in studies of memory during general anaesthesia. In: Sebel P S, Bonke B, Winograd E. (eds) Memory and Awareness in Anaesthesia. Englewood Cliffs, NJ: Prentice Hall, 1993; 31–47

29. Liu W H D, Standen P J, Aitkenhead A R. Therapeutic suggestions during general anaesthesia in patients undergoing hysterectomy. Br J Anaesth 1992; 68: 277–281

30. Merikle P M, Danemann M. Memory for events during anaesthesia: a meta-analysis. In: Bonke B, Bovill J G, Moerman N. (eds) Memory and Awareness in Anaesthesia. Assen: Van Gorcum, 1996: 108–121

31. Dwyer R, Bennett H L, Eger E I, Heilbron D. Effects of isoflurane and nitrous oxide in sub-anesthetic concentrations on memory and responsiveness in volunteers. Anesthesiology 1992; 77: 888–898

32. Chortkoff B S, Bennett H L, Eger E I. Subanesthetic concentrations of isoflurane suppress learning as defined by the category-example task. Anesthesiology 1993; 79: 16–22

33. Block R I, Ghoneim M M, Pathak D, Kumar V, Hinrichs J V. Effects of a subanesthetic concentration of nitrous oxide on overt and covert assessments of memory and associative processes. Psychopharmacology 1988; 96: 324–331

34. Chortkoff B S, Bennett H L, Eger E I. Does nitrous oxide antagonize isoflurane-induced suppression of learning? Anesthesiology 1993; 79: 724–732

35. Hughes J A, Sanders L D, Dunne J A, Tarpey J, Vickers M D. The effect of suggestion during general anaesthesia on postoperative smoking habits. Anaesthesia 1994; 49: 126–128

36. Myles P S, Hendrata M, Layher Y et al. Double-blind, randomized trial of cessation of smoking after audiotape suggestion during anaesthesia. Br J Anaesth 1996; 76: 694–698

37. Bennett H L, Davis H S, Giannini J A. Non-verbal response to intraoperative conversation. Br J Anaesth 1985; 57: 174–179

38. Millar K. Unconscious perception during general anaesthesia [correspondence]. Br J Anaesth 1987; 59: 1334–1335

39. Gonsowski C H, Chortkoff B S, Eger E I, Bennett H L, Weiskopf R B. Subanesthetic concentration of desflurane and isoflurane suppress explicit and implicit memory. Anesth Analg 1995; 80: 568–572

40. Chortkoff B S, Gonsowski C T, Bennett H L et al. Subanesthetic concentrations of desflurane and propofol suppress recall of emotionally charged information. Anesth Analg 1995; 81: 728–736

41. Dwyer R, Bennet H L, Eger E I, Peterson N. Isoflurane anesthesia prevents unconscious learning. Anesth Analg 1992; 75: 107–112

42. Bethune D W, Ghosh S, Gray G et al. Learning during general anaesthesia: implicit recall after methohexitone or propofol infusion. Br J Anaesth 1992; 69: 197–199

43. Block R I, Gonheim M M, Sum Ping S T, Ali M A. Human learning during general anaesthesia and surgery. Br J Anaesth 1991; 66: 170–178

44. Jansen C K, Bonke B, Klein J, van Dasselaar m, Hop W C J. Failure to demonstrate unconscious perception during balanced anaesthesia by postoperative motor response. Acta Anaesthesiol Scand 1991; 35: 407–410

45. Goldmann L, Shah M V, Herbden M W. Memory of cardiac anaesthesia. Anaesthesia 1987: 42: 596–603

46. Winograd E, Sebel P S, Goldmann W P, Clifton C, Lowdon J D. Indirect assessment of memory for music during anesthesia. J Clin Anesth 1991; 3: 276–279

47. Moerman N, Bonke B, Oosting J. Awareness and recall during general anaesthesia. Anaesthesiology 1993; 79: 454–464

48. Russell I F. Conscious awareness during general anaesthesia: relevance of autonomic signs and isolated arm movements as guides to depth of anaesthesia. In : Jones J G. (ed.) Bailliere's Clinical Anaesthesia, vol. 3, no. 3: Depth of Anaesthesia. London: Bailliere Tindall, 1989; 511–532

49. Wang M, Russell I F, Charlton P F C, Conlon J. An experimental simulation of anaesthetic awareness and validation of the isolated forearm technique. In: Sebel P S, Bonke B, Winograd E. (eds) Memory and Awareness in Anaesthesia. Englewood Cliffs, NJ: Prentice Hall, 1993; 434–446

50. Jones J G. Awake during surgery [Correspondence]. The Times 10th April 1995

51. Mehlman M J, Kanoti G A, Orlowski J P. Informed consent to amnestics. J Clin Ethics 1994; 5: 105–109

52. Wang M, Russell I. Memory of intra-operative events [Correspondence]. BMJ 1995; 310: 601

53. Russell I F. Midazolam-alfentanyl: an anaesthetic? An investigation using the isolated forearm technique. Br J Anaesth 1993; 70: 42–46

54. Meyer B C, Blacher R S. A traumatic neurotic reaction induced by succinylcholine chloride. NY State J Med 1961; 61: 1255–1261

55. Tunstall M E. Anaesthesia for obstetric operations. Clin Obstet Gynaecol 1980; 7: 681–698

56. Howard J F. Incidents of auditory perception during anaesthesia with traumatic sequelae. Med J Aust 1987; 146: 44–46

57. Tinnin L. Conscious forgetting and subconscious remembering of pain. J Clin Ethics 1994; 5: 151–152

58. Baddeley A. Working memory. Science 1992; 255: 556–559

59. Richardson J T E. Human memory: psychology, pathology and pharmacology. In: Jones J G. (ed.) Bailliere's Clinical Anaesthesia, vol. 3, no. 3: Depth of Anaesthesia. London: Bailliere Tindall, 1989; 451–472

60. Russell I F, Wang M. Absence of memory for intraoperative information during surgery under adequate general anaesthesia. Br J Anaesth 1997; 78: 3–9

61. Bonebakker A E, Bonke B, Klein J et al. Information processing during general anesthesia: Evidence for unconcious memory. Mem Cogn 1996; 24: 766–776

62. Cork R C, Heaton J F, Campbell C E, Kihlstrom J F. Is there implicit memory after propofol sedation? Br J Anaesth 1996; 76: 492–498

63. Alkire M T, Haier R J, Fallon J H, Barker S J, Shah N K. Positron emission tomography suggest the functional neuroanatomy of implicit memory during propofol anaesthesia. In: In: Bonke B, Bovill J G, Moerman N. (eds) Memory and Awareness in Anaesthesia. Assen: Van Gorcum, 1996; 17–25

64. Millar K, Macrae W J, Thorp J M. Implicit memory as a function of surgery-induced arousal and variation in anaesthetic state. In: Bonke B, Bovill J G, Moerman N. (eds) Memory and Awareness in Anaesthesia. Assen: Van Gorcum, 1996; 36–42

65. Donker A G, Phaf H R, Porcelijn T, Bonke B. Processing familiar and unfamiliar stimuli during general anaesthesia. In: Bonke B, Bovill J G, Moerman N. (eds) Memory and Awareness in Anaesthesia. Assen: Van Gorcum, 1996; 84–93

66. Hughdahl K, Matthiesen J R, Gullestad S. Implicit memory during anaesthesia – attempt at replication. Int J Neurosci 1996; 87: 63–69

67. Kalff A C, Bonke B, Wolters G, Manger F W. Implicit memory for stimuli presented during inhalation anesthesia in children. Psychol Rep 1995; 77: 371–375

68. De Roode A, Jelicic M, Bonke B, Bovill J G. The effect of midazolam premedication on implicit memory activation during alfentanil-nitrous oxide anaesthesia. Anaesthesia 1995; 50: 191–194

69. Van Hooff J C, De Beer N A M, Brunia C H M et al. Information processing during cardiac surgery: an event related potential study. Electroenceph Clin Neurophysiol 1995; 96: 433–452

70. Schwender D, Madler M, Klasing S, Peter K, Pöppel E. Anaesthetic control of 40-Hz brain activity and implicit memory. Consc Cogn 1994; 3: 129–147

71. Andrade J, Munglani R, Jones J G, Baddeley A D. Cognitive performance during anaesthesia. Consc Cog 1994; 3: 148–165

72. Parker C J R, Oates J D L, Boyd A H, Thomas S D. Memory for auditory presented material presented during anaesthesia. Br J Anaesth 1994; 72: 181–184

73. Villemure C, Plourde G, Lussier I, Normansin N. Auditory processing during isoflurane anaesthesia a study with an implicit memory task and auditory evoked potentials. In: Sebel P S, Bonke B, Winograd E. (eds) Memory and Awareness in Anaesthesia. Englewood Cliffs, NJ: Prentice Hall, 1993; 99–106

74. Jelicic M, Bonke B, De Roode A, Bovill J G. Implicit learning during anesthesia. In: Sebel P S, Bonke B, Winograd E. (eds) Memory and Awareness in Anaesthesia. Englewood Cliffs, NJ: Prentice Hall, 1993; 81–84

75. Schwender D, Kaiser A, Klasing S, Peter K, Pöppel E. Midlatency auditory evoked potentials and explicit and implicit memory in patients undergoing cardiac surgery. Anesthesiology 1994; 80: 493–501

76. Cork R C, Kihlstrom J F, Schacter D L. Implicit and explicit memory with isoflurane compared to sufentanil/nitrous oxide. In: Sebel P S, Bonke B, Winograd E. (eds), Memory and Awareness in Anaesthesia. Englewood Cliffs, NJ: Prentice Hall, 1993; 74–80

77. Bonebakker A E, Bonke B, Klein J, Wolters G, Hop W C. Implicit memory during balanced anaesthesia. Anaesthesia 1993; 48: 657–660

78. Westmoreland C L, Sebel P S, Winograd E, Goldmann W P. Indirect memory during anesthesia. Anesthesiology 1993; 78: 237–241

79. Charlton P F C, Wang M, Russell I F. Implicit and explicit memory for word stimuli presented during general anaesthesia without neuromuscular blockade. In: Sebel P S, Bonke B, Winograd E. (eds) Memory and Awareness in Anaesthesia. Englewood Cliffs, NJ: Prentice Hall, 1993; 64–73

80. Jelicic M, Asbury AJ, Millar K, Bonke B. Implicit learning during enflurane anaesthesia in spontaneously breathing patients? Anaesthesia 1993; 48: 766–768

81. Bonke B, Van Dam M E, van Kleef J W, Slijper F M E. Implicit memory tested in children with inhalation anaesthesia. In: Sebel P S, Bonke B, Winograd E. (eds) Memory and Awareness in Anaesthesia. Englewood Cliffs, NJ: Prentice Hall, 1993; 48–56

82. Brown A S, Best M R, Mitchell D B, Haggard L C. Memory under anesthesia: evidence for response suppression. Bull Psychon Soc 1992; 30: 244–246

83. Cork R C, Kihlstrom J F, Schacter D L. Absence of explicit and implicit memory in patients anesthesized with sufentanil/nitrous oxide. Anesthesiology 1992; 76: 892–898

84. Roorda-Hrdlickova V, Wolters G, Bonke B, Phaf R A. Unconscious perception during general anaesthesia, demonstrated by an implicit memory task. In: Bonke B, Fitch W, Millar K. (eds) Memory and Awareness in Anaesthesia. Amsterdam: Swets & Zeitlinger, 1990; 150–156

85. Kihlstrom J F, Schacter D L, Cork R C, Hurt C A, Behr S E. Implicit and explicit memory following surgical anesthesia. Psychol Sci 1990; 1: 303–306

86. Standen P J, Hain W R, Hosker K J. Retention of auditory information presented during anaesthesia. Anaesthesia 1987; 42: 604–608

87. Stolzy S, Couture L J, Edmonds H L. Evidence of partial recall during general anesthesia. Anesth Analg 1986; 65: S154

88. Eich E, Reeves J L, Katz R L. Anesthesia, amnesia, and the memory/awareness distinction. Anesth Analg 1985; 64: 1143–1148

89. Millar K, Watkinson N. Recognition of words presented during general anaesthesia. Ergonomics 1983; 26: 585–594

90. Dubovsky S L, Trustman R. Absence of recall after general anesthesia: implications for theory and practice. Anesth Analg 1976; 55: 696–701

91. Terrell R K, Sweet W O, Gladfelter J H, Stephen C R. Study of recall during anesthesia. Anesth Analg 1969; 48: 86–90

92. Jones J G, Konieczko K. Hearing and memory in anaesthetised patients [Editorial]. BMJ 1986: 292; 1291–1293

93. Barth L, Buchel C G. Klinische Untersuchen uber die narkotische Effektivitat von Stickoxydul. Anaesthesist 1975; 24: 49–55

94. Schwender D, Kaising S, Madler C, Pöppel E, Peter K. Midlatency auditory evoked potentials and cognitive function during general anaesthesia. Int Anaesthesiol Clin 1993; 31: 89–106

95. Thornton C, Barrowcliffe M P, Konieczko K M et al. The auditory evoked response as an indicator of awareness. Br J Anaesth 1989; 63: 113–115

96. Dutton R C, Smith W D, Smith N T. Wakeful response to command indicates memory potential during emergence from general anaesthesia. J Clin Monit 1995; 11: 35–40

Peter McCullagh

CHAPTER

6

Fetal sentience and fetal surgery

Fetal sentience, or the capacity of the fetus to experience painful or unpleasant sensation, has become an issue.[1] Why? Perhaps the most influential reason has been the marked change that has occurred in medical practice in analgesia for neonates undergoing major surgery. In 1988, only 1 in 10 of British anaesthetists administered opioids; by 1996, only 1 in 10 did not.[2] Fetal sentience has also been highlighted by increasing possibilities for *in utero* surgical approaches to correction of congenital abnormalities.

Scientific discussion of fetal sentience has been retarded by the non-availability of technology for detecting it. Journals dealing with fetal development or with pain have largely ignored fetal pain. The inevitable linkage of questions of fetal sentience with abortion has inhibited investigation, if not discussion.[3] Semantics, in particular the definition of pain that is selected, also complicate discussion of fetal sentience.

The meaning attached to 'pain' in specialist literature generally follows the International Association for the Study of Pain, namely 'an unpleasant sensory and emotional experience associated with actual or potential tissue damage'. Recognition of the significance of emotion with its connotations of memory of past experience and apprehension about the future is essential for pain management. However, the selected definition is not only species-specific but also applies fully only to relatively mature subjects. Limitations inherent in this definition, when considering the fetus, led Glover and Fisk to write of 'suffering' and 'distress'[3] while Anand and Hickey, having noted that 'nociceptive activity' rather than pain should be the issue for neonates, observed that 'terms relating to pain and nociception are used interchangeably' in the literature and opted not to distinguish between them.[4]

Apart from the noun used for the grammatical object, the selection of a verb to describe its impact on the subject is likely to convey additional meaning.

Dr Peter McCullagh MD BS DPhil MRCP, Senior Fellow, Developmental Physiology Group, Division of Molecular Medicine, The John Curtin School of Medical Research, The Australian National University, PO Box 334, Canberra, ACT 2601, Australia

Terms such as receive, feel, perceive, experience or appreciate, among others, could all refer to the impact of a noxious stimulus but lend themselves to different interpretations. In this short review which is predominantly concerned with experimental observations, single terms will be used without qualification or implications of particular shades of meaning. Irrespective of the verb used in relation to receipt of the result of application of a noxious stimulus, it is necessary to emphasize that receipt and response, no matter how closely linked, are not synonymous.

None of the preceding limitations to clarifying questions about fetal sentience are insuperable. Irrefutable responses to questions of whether and when a fetus becomes susceptible to unpleasant sensory experience, and of qualitative resemblance between this and pain as experienced by the investigator remain unattainable. Nevertheless, accessible data permit refinement of the questions. Including data published 50 years ago in a volume on recent advances may seem incongruous, but its experimental repetition has been precluded by changed attitudes towards animals and the human fetus.

The work of Anand and colleagues which changed neonatal anaesthetic practice included comprehensive presentation of evidence suggesting sentience in the human neonate and fetus,[4] juxtaposed with accounts of the usual omission of anaesthesia during major surgery, such as ligation of patent ductus arteriosus.[5] Demonstration of hormonal stress responses during surgery in unanaesthetised neonates and their partial mitigation by anaesthesia[6,7] evoked calls for pain relief both on humane grounds and to reduce postoperative complications.[8] Reliability of stress responses as an index of pain, and reduction of postoperative complications following use of opioids, have both been questioned without dissenting from the introduction of adequate neonatal anaesthesia.[9]

AN APPROACH TO ASSESSING FETAL SENTIENCE

The simple answer to whether the fetus feels pain remains as provided in 1985 by Wall, a pioneer of pain research, 'who knows?'[10] Consequently, an epistemological approach (epistemology: the study of what is known and the source of that knowledge) to the question of fetal sentience appears mandatory to me. What is the nature of the data on which knowledge of fetal sentience is based? What are the limitations to that knowledge? What extensions to it might be foreseeable as possible? In response, data on the development of sentient capacity in other species will be examined first followed by information from human fetuses. The question of cerebral cortex complicity in fetal pain/distress will be considered, as also will be implications for existing practice in provision of analgesia during various fetal procedures.

That pain felt by another can only be indirectly inferred by an observer is a truism which, nevertheless, requires emphasis. The observer accepts the truth of a communicative human subject's description of pain (which may be validated against objectively observed behaviour). When the subject lacks communicative capacity, reliance must be placed on observed behaviour and estimated intensity of the potentially painful stimulus. The observer becomes dependent upon the subject's capacity both for memory and communication.

Any account of previous experience presupposes recall. Whilst the interpretation of observations of intra-operative awareness made with the isolated forearm technique is disputed, the use of this technique focuses attention on the discrete nature of awareness and its subsequent recall.[11] The fetus lacks capacity to communicate, whilst ability to recall prenatal experiences, when communication becomes possible, remains unproven. Hence one depends entirely upon observing fetal behaviour and/or inferring potential function from observable structure.

A paradigm, employed to understand the physiology of many organ systems, relies upon predicting function from a knowledge of structure. Inferring capacity of **mature** subjects to experience pain from anatomical structure remains subject to qualifications. However, these become minor in comparison with the difficulties encountered in drawing inferences about subjects with a nervous system still in its developmental stage. Mature characteristics of nociception, such as lack of correlation between stimulus intensity and resultant pain, cortical modification of painful sensation and the existence of alternative pain pathways have rendered disclaimers about 'hard wiring' *de rigueur*.

The construction of structure/function inferences applicable to the incompletely developed nervous system based on analogies with the mature system has been severely criticized on conceptual[12,13] and clinical[14] grounds. Conceptual criticisms based on behavioural psychology, question whether causative relationships between structure and function in the developing nervous system are invariably unidirectional. The expression 'probabilistic epigenesis' has been used to describe the proposition that function *in utero* not only facilitates structural maturation and behavioural development but, in some circumstances, exerts a determinative influence. In contrast, conventional accounts of development, with function constrained by established structure, dismiss functioning by the fetal nervous system as an incidental side effect. Observable function in the immature fetal nervous system is an essential minimum prerequisite before probabilistic epigenesis can be considered. However, demonstration of function does not, of itself, establish that it influences maturation of the nervous system, but at least leaves this possibility open.[13] Appearance of capabilities in the fetal nervous system before development of structures believed to subserve those functions supports probabilistic epigenesis.

Clinical objections to application of neuroanatomical structure/function relationships based on the intact mature nervous system to the incompletely developed system have arisen from studies of anencephalic infants.[14]

EXTRAPOLATION FROM STUDIES OF EXPERIMENTAL ANIMALS TO THE HUMAN FETUS

Data from animal experimentation support some inferences about acquisition of sentience by the human fetus. Nevertheless, whilst the use of animals enables reproducible observations to be made under controlled conditions unobtainable with human subjects, many constraints limit application of these data to human beings. A fundamental limitation is the extent to which pain is a comparable entity in human beings and other species. Descriptions of pain or distress in animals and any concept of fetal pain experience are alike based on conjecture. Melzach and Dennis proposed 'that the primates (probably) and the carnivores (certainly) are comparable to lobotomized people: that they experience the sensory and motivational-emotional components of pain, not the 'suffering' or the 'big pain' that appears to require a cortex like man's capable of understanding death and of generating the anxiety that surrounds illness and injury'.[15] They noted retention of function, throughout evolution, by phylogenetically old, slowly conducting pathways that contribute to multiple alternative pain pathways. Adoption of a pain definition applicable only to the human species could amount to reversion to a Cartesian concept that would now be unacceptable in an animal welfare context.

Apart from considerable inter-species differences that complicate application to humans of data obtained from study of the **mature** nervous system of other species, variations in rate of maturation of different organ systems in fetuses of different species introduces further complexity. A strong temptation, frequently not resisted in assessing capacity for human fetal sentience, is to posit 'equivalence scales' aligning fetuses of different species at a range of gestational ages with other species and so to infer that comparable stages of functional development can be attributed to them. Use of this strategy to infer progress of acquisition of sentient capacity by the human fetus based on extrapolation from another species has little to recommend it. Relative rates of maturation of function by different organ systems in different species do not conveniently obey consistent rules. For example, the two species most utilised in studies of fetal development, sheep and rat, have respective gestation periods of 150 and 22 days. If development of their immune systems is compared, the fetal lamb has matured sufficiently to be resistant to tolerance induction by 70 days, a stage not attained by the rat until several days postnatally. However, when lung maturation is compared, neither species attains a degree of development consistent with survival *ex utero* until close to term. Scales comparing development of either species with the other, or with the human fetus, could be constructed to support any required proposition.

Notwithstanding the limitations inherent in extrapolating between fetuses of different species, studies of the fetal nervous system in experimental animals may be relevant to some questions about human fetuses. Whilst studies of fetal animals have examined responsiveness to tactile rather than noxious stimuli, the capacity of receptors in fetal and neonatal animals to respond to a wider range of stimuli provides some validation for inferring response to noxious stimuli from study of tactile stimulation. Two topics to which experiments with fetal animals have contributed data with potential human application are the development of afferent pathways in the spinal cord and the early stages of formation of the cerebral cortex. The former has resulted from studies in rats: the latter depends upon studies in larger species.

Fitzgerald has recorded from single dorsal root ganglion cells in fetal and neonatal rats detecting responses by day 17 of gestation after mechanical stimulation of the hindlimbs.[16,17] Polymodal nociceptors in the rat were shown to be fully mature at birth having developed *in utero*, presumably in the absence of external stimulation.[18] Descending inhibitory controls developed much later than the afferent tracts, the function of which they modulate in the mature nervous system.[18] Extrapolating to human neonates, Fitzgerald has suggested that 'the lack of descending and segmental inhibition in the neonatal cord implies that there is less endogenous control of noxious inputs. As a result, noxious inputs may have an even more profound effect than in the adult but the reactions will be more diffuse and the effects potentially underestimated'.[19] Examination of human neonates in the light of these experimental results led to the conclusion 'that the preterm infant is, if anything, supersensitive to painful stimuli when compared with the full term infant'.[20] Altered sensitivity to subsequent noxious stimuli would accord with earlier demonstrations of persistent changes in rat spinal cord following stimulation. Injury to the hindpaw of decerebrate rats resulted in persistent decrease in the threshold for response to subsequent stimuli together with increased responsiveness.[21] Altered sensitivity could also have a molecular basis, in permanent alteration in the level of transcription of genes regulating stress responses.[22]

Limited information about early function of the cerebral cortex in fetuses of larger species may be relevant to cortical involvement in fetal sentience. Electrodes on the exposed cortex of fetal lambs detected somesthetic cortical responses following tactile cutaneous stimulation in the trigeminal area from as early as 40 day's gestation. Nevertheless, examination of the fine structure of the hemisphere at this stage failed to reveal connections of ascending tracts with the cortical plate.[23] Fetal lambs with intact placental connection to decerebrate ewes were examined by Meyerson and Persson in the absence of anaesthetic agents. They queried whether preconditions existed for sensory stimulation of the fetus to influence the subsequent functional development of the central nervous system by testing for transmission of impulses to the fetal cortex following tactile skin stimulation over a range of gestational ages.[24] Dissociation between structure and function in the developing nervous system, with absence of structures believed to be essential in mediating the observed function, as in these studies, has been a recurring finding. It could be interpreted either as an example of probabilistic epigenesis or, as a failure of the observer to examine the appropriate structure.

Cerebral cortical involvement in response to **noxious** stimuli has been examined in other species with equivocal outcomes. Cortical neurons in the primary somatosensory monkey cortex appeared to be involved in perceiving the intensity of stimulation.[25] However, cats from which both cerebral hemispheres had been removed (leaving the thalamus exposed) in the perinatal period were observed to 'freeze' rather than to escape[26] when placed on an electrified floor, behaviour consistent with distress or fright.[15]

DIRECT STUDIES OF HUMAN FETAL FUNCTION

Most of the information derived from human fetal experimentation *ex utero* to be considered below was published 4 or 5 decades ago and has not been repeated. Refinement of ultrasound imaging has permitted *in utero* studies which have extended understanding of fetal behaviour and enabled fetal blood sampling. No published studies of the fetal sensory system *ex utero* explicitly tested for **painful** sensation. Nevertheless, implications for nociception of studies of tactile sensation have been extensively quoted. The information summarized below, about fetal responsiveness to tactile stimulation, implies function by intact peripheral afferent and motor nerves. The issue such investigations raise, but cannot address, is whether sensory experience accompanies reflex responses. Many commentators dismiss fetal movements in response to touching, even in fetuses of 30 weeks' gestation,[27] as solely reflex. As noxious stimulation sufficiently intense to evoke pain in a mature subject should also elicit a reflex response, assuming stimulus application to a receptive area and intact motor function, it is impossible, from observing the same response in a non-communicating subject, to determine whether unpleasant sensation accompanies it. Exclusion of sensation concurrent with the reflex requires independent proof that this is impossible because of damage to or immaturity of essential structures. Exclusion, in the human fetus, based on the inference that necessary structures, in particular the cerebral cortex, are insufficiently mature raises questions of **which** structures are essential and **how mature** they must be.

Deferring consideration of cortical participation in pain, substantial limitations, predisposing to false negative outcomes, have been recognised in data obtained from fetal observation *ex utero*. Whereas observations of fetal animals *ex utero* utilised subjects with intact placental connection most human observations arise from isolated fetuses. Hooker noted, 'the period during which one of these young fetuses will respond to stimulation is limited by the progressive anoxia and asphyxia which it is undergoing'.[28] Anoxia soon became apparent, even when the fetus was examined still attached to the placenta during hysterotomy under spinal anaesthesia.[29] Residual effects of maternal anaesthesia could also affect outcomes. In the absence of intact motor function, no indication of fetal sensory function is obtainable, and it may be relevant that sensory nerve endings are almost completely developed in the human fetus before motor ending differentiation begins.[30] Inherent in any extrapolation is the assumption that the development of structures for receiving and transmitting nociceptive stimuli will resemble that of the tactile receptors that were actually examined.

Fetal response to light touch first appeared in the trigeminal nerve distribution at 5.5–7.5 weeks' gestational age, extending to the hands by 9 weeks and most of the body by 11 weeks.[31] (Fetal ages have been reported in the literature either as menstrual age or gestational age. For uniformity, all ages will be expressed in gestational age – menstrual age minus 2 weeks – even when indicated in menstrual age in the cited publications.) Whilst all reports relate to testing with light touch, not noxious stimuli, strong stimulation could elicit responses after the response to light touch had been extinguished by anoxia.[29] The extinction of a later developing (palm) reflex by the simultaneous elicitation of an (earlier developing) reflex response in the trigeminal area was observed by Hooker,[28] implying the functional status of interconnecting tracts in the spinal cord. The cessation of such extinction following double simultaneous stimulation by 12 weeks' gestational age, was attributed to additional maturation.[31,32]

The **observed** fetal responses to tactile stimulation are reflexes. It can be confidently inferred that both sensory and motor nerves passing between the stimulated trigeminal area of skin and the spinal cord are functional by 5.5 weeks. It can not be inferred, from observing reflex responses, that the fetus experiences touch (or any distress if the stimulus is noxious). On the other hand, sensation being **unobservable**, it would be illogical to exclude possible sensation simply because the observed responses are reflexes. At some stage of development, reflex responses certainly will be accompanied by sensation, but no observable change in the nature of the reflex will indicate this. Once peripheral sensory nerves are functioning, inferences about the probability of sentience depend on data about the attained stage of functional maturation of the central nervous system. Two limitations to assessing the likelihood of sentience are the reliability of structure/function correlations during development[12] and the confidence with which analogies with mature structure/function relationships can be constructed.[14]

A striking example of function apparently antedating structure in the human fetus is the appearance of reflex responses from skin lacking observable innervation.[33] 'The interpretation of the physiological activity of a nervous system which has end-organs seemingly so immature as those described but which, nevertheless, gives such positive evidence of being able to respond to light cutaneous stimulation presents a rather perplexing problem'.[33] Perhaps developing subcutaneous nerve plexuses function as a relatively nonspecific receptor initially being superseded later by specialised end organs.[34]

Observations of fetuses *ex utero* illustrate several likely characteristics of the onset of fetal sentience, irrespective of timing. Firstly, capacity for sentience may not develop throughout the body simultaneously. An anatomical 'hierarchy' of appearance of tactile sensation exists. Secondly, capacity for all sensory modalities may not appear simultaneously so that stronger stimuli may evoke responses after light touch fails (or before it acts). Thirdly, the fetal response repertoire may not be limited to stimuli to which term neonates respond. Thus, the fetus is said to respond to sound frequencies too high or low to be detected by the adult ear and to react to Doppler ultrasound.[35] Intuitively, it seems improbable that the fetus suddenly acquires a 'normal' postnatal range of sensitivity. Gradual acquisition of capacity to receive and appreciate an increasing variety of stimuli differentially over the entire body would seem more plausible.

Observations of the responsiveness of the fetus *ex utero* have been complemented by ultrasound examination dating spontaneous fetal movements *in utero* at 5.5–6.5 weeks' gestation. Movements *in utero* are more complex than those elicited by stimulation *ex utero*, but Prechtl has made the point that inferences of intentional behaviour 'go far beyond the available evidence'.[36] On the other hand, there is no *a priori* reason why capacity for sensation should not antedate intentional responses. Recognising reports that function may anticipate structure, Prechtl commented 'minimal neural structures are capable of generating well organized movements' drawing attention to the early stage of synaptic innervation of cervical motor neurons, as assessed anatomically at 7–8 weeks, alongside capacity for a variety of movements.

The most recent data on fetal response to noxious stimuli relate to hormonal stress responses in fetuses following venepuncture of the innervated, intrahepatic portion of the umbilical vein. Elevated blood levels of cortisol and β-endorphin after venepuncture at 20–34 weeks' gestation prompted Giannakoupoulos and his colleagues to refer to 'the possibility that the human fetus feels pain *in utero*, and may benefit from anaesthesia or analgesia for invasive procedures'.[37] An opposing view point has been that stress responses may still be observed in patients receiving adequate analgesia,[9] but whether stress responses occur without distress in subjects **not** receiving analgesics is unknown. Equally unknown is the relative timing of onset in ontogeny of stress responses and capacity for distress. Although the human fetal adrenal is said to function independently of the mother by mid-gestation,[38] it is notable that most adrenal cortex development in sheep[39] and primates[40] occurs in the last third of pregnancy. Haemorrhage, used as a means of stressing fetal lambs, evokes increased cortisol levels only in this period.[39] Similarly, hypoxia evokes β-endorphin increase in fetal lambs only after 130 days.[41] There is no reason why fetal neurological and endocrinological responses to noxious stimuli should develop simultaneously. Stress responses, as monitored by Doppler measurement of cerebral blood flow, have been described recently following puncture of the human fetus at 18 weeks.[42]

STUDIES OF STRUCTURE OF THE FETAL HUMAN NERVOUS SYSTEM

Inferences about capacity for human fetal sentience based on anatomically assessed maturation of the nervous system have been substituted for direct observation of function. The two outstanding limitations are uncertainty about anatomical correlates of every aspect of pain sensation in the mature nervous system and doubts about the validity of functional conclusions based on anatomical comparisons of immature and mature structures. Both relate to cortical involvement in pain sensation at different developmental stages and will be considered subsequently. Data relating to the remainder of the nervous system will be summarized now.

A minimal spinal cord requirement for sentience would be the presence of neurons and synapses in those structures associated with nociception. The degree of structural complexity required to be confident that noxious stimuli would cause distress remains conjectural. A simpler approach is to identify minimum developmental requirements, the absence of which suffices to exclude capacity for distress. As a guide, Wozniak and colleagues studied the spinal cord in human fetuses[43] and suggested 'the formation of synaptic junctions is the most characteristic sign of maturation of the nervous system and implies the beginning of its function'. These workers observed synapse formation proceeding craniocaudally and being well established by the 45 mm stage (approximately 8.5 weeks' gestational age). Okado first detected permanent synapses (as distinct from earlier transitional forms), in the dorsal marginal layer of the cord around 35 day's gestation.[44] Rizvi and colleagues interpreted synapse development in the dorsal marginal zone cord specifically in terms of transmission of painful sensation.[45] Finding well defined synapses in the dorsal marginal zone by 8 weeks' gestation they concluded 'presence of these synapses thus indicates that the morphological substrate for nociception in the marginal zone of the spinal cord exists even in the very early stages of development in man'.

Functional indications that afferent connections first appear in the trigeminal innervation have encouraged its morphological study. Subnucleus caudalis of the nucleus of the spinal tract of the trigeminal nerve, the first part of the trigeminal nuclei to develop, has been associated, on phylogenetic embryologic and clinical grounds, with transmission of facial pain. As it was well developed by 6.5 weeks' gestational age, and was the most primitive part of the fifth cranial nerve, Brown concluded 'it is only to be expected that the various primitive or protopathic types of cutaneous sensory stimuli would be transmitted through it'.[46,47] While the identity of all thalamic nuclei capable of processing painful sensation in the mature brain remains uncertain, it may be relevant to inferences about functional development that the ventral nuclei are well demarcated in the 40 mm fetus[48] (approximately 8 weeks' gestational age).

Antibodies against many small peptides incriminated in neurotransmission have been used to detect them in the fetal spinal cord. Most of the known molecules are detectable by the latter part of the third month. Among others, substance P,[49] enkephalin[50] and neurofilament triplet proteins[51] have been first detected around 10–12 weeks' gestation. The relevance of these data for fetal sentience will remain uncertain until the function of these transmitters becomes clearer and their appearance in the fetus can be quantitated.

THE CEREBRAL CORTEX AND FETAL SENTIENCE

The essentiality of the **mature** cortex for receiving unpleasant sensation remains unresolved. Consequently, a requirement for any specified stage of cortical development for fetal distress remains conjectural. It is an interesting paradox that, whilst the cortex has customarily been said not to be involved in pain sensation, immaturity of the cortex is most frequently advanced as the reason for the non-existence of fetal sentience. In this context several questions seem appropriate. Has the cortex a role in pain sensation in a mature subject? What is that role? To what extent is its fulfilment essential for pain sensation? If an essential cortical role in pain/suffering can be specified, the crucial question becomes: what is the time scale of acquisition of the necessary cortical functions during fetal development?

The traditional belief, adumbrated by Head and Holmes after study of patients with cortical lesions, was that 'pure cortical lesions lead to no change in pain sensation'.[52] A similar conclusion was drawn by Penfield & Boldrey on the basis of electrical stimulation of the cortex during neurosurgery in conscious patients.[53]

Positron emission tomography (PET) has recently demonstrated activity in the cingulate cortex following application of painful heat stimuli. (Background PET activity produced by non-painful heat was subtracted.[54,55]) In interpreting these data, Jones and colleagues suggested that the cingulate cortex was responsible for bringing pain to attention, because patients may become indifferent to chronic pain after cingulate surgery.[54] Cingolomyotomy has been advocated for relief of chronic pain on the basis of interrupting its emotional interpretation. The procedure is said to offer relief but is frequently subject to substantial relapse.[56] PET has also been used to demonstrate involvement of another limbic structure, the amygdaloid complex, in memory of emotionally aversive experience.[57]

The essentiality of an intact cortex for painful experience is challenged by reports of its persistence despite surgical removal of an entire hemisphere.[58] Experiments demonstrating activity in the somatosensory cortex of non-human primates following noxious stimuli have led to suggestions that it might undertake encoding enabling a monkey to perceive the stimulus intensity[25] and that learning about potentially painful exposures might be dependent on the activated cortex.[59]

Paediatricians experienced with anencephalic infants report the retention of capacity for unpleasant sensory experience. Van Assche and colleagues concluded that anencephalic infants with a functional hypothalamohypo-physial system had pain reactions.[60] Shewmon and colleagues unequivocally concluded that anencephalic infants had capacity for pain, and commented on the use of structure/function analogies based on the mature nervous system to infer the sentient capacity of these infants 'it simply begs the question to apply adult-derived neurophysiological principles to this age group in support of the claim that a functioning cortex is necessary for consciousness or pain perception in newborns'.[14]

To summarise, the cortex can be activated in response to noxious stimuli but some form of pain sensation appears to remain in the absence of normal cortical tissue. That is, the presence of a functioning cortex has not been demonstrated to be essential for pain sensation. Intuitively, one might anticipate that functions such as discrimination and localization of pain and appreciation of specific qualities would have a cortical location, whereas distress evoked by a noxious stimulus need not.

Whilst synapses appear in the cortex at a time comparable with those noted above for development of other structures potentially concerned with nociception, their development within the cortical plate itself may be delayed. Molliver and colleagues examined synapse development in a series of human fetuses and found that, from 8.5 weeks' gestation, cortical synapses were consistently present above and below, but never within, the cortical plate.[61] Nevertheless, they commented that 'the presence of cortical synapses at 8.5 weeks of gestation demonstrates that the establishment of neuronal circuitry begins surprisingly early in fetal life'. Synapses were not observed within the plate until 23 weeks. However, given the observation of electrical impulse transmission to the fetal lamb cortex before attainment of the degree of anatomical cortical development believed to be necessary for this, interpretation of the morphological observation becomes less simple.

There have been conflicting interpretations from anatomical studies of the development of thalamic projections to the human fetal cortex. Poliakov[62] and Sidman & Rakic[63] found that many ascending axons from thalamic neurons had already reached the cortical plate by the tenth and eleventh weeks. In contrast, Mrzljak and colleagues[64] placed the commencement of ingrowth of thalamic projections into the cortical plate at 26 weeks. The latter estimate has been adduced as strong evidence for the impossibility of fetal sentience before this stage.[65] To the extent that cortical participation is considered to be essential for pain/nociception, resolution of the uncertainty about timing of thalamocortical conception in the human fetus is clearly important. In view of the comment by Sidman & Rakic that wide variation exists between different cortical regions in the timing of cortical differentiation[63] and given the incrimination of cingulate and limbic structures in pain appreciation, access of thalamic projections to these areas would seem to be the critical issue. Historically, it has been proposed that the phylogenetically primitive limbic system subserves appreciation of noxious stimuli and develops early in ontogeny. PET studies certainly support the conventional attribution of function. To some extent, variation in the reported timing of connection of the thalamus with the cortical plate may reflect differences in assessing the presence of synapses and in deciding what is the significant quantitative level of their occurrence in relation to effective synaptic function. Electron microscopic studies of synapse development within the limbic cortex could be relevant.

Very few studies of the human fetus *ex utero* have been specifically concerned with cortical activity. As with other experimentation on human fetuses *ex utero*, these studies date back several decades. An irregular slow wave EEG pattern occurred in fetuses from as early as the second month.[66,67] It was suggested that electrical activity originated from both the cortex and deeper regions of the fetal brain with the former gradually disappearing with anoxia. Borkowski & Bernstine commented that 'phylogenetically the same type high voltage slow waves with superimposed fast activity has been observed in mature birds, in the mature frog and in the mature rabbit and mature marmot'.[67] More recent reports of EEG examination of fetuses *ex utero* are lacking.

CLINICAL COGNISANCE OF FETAL SENTIENCE

Human fetal surgery has extended beyond purely endoscopic procedures to open correction of congenital diaphragmatic hernia, lung cysts, urinary tract obstructions and sacrococcygeal teratoma.[68] The absence of specific attention to fetal analgesia in accounts of fetal surgery is perhaps not surprising given that, until recently, only a minority of **neonates** undergoing surgery received analgesia.[5] Consideration is more likely to have been given to potential dangers of anaesthesia for the fetus[69] rather than to its need. Significantly, an article titled *Anaesthesia for fetal surgery* omitted any reference to **fetal** anaesthesia but advocated maternal analgesia with local anaesthetic together with sufficient additional medication 'to reduce fetal movement'.[70] An operation description from another centre of fetal surgery again noted only maternal local anaesthetic.[71] A more recent report described the substitution, for maternally administered narcotics, of fetally-administered neuromuscular blocking agents (without any analgesia) to reduce fetal movement during surgery.[72] Again, significantly, the stated objectives were concerned only with immobilization to facilitate surgery.

Anaesthetic practice in relation to termination of pregnancy is subject to considerable geographic variation. A standard textbook published in the UK recommends thiopentone with nitrous oxide and oxygen, diazepam or neurolept agents for vaginal termination, halothane being noted as having the potential disadvantage of relaxing the uterus.[73] Recently, there has been strong advocacy for the use of local, rather than general, anaesthesia for termination of pregnancy.[74]

Key points for clinical practice

- Not everything is knowable. The nature of any sensory experience of any subject incapable of communication, whether because of species, immaturity or disease, can never be known by another.

- Observation of response to a stimulus can provide a guide to a subject's receipt of sensation, with the qualifications that responses do not irrefutably denote sensation and that sensation need not be accompanied by observable response.

- Structure frequently provides a useful indication of functional capability, but this guide becomes of limited value if the nature of the function precludes its independent verification.

- Decisions about provision of analgesia to non-communicating subjects in veterinary or human medicine require a practitioner to determine where the burden of proof of non-sentience falls in any case.

ACKNOWLEDGEMENT

The author acknowledges with gratitude the critical reading of a draft manuscript by David Curtis, Jim Keaney and John McLean.

References

1. Commission of Inquiry into Fetal Sentience. Human sentience before birth. London: HMSO 1996
2. de Lima J, Lloyd-Thomas AR, Howard RF, Sumner E, Quinn TM. Infant and neonatal pain: anaesthetists' perceptions and prescribing patterns. BMJ 1996; 313: 787
3. Glover V, Fisk N. We don't know; better to err on the safe side from mid-gestation. BMJ 1996; 313: 796
4. Anand KJS, Hickey PR. Pain and its effects in the human neonate and fetus. N Engl J Med 1987; 317: 1321–1329
5. Ward Platt MP, Anand KJS, Aynsley-Green A. The ontogeny of the metabolic and stress response in the human fetus, neonate and child. Intensive Care Med 1989; 15: S44–S45
6. Anand KJS, Ward-Platt MP. Neonatal and pediatric stress responses to anesthesia and operation. Int Anesthesiol Clin 1988; 26: 218–225
7. Anand KJS, Hickey PR. Halothane-morphine compared with high-dose sufentanil for anesthesia and postoperative analgesia in neonatal cardiac surgery. N Engl J Med 1992; 326: 1–9
8. Rogers MC. Do the right thing. Pain relief in infants and children. N Engl J Med 1992; 326: 55–56
9. Wolf AR. Treat the babies, not their stress responses. Lancet 1993; 342: 319–320
10. Richards T. Can a fetus feel pain? BMJ 1985; 291: 1220–1221
11. Rusell IF, Wang M. Awareness under anaesthesia. BMJ 1992; 305: 50
12. Gottlieb G. Introduction to behavioural embryology. In: Gottlieb G. (ed.) Behavioural Embryology. New York: Academic Press, 1973; 3–45
13. Gottlieb G. Conceptions of prenatal development: behavioural embryology. Psychol Rev 1976; 83: 215–234

14. Shewmon DA, Capron AM, Peacock WJ, Schulman BL. The use of anencephalic infants as organ sources. A critique. JAMA 1989; 261: 1773–1781

15. Melzach R, Dennis SG. Phylogenetic evolution of pain expression in animals. In: Kosterlitz HW, Terenius LY. (eds) Pain and Society. Weinheim: Verlag Chemie GmbH, 1980; 13–36

16. Fitzgerald M. Spontaneous and evoked activity of fetal primary afferents in vivo. Nature 1987; 326: 603–605

17. Fitzgerald M. Cutaneous primary afferent properties in the hind limb of the neonatal rat. J Physiol 1987; 383: 79–92

18. Fitzgerald M, Koltenberg M. The functional development of descending inhibitory pathways in the dorsolateral funiculus of the newborn rat spinal cord. Dev Brain Res 1986; 24: 261–270

19. Fitzgerald M. Development of pain mechanisms. Br Med Bull 1991; 47: 667–675

20. Fitzgerald M, McIntosh N. Pain and analgesia in the newborn. Arch Dis Child 1989; 64: 441–443

21 Woolf CJ. Evidence of a central component of post-injury pain hypersensitivity. Nature 1983; 306: 686–688

22. Meaney MJ, Bhatnagar S, Diorio J et al. Molecular basis for the development of individual differences in the hypothalamic-pituitary-adrenal stress response. Cell Mol Neurobiol 1993; 13: 321–347

23. Åström KE. On the early development of isocortex in fetal sheep. Prog Brain Res 1967; 26: 1–59

24. Meyerson BA, Persson HE. Early epigenesis of recipient functions in the neocortex. In: Gottlieb G. (ed.) Aspects of Neurogenesis, vol 2. New York: Academic Press, 1974; 171–204

25. Kenshalo DR, Chudler EH, Anton F, Dubner R. SI nociceptive neurons participate in the encoding process by which monkeys perceive the intensity of noxious thermal stimulation. Brain Res 1988; 454: 378–382

26. Bjursten L-M, Norrsell K, Norrsell U. Behavioural repertory of cats without cerebral cortex from infancy. Exp Brain Res 1976; 25: 115–130

27. Tawia S. When is the capacity for sentience acquired during human development? J Mat Fet Med 1992; 1: 153–165

28. Hooker D. Early human fetal behaviour with a preliminary note on double simultaneous fetal stimulation. Res Publ Assoc Res Nerv Ment Dis 1954; 33: 98–113

29. Fitzgerald JE, Windle WF. Some observations on early human fetal movements. J Comp Neurol 1942; 76: 159–167

30. Hewer EE. The development of nerve endings in the human foetus. J Anat 1935; 69: 369–378

31. Humphrey J. Some correlations between the appearance of human fetal reflexes and the development of the nervous system. Prog Brain Res 1964; 4: 93–133

32. Humphrey T, Hooker D. Double simultaneous stimulation of human fetuses and the anatomical pattern underlying the reflexes elicited. J Comp Neurol 1959; 112: 75–102

33. Hogg ID. Sensory nerves and associated structures in the skin of human fetuses of 8 to 14 weeks of menstrual age correlated with functional capability. J Comp Neurol 1941; 75: 371–410

34. Bradley RM, Mistretta CM. Fetal sensory receptors. Physiol Rev 1975; 55: 352–382

35. Valman HB, Pearson JF. The first year of life. What the fetus feels. BMJ 1980; 280: 233–234

36. Prechtl HFR. Ultrasound studies of human fetal behaviour. Early Hum Dev 1985; 12: 91–98

37. Giannakoulopoulos X, Sepulveda W, Kourtis P, Glover V, Fisk NM. Fetal plasma cortisol and β-endorphin response to intrauterine needling. Lancet 1994; 344: 77–81

38. Sippell WG, Partsch CJ, Mackenzie IZ, Aynsley-Green A. The steroid hormonal milieu of the human fetus and mother at 16–20 weeks of gestation. Pediatr Res 1986; 20: 1181

39. Rose JC, Macdonald AA, Heyman MA, Rudolph AM. Developmental aspects of the pituitary-adrenal axis response to haemorrhagic stress in lamb fetuses *in utero*. J Clin Invest 1978; 61: 424–432

40. Pepe GJ, Albrecht ED. Regulation of the primate fetal adrenal cortex. Endocr Rev 1990; 11: 151–176

41. Stark RI, Wardlaw SL, Daniel SS. Characterization of plasma β-endorphin immunoactivity in the fetal lamb: effects of gestational age and hypoxia. Endocrinology 1986; 119: 755–761

42. Texeira J, Fogliani R, Giannakoulopoulos X, Glover V, Fisk N. Fetal haemodynamic stress response to invasive procedures. Lancet 1996; 347: 624

43. Wozniak W, O'Rahilly R, Olszevska B. The fine structure of the spinal cord in human embryos and early fetuses. J Hirnforsch 1980; 21: 101–124

44. Okado N. Onset of synapse formation in the human spinal cord. J Comp Neurol 1981; 201: 211–219

45. Rizvi JA, Wadhwa S, Mehra RD, Bijlani V. Ultrastructure of marginal zone during prenatal development of human spinal cord. Exp Brain Res 1986; 64: 483–490

46. Brown JW. The development of subnucleus caudalis of the nucleus of the spinal tract of V. J Comp Neurol 1958; 110: 105–127

47. Brown JW. The development of the nucleus of the spinal tract of V in human fetuses of 14 to 21 weeks of menstrual age. J Comp Neurol 1956; 106: 393–412

48. Cooper ER. The development of the thalamus. Acta Anat 1950; 9: 201–226

49. Charnay Y, Paulin C, Chayvialle J-A, Dubois PM. Distribution of substance P-like immunoreactivity in the spinal cord and dorsal root ganglia of the human foetus and infant. Neuroscience 1983; 10: 41–55

50. Charnay Y, Paulin C, Dray F, Dubois P-M. Distribution of enkephalin in human fetus and infant spinal cord: an immunofluorescence study. J Comp Neurol 1984; 223: 415–423

51. Marti E, Gibson SJ, Polak JM et al. Ontogeny of peptide and amine-containing neurones in motor, sensory and autonomic regions of rat and human spinal cord, dorsal root ganglia and rat skin. J Comp Neurol 1987; 266: 332–359

52. Head H, Homes G. Sensory disturbances from cerebral lesions. Brain 1911; 34: 102–254

53. Penfield W, Boldrey E. Somatic motor and sensory representation in the cerebral cortex of man as studied by electrical stimulation. Brain 1937; 60: 389–443

54. Jones AKP, Brown WD, Friston LY, Frackowiak RSJ. Cortical and subcortical localization of response to pain in man using positron emission tomography. Proc R Soc Lond [Biol] 1991; 244: 39–44

55. Talbot JD, Marrett S, Evans AC, Meyer E, Bushnell MC, Duncan GH. Multiple representations of pain in human cerebral cortex. Science 1991; 251: 1355–1358

56. Santo JL, Arias LM, Barolat G, Schwartzman RJ, Grossman K. Bilateral cingulumotomy in the treatment of reflex sympathetic dystrophy. Pain 1990; 41: 55–59

57. Cahill L, Haier R, Fallon J et al. Amygdala activity at encoding correlated with long-term free recall of emotional information. Proc Natl Acad Sci USA 1996; 93: 8016–8021

58. Walker AE. Central representation of pain. Res Publ Assoc Res Nerv Ment Dis 1942; 23: 63–85

59. Dong WK, Salonen LD, Kawakami Y et al. Nociceptive responses of trigeminal neurons in SII-7b cortex of awake monkeys. Brain Res 1989; 484: 314–324

60. Van Assche FA. Anencephalics as organ donors. Am J Obstet Gynec 1990; 163: 599–600

61. Molliver ME, Kostovic J, Van der Loos H. The development of synapses in cerebral cortex of the human fetus. Brain Res 1973; 50: 403–407

62. Poliakov GI. Some results of research into the development of the neuronal structure of the cortical ends of the analyzers in man. J Comp Neurol 1961; 117: 197–212

63. Sidman RL, Rakic P. Neuronal migration with special reference to developing human brain: a review. Brain Res 1973; 62: 1–35

64. Mrzljak L, Uylings HBM, Kostovic I, Van Eden CG. Prenatal development of neurons in the human prefrontal cortex. I. A qualitative Golgi study. J Comp Neurol 1988; 271: 355–386

65. Fitzgerald M. Neurobiology of fetal and neonatal pain. In: Wall PD, Melzach R. (eds) Textbook of Pain, 3rd edn. Edinburgh: Churchill Livingstone, 1994; 153–163

66. Okamoto Y, Kirikae T. Electroencephalographic studies on brain of foetus, of children of premature birth and new-born, together with a note on reactions of foetus brain upon drugs. Fol Psych Neurol Jpn 1951; 5: 135–146

67. Borkowski WJ, Bernstine RL. Electroencephalography of the fetus. Neurology 1955; 5: 362–365

68. Flake AW, Harrison MR. Fetal surgery. Annu Rev Med 1995; 46: 67–78

69. Lah F. Anaesthesia and the sick foetus. Anaesth Intensive Care 1990; 18: 327–330

70. Spielman FJ, Seeds JW, Corke BC. Anaesthesia for fetal surgery. Anaesthesia 1984; 39: 756–759

71. Golbus MS, Harrison MR, Filly RA, Callen PW, Katz M. *In utero* treatment of urinary tract obstruction. Am J Obstet Gynecol 1982; 142: 383–388

72. Fan SZ, Susetiol, Tsai MC. Neuromuscular blockade of the fetus with pancuronium or pipecuronium for *intra-uterine* procedures. Anaesthesia 1994; 49: 284–286

73. Atkinson RS, Rushman GB, Lee JA. A Synopsis of Anaesthesia, 10th edn. Bristol: Wright, 1987

74. Penney G. Induced abortion: the next decade. Br J Obstet Gynaecol 1995; 102: 754–756

CHAPTER

7

Shirley M. Alexander Duncan J. Macrae

Stabilisation and transportation of children requiring admission to a PICU

Seriously ill children are not always treated by the right people in the right place. A report commissioned by the British Paediatric Association published in 1993,[1] demonstrated that only 51% of critically ill children received care in paediatric intensive care units (PICUs), the remainder receiving such care in paediatric wards or adult units. There is clear evidence from studies conducted in The Netherlands,[2] the US[3] and the UK[4] that outcome is improved when critically ill children are cared for in large regional paediatric intensive care units. The Trent Victoria study[4] showed that the risk of mortality was significantly higher (odds ratio 2.09) when intensive care was delivered in a fragmented model (Trent, UK) compared to an Australian state with centralised provision.

When paediatric intensive care is regionalised, it is inevitable that transport facilities be established for the safe movement of children from local hospitals to specialist regional PICUs. Appropriate immediate management for the critically ill child is important and the local hospital should have sufficient expertise to provide this.[5] It is good practice for local hospitals to consult specialist staff at the regional centre early in a child's illness, perhaps before a child is in need of specialist intensive care, and to base their initial management of common problems on protocols or clinical guidelines agreed in advance with the regional specialist unit.

Transport teams can contribute very effectively to the extended resuscitation and stabilisation of critically ill children.[6] The UK is currently undergoing a significant expansion in the provision of paediatric intensive care services, and has recently attracted strong support from central government for these services

Dr Duncan J. Macrae BMSc MB ChB FRCA FRCPH, Consultant in Paediatric Intensive Care, Cardiac Intensive Care Unit, Great Ormond Street Hospital for Children NHS Trust, Great Ormond Street, London WC1N 3JH, UK

Dr Shirley M. Alexander MB ChB MRCP, ECMO Research Fellow, Cardiac Intensive Care Unit, Great Ormond Street Hospital for Children NHS Trust, Great Ormond Street, London WC1N 3JH, UK

(NHS Executive[7]). Interestingly, as recently as 1995, Dryden & Morton reported that only 3 out of 19 PICUs routinely provided transport teams to collect patients referred to them.[8] The implementation of the recommendations contained in the recent report to the UK Department of Health[7] is expected to lead to substantial changes in the delivery of intensive care in many parts of the UK and, most importantly, in an improved provision of transport for critically ill children.

This chapter aims to summarise the essentials of the process of transporting critically ill children between hospitals.

AIMS AND ORGANISATION

Most seriously ill children are transported between hospitals because of their need for specialised facilities or treatment which cannot be provided at the referral hospital. The role of a specialised transport team can be summarised as achieving safe delivery of a critically ill child to a regional PICU, whilst providing a continuum of high quality care throughout the transfer; literally providing a mobile paediatric intensive care bed.

A paediatric emergency transport service should be tailored to the administrative and population needs of the region it serves. Factors influencing provision of this service will include the availability of financial resources, location of PICUs and the geographical and demographic variations of the area. The service should be led by a medical director with experience of intensive care and transport medicine, who should have overall responsibility for the administration of the service. On a day-to-day basis, responsibility for the service should rest with the 'on call' consultant intensivist who may not necessarily be the medical director. Clear and concise protocols should be in place covering both administrative and clinical matters in keeping with UK and US guidelines.[9,10] Direct links with the transport providers should be established and a referral system that is well known to all referring hospitals must be in place. The team should have a rapid response time and be accessible 24 hours a day. Transport personnel must be adequately trained in both the theoretical and practical aspects of paediatric intensive care and also in aspects of transport medicine. Training should include familiarisation with operational and safety aspects of the transport vehicles the team will use. In the case of air transports, additional training in relevant aspects of aviation medicine will be required.

WHO SHOULD BE TRANSPORTED?

A request for a child to be transferred to a regional PICU is usually made when a referring paediatrician perceives that further management of the child is beyond, or will soon be beyond, the capabilities and resources of the local institution.[11] Early discussion of potential referrals should be encouraged by regional units, who must be helpful and welcoming in their response to enquiries. Early specialist advice may lead to clinical improvement with potential to reduce morbidity or perhaps prevent the need for transfer to the regional centre. Effective communication between senior doctors in the referral

Table 7.1 Commonest indications for transfer to PICUs by disease category
(cumulative data from references[11-16])

Indication for transport	No of patients	(%)
Respiration	634	(39.8)
CNS	269	(16.9)
Trauma	293	(18.4)
Sepsis	116	(7.3)
CVS	33	(2.1)
Poison	59	(3.7)
Other	190	(11.9)
Total number	**1594**	

hospital and specialist unit are essential in order that an accurate and detailed picture of the critically ill child is obtained, from which relevant advice can be given on the resuscitation and further management of the child. The regional centre should routinely record basic administrative and clinical information when advice or referrals are made. A subjective assessment of the severity of illness of a child must be made at the time of referral as this will guide the urgency of response and composition of the medical team required in any particular case. The most common disorders which necessitate interhospital transport of critically ill children are given in Table 7.1.

Severity of illness scoring

The paediatric risk of mortality score (PRISM) gives a statistical risk of mortality based on 14 physiological and laboratory parameters recorded during the first 24 h of PICU admission, taking into account age and postoperative status. PRISM was constructed in the setting of a PICU with patients being monitored and treated by skilled paediatric intensivists[17] and has subsequently been validated in a range of PICUs mainly in North America. Recently, a simpler mortality predictor, the paediatric index of mortality score (PIM), has been introduced based on 8 variables collected at the time of PICU admission or first contact with a PICU transport team.[18] PIM has yet to be as extensively validated as PRISM, but early assessments with data from Australia and the UK are encouraging. Although PRISM and PIM are useful audit tools for comparison of intensive care unit performance, they cannot, and should not, be used to define severity of illness or risk of mortality in individual cases and certainly cannot be used in isolation to determine the level of response required of a PICU's transport team.[19] Nor is it appropriate to use serial PRISM scoring to imply improvement of stability achieved by transport teams.[20,21] Specialist intensivists must bear in mind that what is relatively low risk in a PICU setting could be extremely high risk in a peripheral hospital where paediatric resources and skills are limited.[19] There is no substitute for the discussion of individual cases at very senior level; a willingness on the part of referral units to discuss cases early; and an understanding in regional PICUs of what is reasonable to expect of particular referral units.

It is well established that the period of transport between hospitals is associated with potential risks to patients and occasionally transport team members.[13–15,22–26] Risks are increased when transport teams: (i) fail to stabilise adequately and prepare patients for transport; (ii) are poorly trained or equipped; (iii) fail to recognise diagnoses such as pneumothorax or clinical deterioration; or (iv) are generally inexperienced and unfamiliar with the transport environment.

There is no clear agreement about what constitutes the optimal escort for the interhospital transport of critically ill children. For organisational and financial reasons, some experts have suggested that a physician is not always required during such transports.[14,27–29] A number of studies have shown that the incidence of new problems or secondary insults during transport is reduced when more experienced personnel are responsible for the conduct of the transport.[6,24] This is especially so if the patient is under one year of age; is intubated and/or has unstable vital signs.[30] In the UK, paediatric emergency transport teams usually consist of consultants in paediatric intensive care or senior trainees with relevant experience accompanied by a qualified children's intensive care nurse. In other healthcare systems, different arrangements apply and specially trained nursing or paramedic led teams operate successfully in parts of the US and Canada,[24,31] particularly in the transport of children with relatively stable conditions.

TRANSPORT VEHICLES

The choice of transport by road, helicopter or fixed wing air ambulance, if all vehicle types are freely available, should be based on factors such as the urgency of the case, weather conditions and geographical location of the referring hospital. In many parts of the world, the transport resources available are limited and frequently there are administrative and cost constraints on the availability of air ambulances. The principal advantages and disadvantages of various modes of transport are set out in Table 7.2.

Macnab and colleagues found that, in all modes of transport, the level of noise and vibration inside infant transport incubators was often in excess of recommended limits.[32] Vibration between 1–80 Hz (such as found in transport vehicles) can cause stress reactions similar to those of mild exercise and high noise levels may contribute to cochlear damage, both of which may be detrimental to the physiologically compromised patient. In addition, vibration may loosen or cause alterations in settings of equipment, and produce artefacts in monitors.[33] Excessive noise levels in helicopters affect the ability of team members to communicate and it is necessary to provide headsets for communication between the medical team and their patient, if conscious, or ear protection to unconscious patients.

It is absolutely essential that, whilst the medical team and transport crew should co-operate in effecting transport of the patient, neither team should exert undue pressure on the other. The medical crew should not be pressurised into leaving a referral hospital before their patient is fully stabilised, nor should an ambulance crew or pilot be persuaded to undertake transport of a patient or transport team if there are potential weather or other operational limitations which should be observed. A system should be in place such that requests for urgent transfer by transport teams are accorded clear priority by

Table 7.2 Advantages and disadvantages of modes of transport

Transport mode	Advantages	Disadvantages

Road ambulance	Rapid mobilisation
	Door to door service
	Ability to stop for
	  procedures
	Inexpensive
	Large working area
	Few weather restrictions
		Slow – 15 mph urban areas
		        – 60 mph rural areas
		Poor suspension
		High incidence of motion sickness

Helicopter	Rapid mobilisation
	Ground speed 150 mph
	Close access to most
	  hospitals possible
		Limited work space
		Limited range (170 miles
		  without refuelling)
		High noise and vibration levels
		Multiple moves for patient
		Landing area required
		Weight limitations
		Night and weather restrictions
		  may apply
		High cost

Fixed wing	Fast ground speed,
	  typically 200 mph
	Fewer weather restrictions
	  than helicopter
	Pressurised at altitude
	Work space usually
	  adequate
		Need for landing strip or airport
		Multiple moves
		Moderately expensive

ambulance, police or air services. The co-operation of other emergency services, including the police, may be helpful to facilitate urgent transfer of patients through congested urban traffic. Rapid airfield access and air traffic clearances should be obtained where appropriate. Transport teams must, however, act responsibly when deciding to travel, using lights and sirens. There are some circumstances where the patient's best interests may well be served by a slow steady transfer and situations where adverse weather or other facts cause unacceptable risks to accrue if a high speed transfer is undertaken.

EQUIPMENT

Paediatric transport teams must equip themselves to deal with a wide range of disorders scaling the age range from neonate to adolescent. Drugs and medical supplies should be stored in equipment boxes according to predetermined lists against which the contents must be checked, before sealing the boxes ready for subsequent use. In compiling a list of contents for such kits, the aim should be to provide the transport team with a sufficient amount of equipment with which to deal with predictable requirements, during transfers and any highly specialist equipment which may not be available at a referring hospital.

Wherever possible, the team should act to conserve their own supplies of easily available equipment, such as syringes and needles, whilst at the referring hospital. Such a policy reduces the required stock and, therefore, volume of equipment boxes, and facilitates restocking of boxes after use.

Hardware used during transport – including monitors, pumps, ventilators and incubators – should be specifically designed for their purpose, be lightweight but robust. They should be able to operate on internal battery or gas supplies for long periods of time but, in addition, be compatible with electrical and gas supplies available in ambulance vehicles. Equipment must be highly reliable and function well in the adverse conditions of the transport environment, including extremes of temperature, conditions of excessive vibration and high radio frequency fields from radio or telephone equipment, as well as being compatible with the safety requirements of the vehicle. This is of particular importance in the areas of electrical safety, mechanical security of heavy loads such as infant incubators, and compatibility of medical equipment with aircraft systems.

A portable monitor should replicate, as closely as possible, the monitoring available in the regional PICU. The facility to store and download physiological data on return to the specialist unit is valuable as are additional filters and artefact rejection systems. The Propaq® monitor (Protocol Systems Inc.) fulfils such criteria and has been widely used in the transport environment.[34-36]

Although some would advise hand ventilation of the child during transport to aid detection in changes in compliance whilst maintaining a close proximity of monitoring,[34] a transport ventilator can be used, safely freeing the physician to undertake other duties.[35,36] Transport ventilators for children must be capable of providing a wide range of ventilator requirements, including high peak and end expiratory pressures, variable inspired oxygen fraction, and alteration of inspiratory and expiratory times. A number of ingenious transport ventilators, such as the Dräger Oxylog® (Dräger Limited) and Babypac® (PneuPac Limited), are gas powered and function independently of external electrical and compressed air supplies, an inherent advantage during transport. Whatever ventilation system is used, an internal or external disconnect alarm is essential and this device should have both audible and visual warnings, since even loud audible alarms may not be detected against the high background noise in some transport vehicles, particularly helicopters.

Portable suction equipment, which may be either electrically or gas driven or controlled via a footpump, must be available throughout the transport. Although rarely required in children, a portable defibrillator should be available; this may well be part of the standard equipment of the ambulance vehicle used rather than special equipment provided by the transport team. Recently, portable blood gas and electrolyte monitors, such as the i-STAT® device (Hewlett Packard Limited), have become available and are invaluable for measurement of pH, PCO_2, PO_2, haemoglobin and common electrolyte values. Before the availability of such devices, more reliance was placed on pre-departure measurements of blood gases and electrolytes and indirect data from end-tidal CO_2 and oximetry measurements during transport. The security of medical decision making is greatly improved during transport with the availability of such portable devices.

Table 7.3 Essential equipment for transport of critically ill children

Monitor

ECG
Pulse oximetry
Blood pressure – cuff and invasive
End-tidal CO_2
Temperature
Small, robust, lightweight, one screen for all parameters, long battery life

Ventilator

Capable of ventilating all ages
Small, portable, lightweight
Economical on gas usage

Portable oxygen supply

Able to supply both high and low pressure metered flow
Enough for twice expected length of journey

Infusion pumps

Long battery life
Small, lightweight

Resuscitation equipment

Stored in boxes or backpack, easy to access without having to unpack

Drugs – including inotropes, sedatives, analgesics, muscle relaxants, anticonvulsants, diuretics, antibiotics

Airway – range of facemasks, oropharyngeal, endotracheal tubes, laryngoscope, tracheostomy kit

Cannulation equipment including for central line insertion and intraosseus needles

Fluids – crystalloid and colloid

Document folder

Observation charts
Inventory
Telephone numbers ± maps
Information for parents including directions for hospital location

Clothing and mobile phone

Warm, waterproof jackets for staff

Mobile phone for independent communication –
note that these may interfere with monitoring equipment

Miscellaneous

Blood gas and electrolyte analyser
Suction – battery operated, portable
Glucometer
Something to keep infant warm

Critically ill children usually require continuous infusions of several drugs during transport. Delivery systems designed for use in base hospitals (where the purpose of the internal batteries is essentially only to take over for short periods in the event of mains electricity failure) are often unsuitable for use outside hospital owing to their size and limited internal battery duration. One possible solution is the use of mini syringe drivers (Graseby, UK) which can handle 10 and 20 ml Luer Lok syringes and are suitable for low volume infusions of inotropic and sedative drugs during transfers. These pumps function for many hours on standard domestic batteries, a supply of which should be included in the transport kit. An alternative for administering maintenance fluids at higher volumes is use of the 'Intermate infusor' system® (Baxter Limited). These infusors are driven by elastometric pressure and are unaffected by ambient pressures, making them suitable for both ground and air transport. The rate at which they deliver fluids is reasonably consistent, although calibration varies with the type of fluid infused. A range of infusors sizes are available, but the infusion rate cannot be altered once commenced except by adding additional infusors or changing the infusor size.

The most sophisticated solution to drug infusion during transport is to use similar large syringe drivers or pumps to those available in the base hospital with the provision of an adequate AC or DC power source and must be sufficiently secure for the duration of the journey. In practice, such facilities are rarely available except in ambulances specifically designed as mobile intensive care units.

Adequate and convenient sources of oxygen are obviously required during interhospital transport. Ideally, all ambulance vehicles, including air ambulances, will be equipped with necessary cylinders to be used during the journey. Small portable or reserve cylinders are required for use when moving patients between vehicles and within hospitals. Oxygen cylinders should always be well restrained in all types of ambulance vehicle. Restrictions apply to the carriage of oxygen in aircraft and requirements must be fully discussed with the air ambulance operator or commercial airline medical and engineering departments. Liquid oxygen systems (Nellcor Puritan Bennett, USA) have also been used during transport, particularly on dedicated vehicles, efficient weight to gas volume characteristics being an advantage.

Finally, the needs of the medical team themselves ought to be considered. Waterproof and warm clothing should be provided for the team. A good quality mobile telephone is essential for independent communication to and from the team avoiding the need to rely on message transfer through ambulance or aircraft radio systems. Some types of mobile telephone, and also strong radio signals such as those from ambulance or aircraft, can interfere with electronic medical equipment and, where possible, equipment should be tested for such interference and monitored closely when used in close proximity to strong radio signals. Teams may also wish to consider providing travel sickness medication for team members. Nutritional needs of the team should be considered during the planning of transports of long duration (Table 7.3).

COMMUNICATION

Effective communication is the key to any successful emergency transport system. Referring hospitals should be giving clear advice about what services are provided by regional units and how these may be accessed. As mentioned previously, paediatricians should be encouraged to discuss potential cases early which may, in some circumstances, avoid unnecessary transfer. From the moment a referral call is made, there should be a continuous dialogue between the medical teams involved and advice on ongoing resuscitation should be made freely available to the referring hospital if required. The transport team must be fully briefed before departure and remain in contact with the base hospital wherever possible during travel. The transport team must have excellent links with their transport provider, so that appropriate vehicles and transport personnel are provided promptly. The referring hospital should be advised of the estimated arrival time of the team and of any delay during the outbound journey.

On arrival at the referring hospital, the team should communicate effectively with the referring hospital medical and nursing staff and also a child's parents. Handover of patient information is greatly facilitated by the availability of a structured referral letter and copies of patient notes and investigations. Requirements for the return transfer must be clearly communicated to the ambulance and associated services including, where necessary, police and, in the case of international transfers, airport and customs organisations.

It should be recognised that, in the area of intensive care, the specialist expertise of the transport team will usually exceed that available in the referring hospital, who are nevertheless striving under often difficult circumstances to do their best for the sick child. Direct or indirect criticism of the actions of a referring hospital team is unhelpful. The transition of responsibility of care between a referring hospital team and the transport team should evolve in favour of the transport team as the handover and extended resuscitation continues. If additional procedures or alternative treatments are thought necessary by the transport team, these should be explained diplomatically to the referring team.

The correct atmosphere for successful paediatric emergency transport can often be fostered by establishing an outreach education programme through which specialist paediatric intensive care staff can be involved in informing and discussing clinical and administrative problems with referring units. It has been observed that the more cases a hospital refers, the better their initial management becomes.[37]

STABILISATION

Preparation for transfer should have been started by referring hospital staff. Even in situations where a child is adequately resuscitated, a transport team must take time to reassess their patient, attach monitoring equipment and perform detailed clinical and administrative checks before departure.

The time taken to prepare patients for transfer is variable, but has been reported to range from 30–500 min[12,38] with longer times needed in patients requiring multiple or more complex interventions. Teams must, however, bear in mind that definitive care cannot usually be provided locally and that it is sufficient to ensure maximum reasonable resuscitation prior to transfer, even if the child remains very unwell, provided there is believed to be a benefit to the child in ultimately receiving care in the regional PICU.

As part of the resuscitation stabilisation process, particular attention should be paid to the airway and respiratory status, vascular access and to haemo-dynamic stability. These are the familiar A, B, C categories of resuscitation

Table 7.4 Indications for intubation

- Impending respiratory failure
- Upper airway obstruction
- Loss of protective airway reflexes
- Need for hyperventilation
- Apnoea – prolonged or recurrent
- Shock – cardiogenic and septic
- Cardiac arrest
- Facial trauma – including facial/airway burns and scalding

algorithms, but are the areas in which most patient morbidity has been found to occur in the hands of inexperienced transport teams.[6,13,14,22,24,39] A key to safe interhospital transport is to anticipate possible preventable complications and to take steps to minimise their occurrence. It is absolutely essential to perform all necessary procedures at the referral hospital, since it is inevitably more difficult to perform clinical assessments and practical procedures in transport vehicles.[40] Whilst it is not possible in this brief review to detail every possible scenario, there are a few important areas which can be highlighted.

Airway and ventilation

'A secure airway is a *sine qua non* of paediatric transport'.[23] If the ability of a child to maintain a clear airway is in doubt, then steps should be taken to secure the airway by tracheal intubation (see Table 7.4).[36,41] Similarly, if ventilation is impaired through obtunded consciousness, central depression or cerebral hypoxia, then ventilation should be instituted. A decision to intubate and ventilate a child for transport, on the basis that a clinical deterioration might occur during transport, is completely justifiable given the difficulties that would be encountered in an emergency undertaking these procedures on the move. Such decisions are not always fully understood either by referring hospital clinicians or senior intensivists comfortably practising in a teaching hospital environment. Intubation and ventilation procedures are among the most common tasks performed by transport teams.[15,23,42–44]

Nasal intubation is generally preferred for transfer of term neonates and older children in the absence of coagulopathy, basal skull fracture or nasal obstruction. Nasal tubes can be fixed more securely, are less prone to kinking, cannot be bitten and cause less discomfort.[36,45]

A chest radiograph should always be obtained prior to departure. Information required from the X-ray include the position of the tip of the tracheal tube which should be verified as located in the mid tracheal position; focal lung disease be identified; pneumothoraces detected and the correct placement of devices such as central lines and thoracostomy tubes determined. Tracheal suction should be undertaken prior to departure and humidification using a condenser humidifier established. Children should be stabilised on the transport ventilator whilst at the referring hospital, initially mimicking settings of the ICU ventilator, and then fine-tuning, based on blood gas analysis.

Circulation

The transport team must seek to stabilise the circulation with the aid of critical care algorithms. Secure vascular access is of paramount importance and the team may require additional peripheral and central venous access. Intraosseus infusions can be established in term neonates and children of any age in emergency situations where venous access is providing difficult or fails.[46] A sufficient supply of fluid appropriate to the expected ongoing requirements of the child during transport, particularly colloid solutions, 4.5% human albumen, or plasma substitutes and/or cross matched blood should be available.

Invasive monitoring of arterial blood pressure is essential during transport of all critically ill children with any potential to become haemodynamically unstable, as it gives a beat-by-beat read out and is less influenced by motion artefacts than noninvasive blood pressure measurement. Clinical assessment of the circulatory system remains an important aspect of the monitoring undertaken by the transport team, particularly in shocked patients. Pulse volume, capillary refill time and peripheral temperature are readily monitored during transport. Auscultation of heart and breath sounds may prove difficult or impossible due to high background noise levels, particularly in helicopters. The use of $ETCO_2$ monitors in such situations is often reassuring to transport personnel, enabling assessment of continued correct placement and patency of the tracheal tube.[47]

CNS injury

Encephalopathies associated with a variety of conditions and head trauma are relatively common causes of referral to PICUs. Management should be focused on preventing secondary insults thereby reducing morbidity and mortality.[25,48] Emphasis should be placed by the transport team on maintaining adequacy of airway, oxygenation and circulation. Whilst the benefit of elective hyperventilation to induce hypocarbia is disputed, there can be no doubt that maintaining oxygenation and preventing hypocarbia is helpful.[45,48] To this end, continuous end-tidal CO_2 monitoring should be used,[49] combined with regular blood gas analysis. In trauma cases where the possibility of cervical spine injury exists, the neck must be immobilised with a collar or appropriate spinal board system.[48,50]

When children present with encephalopathy of unknown cause, care should be taken to consider abnormalities of blood glucose, hypothermia, intoxication with legal or illegal substances, as well as meningitis or encephalitis. In managing the latter, departure or transfer of a critically ill child to a PICU should never be delayed to obtain a lumbar puncture and antibiotics should be given immediately. Seizures should be controlled; this should being undertaken with full cardiovascular monitoring as anti-convulsants frequently induce hypotension in the critically ill shocked child.

All trauma patients should have a primary and secondary survey prior to leaving the referring hospital so that no important injury is missed. Neurosurgical and/or surgical teams at the receiving hospital should be consulted prior to departure, not only to alert them of the potential admission but also to seek their advice on the surgical aspects of management.

Stabilisation and transportation of children

Analgesia and sedation

Accidental extubation or loss of venous access is unacceptable in hospital practice, but potentially disastrous during interhospital transfer. Inadequate sedation or immobilisation are, however, frequently associated with such events.[6,51] All patients undergoing intensive care must receive appropriate levels of sedation and analgesia and many critically ill children will, in addition, benefit during interhospital transfer from the use of muscle relaxant drugs. Analgesics, sedatives and muscle relaxants may be given by bolus injection but are more frequently delivered by continuous infusion, such that levels of sedation and neuromuscular blockade can be carefully titrated. Although paralysis and sedation temporarily interfere with the assessment of neurological status, they may facilitate measures to control raised intracranial pressure by preventing straining and coughing; protect against worsening potential spinal injury and, if suitable agents are used, reversal can be undertaken to facilitate timely neurological assessment on arrival in the regional PICU.

PACKAGING

Just as an inadequately wrapped postal packet fails to reach its destination intact, so does an inadequately prepared child. The team should adopt procedures to protect against all conceivable eventualities and particularly bear in mind the maxims that anything that 'can fall out will fall out' and that 'anything that can conceivably go wrong will go wrong'. A child may be subjected to many moves between trolleys, road vehicles and air ambulances before reaching a final destination, and is particularly vulnerable to physical adverse events and clinical deterioration during such transfers. Dangers can be minimised by taking extra precautions to secure tubes and monitoring devices to the patient. Monitoring devices should be applied in a logical way such that leads come together as an umbilical cord leading between patient and monitor. A similar arrangement can be planned with infusion devices. Such an approach facilitates safe and easy transfer of patients from one vehicle format to another with minimal risk of disruption.

PRE-DEPARTURE CHECK LIST

To ensure that all aspects of patient preparation have been considered and, therefore, minimising adverse events, teams should utilise a pre-departure check list where by both nurse and doctor cross check all items listed.[36,45] An example of types of information which should be checked is seen in Table 7.5.

PARENTS

The families of critically ill children are obviously very distressed at the sudden illness of their child. The transport team must help the family to understand the

Table 7.5 Pre-departure check list

Airway/ventilation

Need intubation?
ETT position correct and secure?
Blood gas satisfactory?
ETT patent – suction handy?
Ventilator settings checked?
Oxygen supply adequate?
Bag and mask handy?

Circulation

Fully resuscitated?
Volume handy for journey if required?
Blood pressure monitored?
Secure venous/arterial access?
Inotropes infusing?

Drugs/fluid

All potentially necessary drugs handy?
All infusions functioning and secure?
Enough drugs and fluids for journey?
Biochemical abnormalities corrected?

Monitors

Functioning and alarms set?
Secured?

Miscellaneous

Nasogastric tube in place, on free drainage?
Urinary catheter in place?
Chest drain connected to Heimlick valve?

Information/communication

Referral letter and investigation results?
Parents fully informed?
Any consent needed for procedure at receiving hospital?
Receiving hospital staff aware of patient and transport details?
Transport providers ready?

reason for transfer of their child and that transfer is being undertaken by an experienced team. Besides their grief, parents of critically ill children often feel guilty or helpless and these feelings are intensified when they do not fully understand their child's illness or the need for transfer.[52] Research has shown that most parents would prefer to accompany their child on transport.[53] Where possible, efforts should be made to accommodate at least one adult member of the family in the vehicle carrying the child,[54] but in practice this may be difficult to achieve, because of lack of space in the transport vehicle for essential members of the medical team, their equipment and the patient. Parents should be given some time with their child prior to departure and be fully informed about the intended destination, how they can get there and what facilities will be available for them at the regional centre which may well be some distance from their home. Where possible, arrangements should be made by the referring hospital for transfer of the parents to the regional PICU.

Inhaled nitric oxide

Inhaled nitric oxide has been shown to be an effective pulmonary vasodilator and to improve ventilation perfusion matching in a wide spectrum of children's diseases. Despite the lack of conclusive evidence that it improves outcome, the therapy is being widely adopted in the management of critically ill children with severe cardiorespiratory failure. The use of inhaled nitric oxide in sub-regional centres can cause very considerable practical difficulties in delivering that child to the appropriate regional centre, since dependence on inhaled nitric oxide therapy requires that it be continued during transport.[55] A number of methods of delivering inhaled nitric oxide during transport have been described[55,56] as have portable nitric oxide scavenging systems.[57] Recently, at least one commercially available nitric oxide delivery system has become available (Aeronox Transport System®, Pulmonox Medical Corporation, Canada). Delivery of inhaled nitric oxide during transport requires provision of small volume cylinders and small portable battery operated nitric oxide analysers. There are several reports of the successful transport of children receiving inhaled nitric oxide.[55,56]

Whilst the environmental risks from low volume spillage of nitric oxide in a well ventilated intensive care environment have been assessed as minimal, care should be taken to ensure that environmental safety is maintained when inhaled nitric oxide is used in confined spaces.

Mobile extracorporeal life support

Advances in extracorporeal technology over the past 20 years have seen the introduction of successful extracorporeal life support (ECLS) programmes using modified heart-lung bypass equipment. Initially, these techniques were successfully applied to neonates with severe respiratory failure, but have subsequently been applied to children and adults with potentially reversible respiratory or cardiorespiratory failure. Although early discussion of cases potentially suitable for ECLS is strongly encouraged so that their early transfer to the ECLS centre may be facilitated, occasionally situations arise where interhospital transfer even by expert teams is deemed too hazardous. In such situations, several ECLS centres have a limited experience of transferring patients on ECLS. These ECLS centres provide a team of personnel including a surgeon and suitably modified portable equipment, travel to the distant location where the patient is cannulated for ECLS. Having stabilised them on mechanical support, careful transfer back to the ECLS centre by road or by air ambulance by ECLS is performed. The logistical and financial implications of such policies are considerable but have been overcome in certain healthcare systems.[58–60]

In our view, the emphasis should remain on early discussion and referral of cases potentially suitable for ECLS which, even when provided only in supraregional ECLS centres, is extremely costly. Resources spent on mobile extracorporeal membrane oxygenation (ECMO) may be better diverted to improving education and communication between referring hospitals and the ECLS centre.

Telemedicine

It is now feasible to establish data links between referring hospitals and even mobile medical teams through which complex signals can be downloaded, facilitating more rapid discussion with a clinical expert at the regional PICU. Transfer of digital radiographs,[61] ultrasound images, physiological data and waveforms, as well as video images, are likely to improve the quality of initial referral consultations between physicians and potentially enable transport teams to download data throughout the transport process and, if necessary, seek additional advice based on that data.

Transport by air

'Aeromedical evacuation presents no problems as long as one remembers that man is adapted for life at or near sea level'

Johnson Jr A (quoted in De Hart R L. (Ed) *Fundamentals of Aerospace Medicine*, 2nd edn. Williams and Wilkins, Bulletin 1996).

The flight environment is physically and physiologically different from that found in ground ambulances or hospitals. Acceleration and deceleration forces are encountered during take off and landing manoeuvres of fixed wing aircraft. These forces become very significant in supine patients when loaded on a stretcher along the longitudinal axis of an aircraft. In a patient whose head is toward the front of an aircraft, blood will pool in the lower limbs during take off, reducing cardiac output, a process which continues during the 'climb out' of initial ascent. Since the physiological changes associated with landing are opposite to those of take off, it is the accepted rule that patients be loaded with head towards the rear of the aircraft. A better alternative would be to load patients across the horizontal axis of aircraft, however, for logistic reasons, this is rarely possible.

Barometric pressure decreases as aircraft ascend. Gas volumes expand as pressure decreases (Boyle's law), doubling at 18 000 ft (5500 m) where atmospheric pressure is half that at sea level. Air ambulance helicopters typically fly at 1000–3000 ft, unpressurised fixed wing aircraft may fly at up to 10 000 ft, whilst pressurised aircraft fly with the cabin pressurised to the equivalent of 6000–8000 ft. Trapped gas anywhere in the body will expand as the aircraft ascends. Expansion of gas in the gut or pleural space is particularly likely to cause patient discomfort or clinical deterioration. Expansion of trapped gas in the middle ear or sinuses will certainly cause pain or discomfort. Air in tracheal tube cuffs will expand. Measures to prevent the predictable effects of altitude include: (i) ensuring nasogastric tubes are patent and open to atmosphere during flight; (ii) pneumothoraces drained; and (iii) tracheal tube cuffs are partially deflated or filled with saline. The characteristics of some transport ventilators can be dramatically affected at altitude.

Although the atmosphere contains approximately 21% O_2 at all altitudes, the oxygen tension (Patm O_2) falls as ambient atmospheric pressure falls. Healthy passengers compensate for cabin altitude hypoxia by imperceptible increases in respiratory rate and heart rate, thus maintaining tissue O_2 delivery. Patients with O_2 respiratory failure, anaemia or cardiac failure who must travel, will require an increased inspired O_2 fraction to compensate for altitude hypoxia. Stable patients with cyanotic congenital heart disease can safely be transported at cabin altitude without adverse effects.[62] In extremely urgent situations, arrangements may be made with air ambulance operators to fly at lower altitudes, or higher cabin pressures, thus minimising altitude effects. A typical large jet or executive jet can easily maintain sea level pressurisation at altitudes well in excess of 10 000 ft. Supplementation of O_2 30–40% provides 'sea level' alveolar O_2 concentration.

In the UK, there are few genuine cases for which air transfer is appropriate. The geographical isolation of the Highlands and Islands of Scotland has seen the logical development of air ambulance provision within the Scottish Ambulance Service. In most other parts of the UK, air transfers between hospitals are undertaken rarely, usually in patients requiring transfer to supraregional centres for highly specialised care, such as ECMO, transplantation or treatment in hyperbaric chambers.

Transport teams in supraregional centres which regularly undertake air transfers should ensure staff are fully familiar with all technical and physiological aspects of this work. Road transfer is usually safer, and may be quicker than attempts at *ad hoc* air transfer joy-rides by unskilled teams in unsuitable aircraft.

Key points for clinical practice

- .All staff responsible for delivery of paediatric care should be skilled in basic and advanced life support techniques.

- Management of critically ill children should be discussed promptly will a regional specialist PICU.

- Interhospital transfer of critically ill children should be undertaken by specialist paediatric emergency transport teams.

- Transport teams should operate according to clear administrative and clinical protocols.

- Patients should not be transferred without prior resuscitation and preparation.

- Clear communication is essential throughout the transport process.

- Air transport presents additional unique problems and should be undertaken only by specially trained personnel.

ACKNOWLEDGEMENT

The authors thank Carolyn Warner, Great Ormond Street Hospital NHS Trust.

References

1. British Paediatric Association. The Care of Critically Ill Children: Report of the Multidisciplinary Working Party on Paediatric Intensive Care. London: BPA, 1993

2. Gemke R J B J. Centralisation of paediatric intensive care to improve outcome. Lancet 1997; 349: 1187–1188

3. Pollack M M, Alexander S R, Clarke N, Ruttimann U E, Tesselaar H M, Bachulis A C. Improved outcomes from tertiary center pediatric intensive care: A statewide comparison of tertiary and nontertiary care facilities. Crit Care Med 1991; 19: 150–159

4. Pearson G, Shann F, Barry P et al. Should paediatric intensive care be centralised? Trent versus Victoria. Lancet 1997; 349: 1213–1217

5. Raffles A. Impact of a specialised paediatric retrieval teams: intensive care provided by local hospitals should be improved. BMJ 1996; 312: 120

6. Edge W E, Kanter R K, Weigle C G M, Walsh R F. Reduction of morbidity in interhospital transport by specialised pediatric staff. Crit Care Med 1994; 22: 1186–1192

7. NHS Executive. Paediatric Intensive Care 'A Framework for the Future'. Report from the National Coordinating Group on Paediatric Intensive Care to the Chief Executive of the NHS Executive, July 1997

8. Dryden C M, Morton N S. A survey of interhospital transport of the critically ill child in the United Kingdom. Paediatr Anaesth 1995; 5: 157–160

9. Paediatric Intensive Care Society. Standards of Paediatric Intensive Care. Bishop's Stotford: Saldose, 1996; 19–29

10. Guidelines Committee of the American College of Critical Care Medicine, Society of Critical Care Medicine and American Association of Critical Care Nurses Transfer Guidelines Task Force. Guidelines for the transfer of critically ill patients. Crit Care Med 1993 ;21: 931–937

11. Mok Q, Tasker R, Macrae D, James I. Impact of a specialised paediatric retrieval teams: impact of specialised paediatric retrieval teams. BMJ 1996; 312: 119

12. Beddingfield F C, Garrison H G, Manning J E, Lewis R J. Factors associated with prolongation of transport times of emergency pediatric patients requiring transfer to a tertiary care center. Pediatr Emerg Care 1996; 12: 416–419

13. Kanter R K, Boeing N M, Hannan W P, Kanter D L. Excess morbidity associated with interhospital transport. Pediatrics 1992; 90: 893–898

14. Kanter R K, Tompkins J M. Adverse events during interhospital transport: physiologic deterioration associated with pretransport severity of illness. Pediatrics 1989; 84: 43–48

15. Owen H, Duncan A W. Towards safer transport of sick and injured children. Anaesth Intensive Care 1983; 11: 113–117

16. Sweeney D B, Turtle M J. Paediatric retrievals in South Australia. Anaesth Intensive Care 1985; 13: 410–414

17. Pollack M M, Ruttimann U E, Geston P R. Pediatric risk of mortality (PRISM) score. Crit Care Med 1988; 16: 1110–1116

18. Shann F, Pearson G, Slater A, Wilkinson K. Paediatric index of mortality (PIM): a mortality prediction model for children in intensive care. Intensive Care Med 1997; 23: 201–207

19. Orr R A, Venkataraman S T, Cinoman M I, Hogue B L, Singleton C A, McCloskey K A. Pretransport pediatric risk of mortality (PRISM) score underestimates the requirement for intensive care or major interventions during interhospital transport. Crit Care Med 1994; 22: 101–107

20. Britto J, Nadel S, Maconochie I, Levin M, Habibi P. Morbidity and severity of illness during interhospital transfer: impact of a specialised paediatric retrieval team. BMJ 1995; 311: 836–838

21. Morrison A, Runcie C. Impact of a specialised paediatric retrieval teams: comparison of teams is difficult. BMJ 1996; 312: 119

22. Barry P W, Ralston C. Adverse events occurring during interhospital transfer of the critically ill. Arch Dis Child 1994; 71: 8–11

23. Henning R, Mcnamara V. Difficulties encountered in transport of the critically ill child. Pediatr Emerg Care 1991; 7: 133–137

24. Macnab A J. Optimal escort for interhospital transport of pediatric emergencies. J Trauma 1991; 31: 205–209

25. Sharples P M, Storey A, Aynsley-Green A, Eyre J A. Avoidable factors contributing to death of children with head injury. BMJ 1990; 300: 87–91

26. Wallen E, Venkataraman S T, Grosso M J, Kiene K, Orr RA. Intrahospital transport of critically ill pediatric patients. Crit Care Med 1995; 23: 1588–1595

27. Rubenstein J S, Gomez M A, Rybicki L, Noah Z L. Can the need for a physician as part of the pediatric team be predicted? A prospective study. Crit Care Med 1992; 20: 1657–1661

28. Beyer J, Land G, Zaritsky A. Nonphysician transport of intubated pediatric patients: a system evaluation. Crit Care Med 1992; 20: 961–966

29. Sacchetti A, Carraccio C, Feder M. Pediatric EMS transport: are we treating children in a system designed for adults only?. Pediatr Emerg Care 1992; 8: 4–8

30. McCloskey K A, Faries G, King W D, Orr R A, Plouff R T. Variables predicting the need for a pediatric critical care transport team. Pediatr Emerg Care 1992; 8: 1–3

31. James A G. Resuscitation, stabilization and transport in perinatology. Curr Opin Pediatr 1993; 5: 150–155

32. Macnab A, Chen Y, Gagnon F, Bora B, Laszlo C. Vibration and noise in pediatric emergency transport vehicles: a potential cause of morbidity? Aviat Space Environ Med 1995; 66: 212–219

33. Schneider C, Gomez M, Lee R. Evaluation of ground ambulance, rotor-wing, and fixed-wing aircraft services. Crit Care Clin 1992; 8: 533–564

34. Doyle E, Freeman J, Hallworth D, Morton N S. Transport of the critically ill child. Br J Hosp Med 1992; 48: 314–319

35. Ferguson S, Spargo P. Reducing the risks of paediatric transport. Br J Hosp Med 1993; 49: 289

36. Macrae D J. Paediatric intensive care transport. Arch Dis Child 1994; 71: 175–178

37. Robb H M, Hallworth D, Skeoch C H, Levy C. An audit of a paediatric intensive care transfer unit. Br J Intensive Care 1992; 2: 371–379

38. Whitfield J M, Buser M K. Transport stabilisation times for neonatal and pediatric patients prior to interfacility transfer. Pediatr Emerg Care 1993; 9: 69–71

39. Manji M, Bion J F. Transporting critically ill patients. Intensive Care Med 1995; 21: 781–783

40. Thomas S H, Stone C K, Bryan-Berge D. The ability to perform closed chest compressions in helicopters. Am J Emerg Med 1994; 12: 296–298

41. McDonald T B, Berkowitz R A. Airway management and sedation for pediatric transport. Pediatr Clin North Am 1993; 40: 381–405

42. Cray S H, Heard C M B. Transport for paediatric intensive care. Measuring the performance of a specialist transport service. Paediatr Anaesth 1995; 5: 287–292

43. Fuller J, Frewen T, Lee R. Acute airway management in the critically ill child requiring transport. Can J Anaesth 1991; 38: 252–254

44. Kronick J B, Frewen T C, Kissoon N et al. Pediatric and neonatal critical care transport: a comparison of therapeutic interventions. Pediatr Emerg Care 1996; 12: 23–26

45. Henning R. Emergency transport of critically ill children: stabilisation before departure. Med J Aust 1992; 156: 117–124

46. Corneli H M. Evaluation, treatment and transport of pediatric patients with shock. Pediatr Clin North Am 1993; 40: 303–319

47. Bhende M S, Karr V A, Wiltsie D C, Orr R A. Evaluation of a portable infrared end-tidal carbon dioxide monitor during pediatric interhospital transport. Pediatrics 1995; 95: 875–878

48. Sarnaik A P, Lieh-Lai M W. Transporting the neurologically compromised child. Pediatr Clin North Am 1993; 40: 337–353

49. Tobias J D, Lynch A, Garrett J. Alterations in end-tidal carbon dioxide during the intrahospital transport of children. Pediatr Emerg Care 1996; 12: 249–251

50. Graneto J W, Soglin D F. Transport and stabilization of the pediatric trauma patient. Pediatr Clin North Am 1993; 40: 365–379

51. Sharples A, O'Neill M, Dearlove O. Impact of a specialised paediatric retrieval teams: children are still transferred by non-specialised teams. BMJ 1996; 312: 120

52. Frischer L, Gutterman D L. Emotional impact of parents of transported babies. Crit Care Clin 1992; 8: 649–660

53. Macnab A J. Paediatric inter-facility transport: the parents' perspective. Soc Work in Health Care 1992; 17: 21–29.

54. Bristow A, Toff N. A report – recommended standards for UK fixed wing medical air transport systems and for patient management during transfer by fixed wing aircraft. J R Soc Med 1992; 85: 767–771

55. Goldman A P, Tasker R C, Cook P, Macrae D J. Transfer of critically ill patients with inhaled nitric oxide. Arch Dis Child 1995; 73: 480

56. Kinsella J P, Schmidt J M, Griebel J, Abman S H. Inhaled nitric oxide treatment for stabilization and emergency medical transport of critically ill newborns and infants. Pediatrics 1995; 95: 773–776

57. Dhillon J S, Kronick J B, Singh N C, Johnson C C. A portable nitric oxide scavenging system designed for use on neonatal transport. Crit Care Med 1996; 24: 1068–1071

58. Bennet J B, Hill J G, Long III W B, Bruhn P S, Haun M M, Parsons J A. Interhospital transport of the patient on extracorporeal cardiopulmonary support. Ann Thorac Surg 1994; 57: 107–111

59. Day S E, Chapman R A. Transport of critically ill patients in need of extracorporeal life support. Crit Care Clin 1992; 8: 581–596

60. Faulkner S C, Taylor B J, Chipman C W et al. Mobile extracorporeal membrane oxygenation. Ann Thorac Surg 1993; 55: 1244–1246

61. Yamamoto L G, Ash K M, Boychuk R B et al. Personal computer teleradiology interhospital image transmission of neonatal radiographs to facilitate tertiary neonatology telephone consultation and patient transfer. J Perinatol 1996; 16: 292–298

62. Harinck E, Hutter P A, Hoorntje T M et al. Air travel and adults with cyanotic congenital heart disease. Circulation 1996; 93: 272–276

Peter C. Roberts   Richard J. Beale

'The Golden Hour'

The concept of preventable trauma deaths has been documented in retrospective post-mortem studies from the 1960s,[1] but it was not until the early 1970s and the Emergency Medical Services System Act of 1973 that trauma systems were developed in the USA. The states that subsequently adopted such systems reported a dramatic reduction in preventable trauma deaths,[2-9] with some achieving incidence as low as 0–2%, but the avoidable fatality rate when trauma was managed outside of designated trauma centres remained high at 20–40%.[1] In England and Wales, a retrospective study of trauma deaths reported a similarly high incidence,[10] and analysis of the subgroup of individuals dying without central nervous system injury revealed a staggering 63% incidence of avoidable mortality.

In 1979, the American College of Surgeons adopted the Advanced Trauma Life Support (ATLS) course that had been developed in Nebraska, USA following an air tragedy in 1976 that revealed inadequacies in the standards of trauma care. In the mid 1980s, the American College of Surgeons defined criteria for the designation of trauma centres,[11] and outlined the components of a comprehensive system of care.[12] In an article published in *Scientific American* in 1983 entitled *Trauma*, Trunkey identified three separate peaks of trauma deaths: immediate, early and late.[13] Those in the early group were targeted as preventable. In the same article, Trunkey indicated that the time which elapsed between an injury and definitive surgical care was a critical factor in determining the survival rate of trauma victims. This time period later became known as 'the Golden Hour'. In 1988, the Advanced Trauma Life Support (ATLS) programme was implemented by the Royal College of Surgeons of England, but it remains unclear whether trauma care will eventually be

Peter C. Roberts, Departments of Intensive Care and Anaesthetics, Guy's Hospital, London Bridge, London SE1 9RT, UK

Richard J. Beale MBBS FRCA, Senior Lecturer, Departments of Intensive Care and Anaesthetics, Guy's Hospital, London Bridge, London SE1 9RT, UK

regionalised in the UK. Certainly, the institution of a trauma system has resulted in improved performance in countries other than the USA. A prospective study from Sydney, Australia showed a decrease in mortality in patients with an injury severity score of greater than 15 following the adoption of one such system, with the overall death rate falling from 31% to 11%, and the number dying from exsanguination falling from 9.4% to 1.3%.[14] It was noted in this study that the major causes of mortality from trauma were haemorrhage and head injury.

The ATLS protocols for resuscitation and diagnosis prior to directed surgical intervention now form the foundations of modern trauma care, and it is widely accepted that the former should be complete, and definitive surgical intervention commenced, within one hour of injury. It is clear that a rapid and well ordered approach lending itself to defined protocols is required if this is to be achieved; something which is only likely to occur in practised and disciplined units. The argument in support of regional trauma units is furthered by improved surgical outcome in units dealing with increased numbers of patients.[9,15,16] Nevertheless, many of the details of treatment are contested even now, and the principal objective of this short account is to introduce some of these arguments, and approach some new developments that may, in time, show benefit in the early management of trauma patients.

SCENE TRIAGE, BASIC LIFE SUPPORT (BLS) AND ADVANCED LIFE SUPPORT (ALS)

If prehospital resuscitation efforts fail in the event of a cardiorespiratory arrest occurring outside hospital, further resuscitation attempts in the emergency department are usually futile,[17,18] and this gloomy prognosis is certainly no better in those suffering trauma induced cardiac arrest. The cost implications of attempted resuscitation of this group of patients were presented in a retrospective review of all trauma patients in Hillsborough County, Florida, USA between 1 October, 1989 and 31 March, 1991.[19] A total of 12 462 patients' records were reviewed, and 410 of these suffered prehospital cardiopulmonary arrest of traumatic aetiology. Those suffering injuries incompatible with life or who had prolonged absence of vital signs were excluded. There remained a group of 138 patients suffering cardiopulmonary arrest at-scene or in transport to county trauma centres. Whilst the breakdown of the treatments received by this group is interesting, it is more salient that no individual survived to leave ICU, with the ICU stay ranging from two hours to 10 days. The conclusion was that those individuals without vital signs at the scene have no chance of surviving and returning to a premorbid lifestyle regardless of the mechanism of injury, scene time or transport time. The appropriateness of prolonged resuscitative efforts in this group of patients must be seriously questioned.

Resuscitative thoracotomy is clearly a desperate measure and should be distinguished from emergency thoracotomy and definitive procedures. It extends at-scene and transport time if conducted outside hospital and may contribute to mortality.[20] Roadside thoracotomy performed by medical teams arriving with a helicopter emergency service has been shown to be of no benefit and a policy of 'scoop and run' is advocated.[21] When conducted in blunt trauma, thoracotomy is generally unsuccessful irrespective of timing and location.[20–23,39] The weight of evidence suggests that those patients who lose their vital signs outside hospital following either penetrating or blunt trauma will die, and that thoracotomy will not improve resuscitation outcome. The group of patients in which this procedure has been justified are those suffering penetrating thoracic trauma and either experiencing cardiac arrest or rapid progressive deterioration of vital signs in the emergency room or shortly before arrival there. The reported survival is as high as 26% in this group and even 40% in those suffering stab wounds.[24]

There remains controversy regarding the value of various components of prehospital advanced life support (ALS) as opposed to basic life support (BLS) of injured patients. There are studies of blunt and penetrating trauma that support the institution of prehospital ALS.[25–30] Most are retrospective reviews and inadequately controlled. These studies fail universally to demonstrate an improved outcome from the deployment of ALS protocols but have shown improved trauma scores and blood pressures on hospital admission. Potter and colleagues[30] prospectively studied trauma cases in two Australian cities; Sydney metropolitan area in which ALS was employed and the Brisbane and Gold Coast metropolitan area where only BLS was instituted, and were unable to demonstrate an improvement in overall outcome, ITU and hospital stay, or disability after head injury from the use of in-field ALS. There was, however, a lower mortality rate within the first 24 h in the ALS (Sydney area) patients compared with the BLS (Brisbane/Gold Coast area) patients. Other studies have questioned the use of ALS.[31–37] Once again, many of these are retrospective reviews and inadequately controlled. Gerwin and Ivatury[31,33] in their studies of penetrating cardiac and thoracic trauma, and Smith[32] concluded that ALS at-scene delayed transport to hospitals and adversely affected outcome. Kaweski and Martin[35,36] argued that prehospital fluid administration did not improve outcome and may increase mortality. Mattox and colleagues[34] showed a detrimental effect of MAST (military anti-shock trousers) in patients with mild to moderate hypotension, and in their prospective study only those with at-scene systolic blood pressures of less than 50 mmHg benefited from this compression device. Cayten and colleagues[37] could not demonstrate an outcome difference in their retrospective study and concluded that ALS was not beneficial in patients with total prehospital times of less than 35 min. They did, however, demonstrate improved trauma scores and blood pressures in the ALS group on hospital admission and a lower than predicted survival in the penetrating injury subset receiving prehospital ALS.

Many of the opponents of paramedic ALS cite increased at-scene times and prehospital delay as detrimental to patient outcome.[31–33] The majority of evidence suggests that field times are unaltered by the implementation of ALS protocols, and many studies show scene times of 8–12 min in this group,[26,27,33,38,41] with almost all finding times of less than 20 min. Although the value of in-field fluid resuscitation is certainly questionable, the role of airway management and placement of endotracheal tubes by paramedics is altogether better supported. Intubation has been shown to improve patient survival[27,32,33] and to prolong the average period over which cardiopulmonary resuscitation may have a successful outcome from 4.2 min in the non-intubated to 9.4 min.[39]

Table 8.1 Outcome of patients with penetrating torso injuries, according to treatment group

Variable	Immediate resuscitation	Delayed resuscitation	P value
Survival to discharge (%) No. of patients/total no. patients	193/309 (62%)*	203/289 (70%)**	0.04
Estimated intraoperative blood loss (ml)	3127 ± 4937	2555 ± 3546	0.11
Length of hospital stay (days)	14 ± 24	11 ± 19	0.006
Length of ICU stay (days)	8 ± 16	7 ± 11	0.3

*95% confidence interval, 57–68%; **95% confidence interval, 65–75%. Table from Bickell et al,[41] with permission (© *1994 Massachusetts Medical School. All rights reserved*).

Aggressive early fluid resuscitation in the presence of haemorrhage has been advocated[40] and large volumes of crystalloid, colloid and blood are often infused into trauma patients in an attempt to restore normal blood pressures prior to surgical intervention. Early animal models used to justify this approach are based on controlled or graded haemorrhage and do not replicate the uncontrolled haemorrhage that occurs in trauma victims.[44,46] This approach is now increasingly being challenged. There are escalating numbers of animal studies showing improved survival and decreased haemorrhage volumes in uncontrolled haemorrhage models treated with limited fluid resuscitation, and thus maintaining deliberate hypotension.[43–48] Kowalenko and colleagues[43] used a swine model of severe haemorrhage (40 ml/kg) and aortotomy (to provide continued uncontrolled bleeding) to show a 1 h survival of 12.5% in control pigs not receiving resuscitation. Those pigs administered fluid to maintain normotension (MAP = 80 mmHg) had a one hour mortality of 62.5%, while those administered fluids permitting hypotension (MAP = 40 mmHg) had a lower mortality of 12.5%. A prospective study by Bickell and colleagues[41] of 598 hypotensive adults with penetrating torso injuries showed a significantly raised mortality in the group receiving immediate fluid resuscitation compared with those whose fluid resuscitation was delayed until the commencement of surgery (Table 8.1). The individuals receiving delayed fluid resuscitation in this study had no higher incidence of renal failure or other complications associated with hypovolaemia and their ITU and hospital stay were not increased. In a retrospective review of 1727 children suffering from trauma induced hypotension, Cooper and colleagues[42] found no survival benefit of prehospital fluid administration in profoundly hypotensive children, and a detrimental effect of fluid in the mild to moderate hypotension group. These patients had been matched for injury severity, degree of hypotension and age and had suffered both blunt and penetrating injuries.

The overall interpretation of these studies is complex, and it remains likely that those individuals suffering rapid uncontrolled haemorrhage, with all but the shortest prehospital times, will benefit from some volume replacement, especially as the untreated 1 h survival in this group is predicted as 'low'.[49] Similarly, those enduring prolonged prehospital times, either because of difficult extrication or long distances to medical centres, are likely to benefit. It is noticeable that the prehospital times for patients in Bickell's study were short (at-scene times of approximately 8 min and transport times of 12–13 min on average). However, this group of patients with penetrating injuries benefits from a policy of 'scoop and run'. Evidence suggests that attempts to restore 'normal' blood pressures are ill advised and that those receiving prehospital fluid resuscitation should be subjected to a restricted volume replacement to obtain mean arterial pressures of 40–60 mmHg.[45] This policy of permissive hypotension is convincing in individuals suffering penetrating torso injuries and subject to short prehospital times. It has yet to be tested in victims of blunt trauma, those suffering concomitant head injuries and those subject to prolonged prehospital times.

CRYSTALLOID, COLLOID AND HYPERTONIC SOLUTIONS

During the 1970s and early 1980s, there were a number of studies comparing crystalloid and colloidal fluids in hypovolaemia, but consensus is still lacking. One logical conclusion from this is that there simply is no advantage to either solution over the other.[50,51] Whilst it is clear that larger volumes of crystalloid solution than colloid will be required to expand the plasma volume by a set amount and that this infusion may take longer, concern has been expressed regarding anaphylactic reactions to colloids and anticoagulatory actions of these solutions as well as their eventual elimination and excretion pathways. Those supporting the use of colloids are equally critical of the crystalloid induced decreases in colloid oncotic pressure and increased extravascular volume, pulmonary and cerebral oedema. The studies conducted, however, fail to repudiate or support this view. Following the development of statistical methods of assimilating data from similarly designed studies, Velanovich performed a meta-analysis of studies comparing colloid and crystalloid resuscitation.[52] He chose only to consider those studies reporting mortality in humans. Although many of the studies he reviewed involved very small numbers, his analysis showed that in the four studies of trauma victims there was a 12.3% difference in mortality rate in favour of crystalloid solutions.

In 1980, a study by Velasco and colleagues[53] marked the beginning of investigation in earnest of hypertonic solutions in the treatment of haemorrhagic shock. In a canine model of fixed lethal haemorrhage, they demonstrated that 5 ml/kg of 7.5% NaCl (2400 mOsm/l), a volume one-tenth of the blood lost in haemorrhage, immediately restored haemodynamic indices and improved survival without further transfusion. The efficacy of 7.5% NaCl in resuscitating animal models subjected to otherwise lethal haemorrhage was subsequently confirmed by other investigators,[54,55] but the effect was reported to be transient in these studies and lasted less than an hour.

In 1985, Smith and colleagues[56] demonstrated that the duration of the resuscitative effects of hypertonic saline could be extended by the addition of dextran to the solution. Subsequent investigations employing animal models (pigs, sheep and dogs) of fixed volume or pressure haemorrhage showed that survival is further improved by hypertonic saline/dextran solutions compared with hypertonic saline, dextran or normal saline alone and confirmed the sustained improvements in haemodynamic indices reported.[57–60] The most commonly investigated hypertonic/hyperoncotic solution is 7.5% NaCl/6% Dextran 70, termed hypertonic saline/dextran (HSD), although other solutions have also been investigated.[61–63] These studies show a dose response to hypertonicity and oncotic power and stress the importance of sodium in hypertonic solutions. Although dextran is used frequently as the colloidal component, it is likely that other oncotically active agents would be effective in combination with 7.5% NaCl.[64] The optimal dose and combination of salt and colloid remains unidentified. The initial choice of concentrations in HSD was arbitrary, but has since been vindicated and proved highly effective. There are limitations to the degree of hypertonicity and oncotic values that can be employed as intravascular haemolysis has been shown to occur with infusion of near saturated solutions of 25% NaCl/24% dextran in pigs.[63]

Whilst demonstrating the dramatic plasma volume expanding potential of small volumes of hyperosmotic/hyperoncotic solutions, the studies above were not representative of the clinical scenario. Chudnofsky and colleagues[65] used a porcine model of continuous rate of haemorrhage and Prist and colleagues[66] employed a continuous pressure driven haemorrhage in dogs to represent the haemorrhage experienced in trauma victims. These studies introduce the concept of initial resuscitation by infusion of HSD and subsequent infusion of isotonic crystalloids (normal saline or lactated Ringer's solution) in the presence of continued bleeding. In both studies, survival was increased in those animals resuscitated with a combination of HSD and isotonic crystalloid compared with isotonic crystalloid alone[65] or unresuscitated animals, animals infused HSD or lactated Ringer's solution.[66] Nevertheless, in the latter study employing a pressure driven haemorrhage model, the volume of haemorrhage was increased in the fluid resuscitated groups and worst in the group receiving HSD and lactated Ringer's solution. Bickell and colleagues,[67] using their established porcine model of uncontrolled haemorrhage in animals subjected to aortotomy, demonstrated once again that fluid resuscitation in this model increased the volume of haemorrhage and decreased survival compared with unresuscitated animals. Their studies were designed to represent the pattern of bleeding in trauma victims prior to surgical intervention and thus follow the animals for 2 h only.

Studies conducted in patients, both prehospital[68,70–72] and in the emergency room,[69] using hypertonic saline and hypertonic saline/Dextran 70 solution as a resuscitation fluid in haemorrhagic shock have failed to demonstrate an improvement in outcome when compared with isotonic crystalloid resuscitation, although any trends expressed favoured the use of hypertonic solutions. It should be noted that, in these studies, haemodynamic indices were restored more rapidly in those individuals receiving hypertonic resuscitation. In this clinical setting, no advantage could be found in adding dextran to hypertonic saline as resuscitation is a continuous process and not conducted with a single bolus infusion as in the majority of animal models. Initial fears of hypernatraemia and coma, coagulation defects, anaphylaxis and subsequent problems in typing blood appear not to have been substantiated in the human studies conducted. The use of small volume hypertonic resuscitation and its actions involving the microcirculation and immune system have been reviewed by several authors.[64,73,74]

The subset of trauma patients which have shown an outcome benefit with initial hypertonic/hyperoncotic resuscitation and subsequent isotonic fluid administration are those individuals suffering haemorrhagic shock and severe head injury (Glasgow Coma Scale ≤ 8).[68,71] In their retrospective study of hypotensive trauma patients, Vasser and colleagues[71] showed a 34% survival in those patients receiving prehospital hypertonic solutions and a 12% survival in those resuscitated with lactated Ringer's alone in the group with concomitant head injury and GCS ≤ 8. The rapid restoration of haemodynamic indices experienced with small volume hypertonic resuscitation may serve to reduce secondary injury in these individuals, however, there are more specific cerebral effects to consider. Animal studies have shown that hypertonic solutions used to resuscitate hypotension reduce cerebral water content and intracranial pressure both in animals without head injury[75–77] and in models of intracranial injury.[78–82] Freshman and colleagues[83] found in sheep, subjected to raised intracranial pressure using an epidural balloon, that a 250 ml bolus of 7.5% NaCl was equally effective in reducing ICP to pre-intervention levels when compared with the same volume of 20% mannitol.

With some authors reporting higher mortality and increased bleeding in trauma patients receiving fluids prior to surgical intervention, the future choice of intravenous fluids is uncertain. Unquestionably, one group of individuals which has been shown to have an unfavourable outcome if permitted to remain hypotensive is that with concomitant head injury. Similarly, those patients who will suffer a hypovolaemic cardiac arrest if unresuscitated must benefit from intravenous volume replacement. With this in mind, caution should be exercised when practising permissive hypotension and withholding fluid resuscitation. As the fluid volumes infused in the prehospital phase are often inadequate,[32] there remains a role for small volume resuscitation with hypertonic solutions.

OXYGEN CARRYING SOLUTIONS

It is intuitively attractive that resuscitation fluids should improve or maintain oxygen carriage and delivery, and experimental solutions are now available to do this. There is, however, considerable reserve afforded before anaemia from haemorrhage reduces tissue O_2 consumption, and hypovolaemia and hypotension are a more immediate threat to life. Gould and colleagues suggested a haemoglobin of 3.5 g/dl was critical, and an oxygen extraction ratio of ≥ 50%.[84] Nevertheless, in those trauma victims who suffer rapid haemorrhage and prolonged prehospital times, oxygen carrying solutions may prove beneficial, and have the advantages of long shelf-lives and no requirement for crossmatching. The solutions currently being developed can be divided into perfluorocarbons, haemoglobin solutions and liposome-encapsulated haemoglobin solutions, and have recently been subject to review.[85]

Perfluorocarbons are biologically inert liquids that are immiscible in water and are, therefore, prepared as emulsions for intravenous use. They are exhaled via the lungs as well as being taken up by the reticulo-endothelial system prior to progressive excretion. Plasma half-life has been loosely reported as 12–24 h.[86–88] Oxygen is dissolved and not bound, but their O_2

solubilities are high, and the O_2 content is linearly related to the pO_2 value and the concentration of fluorocarbon. Surfactants are employed to maintain small particle size, thus enabling higher perfluorocarbon concentrations and larger surface area for oxygen exchange. A first generation product, Fluosol-DA 20™, is approved for use in the USA to perfuse coronary arteries during angioplasty. It is licensed to be used up to a maximum dose of 40 ml/kg, and has been used in severely anaemic patients who are unable or unwilling to receive blood in the peri-operative period or during haemorrhage.[84,87,88,90,91] Fluosol-DA 20™ has only 20% emulsified fluorocarbon by weight, and thus has a limited oxygen carrying capacity. There are still concerns about the fate of the surfactant polymer used, its pulmonary actions and its ability to maintain small particular size and shelf-life. Currently Fluosol-DA is stored frozen and thawed out immediately prior to use. Second generation perfluorocarbons are being developed that utilise egg yolk phospholipids, used in parenteral nutrition, as emulsifiers. These have much higher shelf stability and concentration of perfluorocarbon and, thus, oxygen solubility. One such product, perfluorooctylbromide (PFOB), is 90% emulsified fluorocarbon by weight and is reported to have a refrigerated shelf-life of greater than 4 years.

Stromal free haemoglobin solutions were first used in humans in the 1940s.[92] Haemoglobin liberated from red cells dissociates into monomers and dimers consisting of α and β chains. These smaller sub-units of haemoglobin tetramers are filtered by the kidneys, reducing their intravascular half-lives and causing renal damage as they precipitate in the acidic ascending limb of the loop of Henle. Cross-linking, conjugation, polymerisation and formation of microspheres are all techniques which have been developed to extend intravascular life and reduce the toxicity of stromal free haemoglobin solutions. Cross-linked, polymerised and conjugated haemoglobin solutions have been successful in sustaining asanginous animal models through exchange transfusion. Microspheres are in earlier stages of development, but may have an O_2 carrying capacity superior to that of blood. Currently, five haemoglobin solutions are undergoing patient safety trials (Table 8.2).[93] Two are cross-linked and three polymerised; the source of haemoglobin is human, bovine and recombinant.

The shelf-lives of these products are reported as one year when frozen, and they have circulation times of approximately 6–8 h, with their uptake and breakdown being largely through the reticulo-endothelial system. Most haemoglobin solutions have demonstrated a vasopressor effect increasing systemic and pulmonary vascular resistance and, although the aetiology of this effect remains unknown, it is postulated that it is secondary to nitric oxide binding by free haemoglobin.

Liposome-encapsulated haemoglobin solutions were proposed in 1957 by Chang in his thesis, and their development and progress were reviewed in 1990.[94] Although still experimental, and having been used in animals only, it is proposed that encapsulation of haemoglobin molecules within a liposome will decrease filtration and toxicity and extend circulation times. It is also possible to manipulate the oxygen binding/unbinding characteristics by the inclusion of 2,3 DPG and similar adjuncts within the liposome and, by maintaining the tetrameric structure, the haemoglobin sub-units exhibit co-operativity. In animals, these solutions have demonstrated circulation half-lives of 16–20 h

Table 8.2 Hemoglobin-based red cell substitutes

Company	Corporate partner	Product	Type	FDA trial status
Baxter	None	HemAssist Diaspirin cross-linked	Human	Phase III, trauma, surgical, cardiac
Northfield	Pharmacia	PolyHeme Glutaraldehyde polymerized	Human	Late Phase II, trauma, surgical
Hemosol	Fresenius	HemoLink O-raffinose polymerized	Human	Early Phase II, surgical
Biopure	B. Braum Melsungen	Hemopure Gluteraldehyde polymerized	Bovine	Late Phase II, cardiac, surgical, trauma
Somatogen	Eli Lilly & Co	Optro Recombinantly cross-linked	Recombinant	Late Phase II, surgical

From[93] [Cohn S M. Is blood obsolete? J Trauma 1997; 42: 730–732] with the permission of the publishers Williams & Wilkins.

and have been successful in sustaining life, but there are concerns over toxicity and the effects of the liposomes within the reticulo-endothelial system that will have to be overcome.

PREVENTION OF SECONDARY CEREBRAL INJURY

The Brain Trauma Foundation recently published the American Association of Neurological Surgeons' guidelines for the management of severe head injury in July 1995,[95] after review of the world literature. The evidence surrounding many hotly-debated issues in the management of head injured patients was scrutinised by an expert panel before a comprehensive draft of recommendations was produced. These have been ranked as standards, guidelines and options in accordance with the strength of supporting evidence. They should now form the basis of management of head injuries.

Predictors of mortality in head injury are age, Glasgow Coma Score, motor response, reactivity of pupils, hypotension, raised intracranial pressure, failure of intracranial pressure to respond to treatment when raised, computed tomography findings of cerebral oedema and intraventricular blood, and the degree of midline shift.[98] Hypoxia isolated from other variables was also associated with prognosis in a study by Chestnut and colleagues of 717 individual cases (Table 8.3).[97] Those individuals suffering head injury and concomitant hypotension have unequivocally demonstrated higher mortality figures than normotensive patients.[96–102] Although it is unclear as to the exact figure that represents hypotension, these studies employed systolic blood pressures of less than 80 mmHg[96] to 95 mmHg,[102] with the majority,[97–101] including Pigula and colleagues' study in children,[100] using 90 mmHg. Ideally, any definition of hypotension should encompass the individual's previous physiological state and not exist as a single absolute value, and it may also be

Table 8.3 Traumatic Coma Data Bank (TCDB) data: outcome by secondary insult at time of arrival at TCDB hospital ER for non-mutually exclusive insults

Secondary insults	Number of patients	Percentage of total patients	Outcome percentage		
			Good or moderate	Severe or vegetative	Dead
Total cases	699*	100.0	42.9	20.5	36.6
Neither	456	65.2	51.1	21.9	27.0
Hypoxia	130	18.6	29.2	20.8	50.0
Hypotension	165	23.6	19.4	15.8	64.8
Both	52	7.4	5.8	19.2	75.0

Hypoxia = $PaO_2 < 60$ mmHg; hypotension = SBP < 90 mmHg.
*The total number of patients is 699 instead of 717 because of missing admission data on blood pressure or arterial blood gas values in 18 patients.
Table from Chestnut,[97] with permission.

more appropriate to use a figure of mean arterial pressure as opposed to systolic pressure. In a large prospective evaluation of trauma victims suffering severe head injury, hypotension was reported in 34.6% of cases and was associated with a 150% increase in mortality.[97] The duration of hypotensive events inversely correlates with the Glasgow outcome score.[99] In their study of intra-operative hypotension and head injury, Pietropaoli and colleagues[99] suggested that a period of hypotension greater than 5 min duration was detrimental to outcome, and they encouraged aggressive management of blood pressure. Pigula and colleagues[100] found that hypotension in children suffering head injury abrogated the protection afforded them by age, and worsened their outcome to that predicted for adults. In trauma victims, hypoxia is more common than hypotension and occurs in 45.6% of individuals.[97] It is described in many studies as an arterial pO_2 of less than 60 mmHg[97,98,100–102] and also has a significant effect on outcome from head injury.[97,102] A combination of hypoxia and hypotension was shown to be of greater detriment than either variable alone.[97]

In the only prospective, randomised, controlled study to date, retrospective subgroup analysis of those individuals suffering head injury revealed improved blood pressures and improved survival in the group receiving hypertonic fluid resuscitation for hypotension.[71] This may have resulted from improved haemodynamics, or from a separate effect of the hypertonic solution.

Hyperventilation has been employed in the management of head injury for many years and lowers intracranial pressure by cerebral vasoconstriction and decreasing cerebral blood flow. This approach has recently been criticised. Cerebral blood flow is decreased following head injury, particularly during the first 24 h,[103,104] and may fall near or below levels at which ischaemia occurs in up to one-third of cases during the first 6 h post injury.[103] Subsequently, individuals often develop hyperaemia or normal cerebral blood flow and those who exhibit early or continued ischaemia may reflect a worse clinical outcome.[103] Aggressive hyperventilation results more consistently in a further decrease in cerebral blood flow than in a reduction in intracranial pressure, with an adverse effect on arterial–jugular venous oxygen content difference and cerebral oxygen delivery.[105] A prospective, randomised study by Muizelaar and colleagues[106] investigated the use of hyperventilation for 5 days following injury and demonstrated fewer good neurological outcomes at 3 and 6 months in the group of patients which was hyperventilated. Hyperventilation used continuously has been shown to have a progressively diminishing effect such that cerebral vessel diameter has returned to baseline levels at 20 h, and subsequent elevation of pCO_2 values to normocapnia may result in rebound rises in intracranial pressure.[107] It is recommended, therefore, that prolonged and prophylactic hyperventilation should be avoided.[95] Similarly, aggressive hyperventilation ($PaCO_2 \leq 25$ mmHg) cannot be advised as it significantly reduces cerebral blood flow to levels that are judged to cause ischaemia (18.6 ± 4.4 ml/100 g/min).[105]

Mannitol has been advocated as the agent of choice in the control of intracranial pressure following severe head injury.[108] It is usually administered as a bolus infusion of 0.25–1.0 g/kg. It consistently lowers intracranial pressure and improves cerebral perfusion pressures and blood flow in head injured patients.[109,110] Mannitol is well known to be an osmotic diuretic, but the degree of diuresis is unrelated to its effect on intracranial pressure or cerebral perfusion pressure.[111] Although intuitively attractive, the concept of mannitol producing an osmotic gradient between the blood and brain and thus decreasing brain water content has been questioned.[111] Pollay and colleagues showed there was no correlation between the duration of the blood–brain osmotic gradient induced by mannitol and the duration of the effect of mannitol in reducing intracranial pressure.[112] In the light of the evidence from studies demonstrating little, if any, change in brain oedema and water content after the administration of mannitol, other mechanisms for its beneficial actions have been postulated. It now seems likely that the early effect of mannitol in lowering intracranial pressure is due to a reduction in blood viscosity and haematocrit. These rheological effects result in improved cerebral blood flow and O_2 delivery which, in turn, via autoregulatory mechanisms, cause reflex cerebral vasoconstriction and decreased cerebral blood volume.[109–111] These same studies showed that mannitol is most effective in individuals with low cerebral perfusion pressure (70 mmHg) and intact cerebral autoregulation.

Concern has been expressed that mannitol aggravates hypotension in haemorrhagic shock and, therefore, interferes with resuscitative efforts. This is largely unsubstantiated and mannitol has been advocated for the resuscitation of combined haemorrhagic shock and head injury and exhibits improved haemodynamics in animal models and humans.[56,113,114] There is evidence, however, that transient hypotension and increases in intracranial pressure result from rapid infusion (< 5 min) of mannitol boluses.[115] It is, therefore, recommended that administration be over 15–30 min. In cases of prolonged administration of mannitol, the diuretic effect may lead to dehydration, volume contraction and haemoconcentration. Not only is this detrimental, but it may lead to subsequent doses failing to control intracranial pressure, and hydration and normovolaemia must be maintained.[111] An animal model of cryogenic cerebral injury indicated a progressive accumulation of mannitol in the oedematous brain tissue following multiple doses, with a reversal of the osmotic gradient to favour oedema formation.[116] It is probable, therefore, that the effects of prolonged mannitol administration and of a single bolus differ and, while there is adequate evidence supporting bolus dose mannitol to lower intracranial pressure, there is limited support for its long term use and efficacy.

The American Association of Neurological Surgeons' guidelines[95] also consider the use of prophylactic anticonvulsants, barbiturates and glucocorticoids in severe head injury. In their review, the panel recommends that prophylactic phenytoin or carbamazepine are effective in preventing 'early' (within 7 days) post-traumatic seizures, but that there is insufficient evidence to suggest an improvement in outcome. The use of glucocorticoids is not supported in head injury, and neither is the use of barbiturates outside of an intensive care setting, as detrimental respiratory and haemodynamic sequelae are common.

The recommendations for the immediate management of severe head injuries are the restoration of circulating blood volume, perfusing blood pressure, oxygenation and ventilation as a priority. Specific treatment modalities that lend themselves to the first hour after injury, both prehospital and in the casualty department resuscitation room, are mannitol and hyperventilation. It is recommended that these should only be administered if there are signs of transtentorial herniation or progressive neurological deterioration not attributable to extracranial aetiology.[95]

HYPOTHERMIA

Animal models of brain injury have shown hypothermia to be beneficial in reducing tissue injury and oedema and improving outcome. In patients, mild hypothermia has been used in the treatment of uncontrollable intracranial hypertension secondary to brain injury.[117] Moderate hypothermia induced in patients as a protective measure early in the course of head injury management has shown encouraging results.[118,119] Marion and colleagues,[119] in a prospective randomised study of 82 patients presenting with closed head injury and a GCS < 8, investigated the effects of cooling patients to a temperature of 32–33°C for 24 h within an average of 10 h from injury. Whilst the overall outcomes were not significantly altered by cooling, the sub-group presenting with GCS of 5–7 demonstrated improved neurological outcome (measured by the Glasgow outcome score) at 3, 6 and 12 months. The hypothermia group demonstrated a lower mean intracranial pressure and cerebral blood flow, and a higher cerebral perfusion pressure during the initial period of induced cooling. The exact mechanism of protection is undetermined, but it is known that cerebral cooling produces a linear reduction in cerebral metabolism and O_2 consumption.[120] Marion[119] measured a highly significant decrease in the excitatory neurotransmitter glutamate within the cerebrospinal fluid with moderate hypothermia, and proposed that this transmitter is involved in the beneficial effects of hypothermia. A study in a rat model of uncontrolled haemorrhage has suggested that outcome is improved by hypothermia (30°C) either alone or in combination with hypotensive fluid resuscitation.[47]

The body of opinion concerning trauma patients without head injury supports the maintenance of normothermia, since increased mortality is associated with a falling core temperature in trauma victims,[121] although it is unclear whether hypothermia is instrumental or merely an associated observation. It is well established that temperatures below 35°C cause

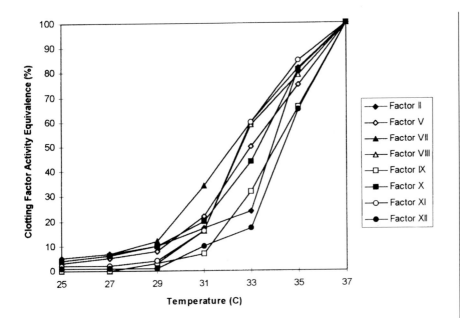

Fig. 8.1 Plot of functional effects of hypothermic plasma clotting conditions expressed as equivalent clotting times produced by specific clotting factor deficiencies under normothermic conditions. Figure from Johnston,[123] with permission.

prolongation of coagulation, and that temperatures below 33°C produce a coagulopathy equivalent to significant factor deficiency states (< 50% normal activity) despite normal clotting factor levels.[122,123] In their study, Gubler and colleagues[122] demonstrated an incremental platelet dysfunction with decreasing temperature below 35°C. The severity of hypothermia induced coagulopathy is often underestimated or missed as screening is conducted at 37°C and does not reveal this functional defect.

There has yet to be an advantage demonstrated in humans from permitting hypothermia in trauma cases without head injury, and, in these cases, normothermia is justified in order to promote haemostasis and wound healing. In head injury there is mounting support for controlled cooling of patients to preserve or improve neurological outcome, and Marion and colleagues[119] experienced no increased complication rate nor bleeding in the group of patients that they cooled to 33°C for 24 h.

CONCLUSIONS

The improvement in the structure of trauma management has resulted in a more thorough approach to these patients. Haemorrhage and head injury are the leading causes of mortality in this group and frequently co-exist, and the fundamental aim in the management of haemorrhage is surgical control. Whilst hypotension may benefit a specific group of patients; it is clearly detrimental to those suffering significant head injury. Conversely, moderate hypothermia may improve neurological outcome but induces a functional coagulopathy and may increase haemorrhage.

There is debate as to the efficacy of deploying paramedic teams to administer fluids at-scene, but the patients requiring airway support and ventilation benefit from early intervention. It is likely that the availability of ALS at-scene is beneficial to those severely injured patients experiencing prolonged prehospital times, and most authors still support a policy of early fluid resuscitation providing it does not delay transfer for definitive surgical intervention. In the absence of head injury this resuscitation may be limited permitting moderate hypotension. Those patients experiencing rapid and uncontrolled haemorrhage outside of hospital, or suffering concomitant head injury and haemorrhage, may be better resuscitated with hypertonic solutions.

The primary goal in the management of head injury is the restoration of cerebral perfusion pressure and oxygen delivery. Subsequent to injury and prior to surgical intervention and monitoring, this is best established by avoiding hypotension, hypovolaemia and arterial hypoxia. Administration of mannitol and moderate hyperventilation should be reserved for those individuals demonstrating clear signs of transtentorial herniation in the absence of other monitoring.

Future resuscitation may be improved by the availability of oxygen carrying solutions with long shelf-lives and no necessity to crossmatch, although frequently it is not anaemia that proves fatal.

Ultimately, the value of these and other developments in the immediate treatment of trauma depend upon the organisation of the healthcare delivery system. In the UK, at least, there is still some way to go.

References

1. Cales R H, Trunkey D D. Preventable trauma deaths: a review of trauma care systems development. JAMA 1985; 254: 1059–1063
2. Cales R H. Trauma mortality in Orange County: the effect of implementation of a regional trauma system. Ann Emerg Med 1984; 13: 1–10
3. Guss D A, Meyer F T, Neuman T S et al. The impact of a regionalized trauma system on trauma care in San Diego County. Ann Emerg Med 1989; 18: 1141–1145
4. Kane G, Wheeler N C, Cook S et al. Impact of the Los Angeles County trauma system on the survival of seriously injured patients. J Trauma 1992; 32: 576–583
5. Mullins R J, Veum-Stone J, Helfand M et al. Outcome of hospitalized injured patients after institution of a trauma system in an urban area. JAMA 1994; 271: 1919–1924
6. Shackford S R, Hollingworth-Fridlund P, Cooper G F et al. The effect of regionalization upon the quality of trauma care as assessed by concurrent audit before and after institution of a trauma system: a preliminary report. J Trauma 1986; 26: 812–820
7. Smith J S, Martin L F, Young W W et al. Do trauma centers improve outcome over non-trauma centers? The evaluation of regional trauma care using discharge abstract data and patient management categories. J Trauma 1990; 30: 1533–1538
8. Smith R F, Frateschi L, Sloan E et al. The impact of volume on outcome in seriously injured trauma patients: two years' experience of the Chicago trauma system. J Trauma 1990; 30: 1066–1076
9. West J G, Cales R H, Gazzaniga A B. Impact of regionalization: the Orange County experience. Arch Surg 1983; 118: 740–744
10. Anderson I O, Woodford M, de Dombal F T, Irving M A. A retrospective study of 1000 deaths from injury in England and Wales. BMJ 1988; 296: 1305–1308
11. Committee on Trauma. Hospital and prehospital resources for the care of the injured patient. Bull Am Coll Surg 1986; 71: 4–12
12. Hospital and prehospital resources for optimal care of the injured patient and appendices A–J. Chicago: American College of Surgeons, 1987

13. Trunkey D D. Trauma. Sci Am 1983; 249: 20–27.

14. Hill D A, West R H, Roncal S. Outcome of patients with haemorrhagic shock: an indicator of performance in a trauma centre. J R Coll Surg Edinb 1995; 40: 221–224

15. Hannan E L, O'Donnell J F, Kilburn Jr H et al. Investigation of the relationship between volume and mortality for surgical procedures performed in New York hospitals. JAMA 1989; 262: 503–510

16. Luft H S, Bunker J P, Enthoven A C. Should operations be regionalized? The empirical relationship between surgical volume and mortality. N Engl J Med 1979; 301: 1364–1369

17. Gray W A, Capone R J, Most A S. Unsuccessful emergency resuscitation – are continued efforts in the emergency department justified? N Engl J Med 1991; 325: 1393–1398

18. Kellerman A L, Staves D R, Hackman B B. In-hospital resuscitation following unsuccessful prehospital advanced cardiac life support: heroic effort or an exercise in futility? Ann Emerg Med 1988; 17: 589–594

19. Rosemurgy A S, Norris P A, Olson S M et al. Prehospital traumatic cardiac arrest: the cost of futility. J Trauma 1993; 35: 468–473

20. Clevenger F W, Yarbrough D R, Reines H D. Resuscitative thoracotomy: the effect of field time on outcome. J Trauma 1988; 28: 441–445

21. Purkiss S F, Williams M, Cross F W et al. Efficacy of urgent thoracotomy for trauma in patients attended by a helicopter emergency service. J R Coll Surg Edinb 1994; 39: 289–291

22. Vij D, Simoni E, Smith R F et al. Resuscitative thoracotomies for patients with traumatic injury. Surgery 1983; 94: 554–561

23. Bodai B I, Smith J P, Blaisdell F W. The role of emergency thoracotomy in blunt trauma. J Trauma 1982; 22: 487–491

24. Washington B, Wilson R F, Steiger Z, Bassett J S. Emergency thoracotomy: a four year review. Ann Thorac Surg 1985; 40: 188–191

25. Aprahamian C, Thompson B M, Towne J G, Darin J C. The effect of a paramedic system on mortality of major open intra-abdominal vascular trauma. J Trauma 1983; 23: 687–690

26. Jacobs L M, Sinclair A, Beiser A, D'Agostino R B. Prehospital advanced life support: benefits in trauma. J Trauma 1984; 24: 8–13

27. Pons P T, Honigman B, Moore E E et al. Prehospital advanced trauma life support for critical penetrating wounds to the thorax and abdomen. J Trauma 1985; 25: 828–832

28. Cwinn A A, Pons P T, Moore E E et al. Prehospital advanced trauma life support for critical blunt trauma victims. Ann Emerg Med 1987; 16: 399–407

29. Reines D H, Bartlett R L, Chudy N E et al. : Is advanced life support appropriate for victims of motor vehicle accidents: the South Carolina highway trauma project? J Trauma 1988; 28: 563–570

30. Potter D, Goldstein G, Fung S C, Selig M. A controlled trail of prehospital advanced life support in trauma. Ann Emerg Med 1988; 17: 582–588

31. Gerwin A S, Fisher R P. The importance of prompt transport in salvage of patients with penetrating heart wounds. J Trauma 1982; 22: 443–448

32. Smith J P, Bodai B I, Hill A S, Frey C F. Prehospital stabilization of critically injured patients: a failed concept. J Trauma 1985; 25: 65–70

33. Ivatury R R, Nallathambi N N, Roberge R J et al. Penetrating thoracic injuries: in-field stabilization vs prompt transport. J Trauma 1987; 27: 1066–1073

34. Mattox K L, Bickell W, Pepe P E et al. Prospective MAST study in 911 patients. J Trauma 1989; 29: 1104–1112

35. Kaweski S M, Sise M J, Virgilio R W. The effects of prehospital fluids on survival in trauma patients. J Trauma 1990; 30: 1215–1219

36. Martin R R, Bickell W H, Pepe P E et al. Prospective evaluation of pre-operative fluid resuscitation in hypotensive patients with penetrating truncal injury: a preliminary report. J Trauma 1992; 33: 354–362

37. Cayten C G, Murphy J G, Stahl W M. Basic life support versus advanced life support for injured patients with an injury severity score of 10 or more. J Trauma 1993; 35; 460–466

38. Honigman B, Rohweder K, Moore E E et al. Prehospital advanced trauma life support for penetrating cardiac wounds. Ann Emerg Med 1990; 19: 145–150

39. Durham L A, Richardson R J, Wall M J et al. Emergency center thoracotomy: impact of prehospital resuscitation. J Trauma 1992; 32: 775–779

40. American College of Surgeons, Committee on Trauma. Advanced trauma life support program (Instructor manual). Chicago: American College of Surgeons, 1993; 75–110

41. Bickell W H, Wall M J, Pepe P E et al. Immediate versus delayed fluid resuscitation for hypotensive patients with penetrating torso injuries. N Engl J Med 1994; 331: 1105–1109

42. Cooper A, Barlow B, DiScala C et al. Efficacy of prehospital volume resuscitation in children who present in hypotensive shock [Abstract]. J Trauma 1993; 35: 160

43. Kowolenko T, Stern S, Dronen S, Wang X. Improved outcome with hypotensive resuscitation of uncontrolled hemorrhagic shock in a swine model. J Trauma 1992; 33: 349–353

44. Bickell W H, Bruttig S P, Millnamow G A et al. The detrimental effects of intravenous crystalloid after aortotomy in swine. Surgery 1991; 110: 529–536

45. Stern S A, Dronen S C, Birrer P, Wang X. Effect of blood pressure on hemorrhage volume and survival in near-fatal hemorrhage model incorporating a vascular injury. Ann Emerg Med 1993; 22: 155–163

46. Capone A C, Safar P, Stezoski S W et al. Improved outcome with fluid restriction in treatment of uncontrolled hemorrhage . J Am Coll Surg 1995; 180: 49–56

47. Kim S-H, Stezoski S W, Safar P et al. Hypothermia and minimal fluid resuscitation increase survival after uncontrolled hemorrhagic shock in rats. J Trauma 1997; 42: 213–222

48. Sakles J C, Sena M J, Knight D A, Davis J M. Effect of immediate fluid resuscitation on the rate, volume, and duration of pulmonary vascular hemorrhage in a sheep model of penetrating thoracic trauma. Ann Emerg Med 1997; 29: 392–399

49. Wears R L, Winton C N. Load and go versus stay and play: analysis of prehospital i.v. fluid therapy by computer simulation. Ann Emerg Med 1990; 19: 163–168

50. Tranbaugh R F, Lewis F R. Crystalloid versus colloid for fluid resuscitation of hypovolaemic patients. Adv Shock Res 1983; 9: 203–216

51. Vigilio R W, Rice C L, Smith D E et al. Crystalloid versus colloid resuscitation: is one better? Surgery 1979; 85: 129–139

52. Velanovich V. Crystalloid versus colloid fluid resuscitation: a meta-analysis of mortality. Surgery 1989; 105: 65–71

53. Velasco I T, Pontieri V, Rocha e Silva M. Hyperosmotic NaCl and severe hemorrhagic shock. Am J Physiol 1980; 239: H664–H673

54. Nakayama S, Sibley L, Gunther R A et al. Small volume resuscitation with hypertonic saline (2400 mOsm/liter) during hemorrhagic shock. Circ Shock 1984; 13: 149–159

55. Bitterman H, Triolo J, Lefer A M. Use of hypertonic saline in the treatment of hemorrhagic shock. Circ Shock 1987; 21: 271–283

56. Smith J G, Kramer GC, Peron P et al. A comparison of several hypertonic solutions for resuscitation of bled sheep. J Surg Res 1985; 39: 517–528

57. Maningas P A, DeGuzman L R, Tillman F J et al. Small volume infusions of 7.5% NaCl in 6% Dextran 70 for the treatment of severe hemorrhagic shock in swine. Ann Emerg Med 1986; 15: 1131–1137

58. Wade C E, Hannon J P, Bossone C A et al. Resuscitation of conscious pigs following hemorrhage: comparative efficacy of small volume resuscitation. Circ Shock 1989; 29: 193–204

59. Velasco I T, Rocha e Silva M, Oliveira M A et al. Hypertonic and hyperoncotic resuscitation from severe hemorrhagic shock in dogs: a comparative study. Crit Care Med 1989; 17: 261–264

60. Walsh J C, Kramer G C. Resuscitation of hypovolaemic sheep with hypertonic saline/dextran: the role of dextran. Circ Shock 1991; 34: 336–343

61. Rocha e Silva M, Velasco I T, Nogueira D A et al. Hyperosmotic sodium salts reverse severe hemorrhagic shock: other solutes do not. Am J Physiol 1987; 253: H751–H762

62. Halvorsen L, Gunther R A, Dubick M A, Holcroft J W. Dose response characteristics of hypertonic saline/dextran solutions. J Trauma 1991; 31: 785–794

63. Pascual J M, Runyon D E, Watson J C et al. Resuscitation of hypovolaemia in pigs using near saturated sodium chloride solution in dextran. Circ Shock 1993; 40: 115–124

64. Vasser M J, Holcroft J W. Use of hypertonic-hyperoncotic fluids for resuscitation of trauma patients. J Intensive Care Med 1992; 7: 189–198

65. Chudnofsky C R, Dronen S C, Syverud S A et al. Intravenous fluid therapy in the prehospital management of hemorrhagic shock: improved outcome with hypertonic saline/6% Dextran 70 in a swine model. Am J Emerg Med 1989; 7: 357–363

66. Prist R, Rocha e Silva M, Velasco I T, Loureiro M I. Pressure driven hemorrhage: a new experimental design for the study of crystalloid and small volume hypertonic resuscitation in anesthetized dogs. Circ Shock 1992; 36: 13–20

67. Bickell W H, Bruttig S P, Millnamow G A et al. The use of hypertonic saline/dextran versus lactate Ringer's solution as a resuscitation fluid following uncontrolled aortic hemorrhage in anesthetized swine. Ann Emerg Med 1992; 21: 1077–1085

68. Vasser M J., Perry C A, Gannaway W L, Holcroft J W. 7.5% Sodium chloride/dextran for resuscitation of trauma patients undergoing helicopter transport. Arch Surg 1991; 126: 1065–1072

69. Younes R N, Aun F, Accioly C Q et al. Hypertonic solutions in the treatment of hypovolaemic shock: a prospective, randomized study in patients admitted to the emergency room. Surgery 1992; 111: 380–385

70. Mattox K L, Maningas P A, Moore E E et al. Prehospital hypertonic saline/dextran infusion for post-traumatic hypotension – the USA multicenter trial. Ann Surg 1991; 213: 482–491

71. Vasser M J, Fischer R P, O'Brien P E et al and the multicenter group for the study of hypertonic saline in trauma patients. A multicenter trial for resuscitation of injured patients with 7.5% sodium chloride: the effect of added Dextran 70. Arch Surg 1993; 128: 1003–1013

72. Vasser M J, Perry C A, Holcroft J W. Prehospital resuscitation of hypotensive trauma patients with 7.5% NaCl with added dextran: a controlled trial. J Trauma 1993; 34: 622–632

73. Dubick M A, Wade C E. A review of the efficacy and safety of 7.5% NaCl/6% Dextran 70 in experimental animals and in humans. J Trauma 1994; 36: 323–330

74. Kreimeier U, Frey L, Messmer K. Small volume resuscitation. Curr Opin Anaesthesiol 1993; 6: 400–408

75. Schmoker J D, Zhuang J, Shackford S R. Hypertonic fluid resuscitation improves cerebral oxygen delivery and intracranial pressure after hemorrhagic shock. J Trauma 1991; 31: 1607–1613

76. Prough D S, Johnson J C, Poole G V et al. Effects on intracranial pressure of resuscitation from hemorrhagic shock with hypertonic saline versus lactated Ringer's solution. Crit Care Med 1985; 13: 407–411

77. Prough D S, Johnson J C, Stump D A et al. Effects of hypertonic saline versus lactated Ringer's solution on cerebral oxygen transport during resuscitation from hemorrhagic shock. J Neurosurg 1986; 64: 627–632

78. Gunnar W, Jonasson O, Merlotti G et al. Head injury and hemorrhagic shock: studies of the blood brain barrier and intracranial pressure after resuscitation with normal saline solution, 3% saline solution, and Dextran 40. Surgery 1988; 103: 398–407

79. Battistella F D, Wisner D H. Combined hemorrhagic shock and head injury: effects of hypertonic saline (7.5%) resuscitation. J Trauma 1991; 31: 182–188

80. Wisner D H, Schuster L, Quinn C. Hypertonic saline resuscitation of head injury: effects of cerebral water content. J Trauma 1990; 30: 75–78

81. Ducey J P, Mozingo D W, Lamiell J M et al. A comparison of the cerebral and cardiovascular effects of complete resuscitation with isotonic and hypertonic saline, hetastarch, and whole blood following hemorrhage. J Trauma 1989; 29: 1510–1518

82. Anderson J T, Wisner D H, Sullivan P E et al. Initial small volume hypertonic resuscitation of shock and brain injury: short and long term effects. J Trauma 1997; 42: 592–601

83. Freshman S P, Battistella F D, Matteucci M, Wisner D H. Hypertonic saline (7.5%) versus mannitol: a comparison for treatment of acute head injuries. J Trauma 1993; 35: 344–348

84. Gould S A, Rosen A L, Sehgal L R et al. Fluosol-DA as a red-cell substitute in acute anemia. N Engl J Med 1986; 314: 1653–1656

85. Dietz N M, Joyner M J, Warner M A. Blood substitutes: fluids, drugs, or miracle solutions? Anesth Analg 1996; 82: 390–405

86. Waxman K. Perfluorocarbons as blood substitutes. Ann Emerg Med 1986; 15: 1423–1424

87. Tremper K K, Friedman A E, Levine E M et al. The preoperative treatment of severely anemic patients with a perfluorochemical oxygen-transport fluid, Fluosol-DA. N Engl J Med 1982; 307: 277–283

88. Spence R K, McCoy S, Costabile J et al. Fluosol-DA 20 in the treatment of severe anemia: randomized, controlled study of 46 patients. Crit Care Med 1990; 18: 1227–1230

89. Gould S A, Sehgal L R, Rosen A L et al. Assessment of a 35% fluorocarbon emulsion. J Trauma 1983; 23: 720–724

90. Mitsuno T, Ohyanagi H, Naito R. Clinical studies of a perfluorochemical whole blood substitute (Fluosol-DA). Summary of 186 cases. Ann Surg 1982; 195: 60–69

91. Waxman K, Tremper K K, Cullen B F, Mason R. Perfluorocarbon infusion in bleeding patients refusing blood transfusions. Arch Surg 1984; 119: 721–724

92. Amberson W R, Jennings J J, Rhode C M. Clinical experience with hemoglobin-saline solutions. J Appl Physiol 1949; 1: 469–489

93. Cohn S M. Is blood obsolete? J Trauma 1997; 42: 730–732

94. Rabinovici R, Rudolph A S, Ligler F S et al. Liposome-encapsulated hemoglobin: an oxygen-carrying fluid. Circ Shock 1990; 32: 1–17

95. Bullock R, Chestnut R M, Clifton G et al. The American Association of Neurological Surgeons' guidelines for the management of severe head injury. The Brain Trauma Foundation, July 1995. Eur J Emerg Med 1996; 3: 109–127

96. Marmarou A, Anderson R L, Ward J D et al. Impact of ICP instability and hypotension on outcome in patients with severe head trauma. J Neurosurg 1991; 75: S59–S66

97. Chestnut R M, Marshall L F, Klauber M R et al. The role of secondary brain injury in determining outcome from severe head injury. J Trauma 1993; 34: 216–222

98. Fearnside M R, Cook R J, McDougall P et al. The Westmead Head Injury Project outcome in severe head injury. A comparative analysis of prehospital, clinical and CT variables. Br J Neurosurg 1993; 7: 267–279

99. Pietropoali J A, Rogers F B, Shackford S R et al. The deleterious effects of intra-operative hypotension on outcome in patients with severe head injury. J Trauma 1992; 33: 403–407

100. Pigula F A, Wald S L, Shackford S R et al. The effect of hypotension and hypoxia on children with severe head injuries. J Pediatr Surg 1993; 28: 310–316

101. Wald S, Fenwick J, Shackford S R. The effects of secondary insults on mortality and long term disability of severe head injury in a rural region without a trauma system. J Trauma 1993; 34: 377–382

102. Miller J D, Becker D P. Secondary insults to the injured brain. J R Coll Surg Edinb 1982; 27: 292–298

103. Bouma G J, Muizelaar J P, Choi S C et al. Cerebral circulation and metabolism after severe traumatic brain injury: the elusive role of ischemia. J Neurosurg 1991; 75: 685–693

104. Marion D W, Darby J, Yonas H. Acute regional cerebral blood flow changes caused by severe head injuries. J Neurosurg 1991; 74: 407–414

105. Obrist W D, Langfitt T W, Jaggi J L et al. Cerebral blood flow and metabolism in comatose patients with acute head injury. J Neurosurg 1984; 61: 241–253

106. Muizelaar J P, Marmarou A, Ward J D et al. Adverse effects of prolonged hyperventilation in patients with severe head injury: a randomized clinical trial. J Neurosurg 1991; 75: 731–739

107. Muizelaar J P, Van der Poel H G, Li Z et al. Pial arteriolar vessel diameter and CO_2 reactivity during prolonged hyperventilation in the rabbit. J Neurosurg 1988; 69: 923–927

108. Miller J D, Piper I R, Dearden N M. Management of intracranial hypertension in head injury: matching treatment with cause. Acta Neurochir 1993; 57 (Suppl.): 152–159

109. Muizelaar J P, Lutz H A, Becker D P. Effect of mannitol on ICP and CBF and correlation with pressure autoregulation in severely head injured patients. J Neurosurg 1984; 61: 700–706

110. Mendelow A D, Teasdale G M, Russell T et al. Effect of mannitol on cerebral blood flow and cerebral perfusion pressure in human head injury. J Neurosurg 1985; 63: 43–48

111. Rosner M J, Coley I. Cerebral perfusion pressure: a hemodynamic mechanism of mannitol and the postmannitol hemogram. Neurosurgery 1987; 21: 147–156

112. Pollay M, Fullenwider C H, Roberts P A, Stevens F A. The effect of mannitol and furosemide on the blood-brain barrier osmotic gradient and intracranial pressure. J Neurosurg 1983; 59: 945–950

113. Israel R S, Marx J A, Moore E E, Lowenstein S R. Hemodynamic effect of mannitol in canine model of concomitant increased intracranial pressure and hemorrhagic shock. Ann Emerg Med 1988; 17: 560–566

114. Feldman J A, Fish S. Resuscitation fluid for a patient with head injury and hypovolemic shock. J Emerg Med 1991; 9: 465–468

115. Ravussin P, Archer D P, Tyler J L et al. Effects of rapid mannitol infusion on cerebral blood volumes: a positron emission tomographic study in dogs and man. J Neurosurg 1986; 64: 104–113

116. Kaufmann A M, Cardoso E R. Aggravation of vasogenic cerebral edema by multiple dose mannitol. J Neurosurg 1992; 77: 584–589

117. Shiozaki T, Sugimoto H, Taneda M et al. Effect of mild hypothermia on uncontrollable intracranial hypertension after severe head injury. J Neurosurg 1993; 79: 363–368

118. Clifton G L, Allen S, Barrodale P et al. A phase 2 study of moderate hypothermia in severe brain injury. J Neurotrauma 1993; 10: 263–271

119. Marion D W, Penrod L E, Kelsey S F et al. Treatment of traumatic brain injury with moderate hypothermia. N Engl J Med 1997; 336: 540–546

120. Bering Jr E A. Effect of body temperature change on cerebral oxygen consumption of the intact monkey. Am J Physiol 1961; 200: 417–419

121. Jurkovich G J, Greiser W B, Luterman A, Curreri P W. Hypothermia in trauma victims: an ominous predictor of survival. J Trauma 1987; 27: 1019–1024

122. Gubler K D, Gentilello L M, Hassantash S A, Maier R V. The impact of hypothermia on dilutional coagulopathy. J Trauma 1994; 36: 847–851

123. Johnston T D, Chen Y, Reed R L. Functional equivalence of hypothermia to specific clotting factor deficiencies. J Trauma 1994; 37: 413–417

Hugh Montgomery Mervyn Singer

CHAPTER 9

Non-invasive monitoring of cardiac output

Measurement of cardiac output has traditionally been the poor relation to pressure monitoring because of the perceived risks, complexity and expense of pulmonary artery catheterisation.[1-3] The latest National Confidential Enquiry into Perioperative Deaths[4] highlighted how only a small minority of the reviewed patients had intraoperative pulmonary artery catheter monitoring yet over three-quarters were classified as being ASA Grade III or higher. No mention was made as to whether cardiac output was actually measured during the operation. The onset of significant haemodynamic deterioration and organ dysfunction is often the cue for its introduction; this belated insertion may partly explain the difficulty in demonstrating any benefit in the critically ill patient. Indeed, a recently published retrospective analysis has actually suggested possible detriment.[5] This paper has generated considerable debate as to when, how and in whom this invasive approach should be used. It has also given added impetus to the development of alternative flow monitoring techniques that are either non- or minimally invasive and, with advances in technology, increasingly reliable and user-friendly. Many of these techniques also provide additional information on circulatory status, e.g. cardiac preload, ventricular contractility and extravascular lung water, which can further assist therapeutic decision making. The particular benefits that could arise from noninvasive flow assessment are early identification and either prevention, or faster correction, of circulatory derangements before a significant tissue oxygen debt has been allowed to develop. This proactive philosophy may impact significantly upon postoperative outcome.[6,7]

Dr **Mervyn Singer** MBBS MD FRCP, Senior Lecturer in Intensive Care, Bloomsbury Institute of Intensive Care Medicine, University College London Medical School, Rayne Institute, University Street, London WC1E 6JJ, UK

Dr **Hugh Montgomery** MBBS BSc MD MRCP, Lecturer in Intensive Care, Bloomsbury Institute of Intensive Care Medicine, University College London Medical School, Rayne Institute, University Street, London WC1E 6JJ, UK

Any blinding enthusiasm for non-invasive techniques should be tempered by awareness of the limitations of both the machine and the technology being utilised. Not infrequently, poor equipment design, over-stated abilities and/or inadequate user education have generated unfavourable studies. This may contribute more to an understandable wariness on the part of the clinician rather than to any inherent problem with the technique itself which is often discredited in the process. It thus behoves prospective users to familiarise themselves fully with both theory and practice underlying a particular device, to develop sufficient expertise to recognise unreliable or erroneous signals, and to be aware of any limitations. All technologies have flaws, and data derived from different methods do not necessarily correlate well. Techniques may often be better at monitoring change rather than delineating absolute output itself. This chapter will provide a brief overview of currently available technology, highlighting some of the recognised pitfalls.

DOPPLER ULTRASONOGRAPHY

The velocity of a moving object can be calculated from the shift in reflected frequency of a sound wave of known frequency.

$$V = (Df \times C)/(2f_t \times \cos \theta) \hspace{3cm} \text{Eq. 1}$$

where v = velocity of the moving blood corpuscles; Df = Doppler frequency shift; C = sound velocity in tissue; f_t = transmitted frequency; and θ = angle between ultrasound beam and the flow direction.

For blood flow measurement, high frequency ultrasound waves are directed at moving erythrocytes. These Doppler frequency shift signals can undergo fast Fourier transform spectral analysis and be displayed in real time as velocity–time waveforms on a monitor (Fig. 5.1).

Doppler measurement of aortic blood flow was first described in the 1960s, initially via a transthoracic approach and then from a probe placed in the suprasternal notch directed at either the ascending or arch portions of the aorta.[8,9] Validations performed against reference techniques, such as thermodilution, have confirmed its accuracy.[10] It is quick, easy to perform,

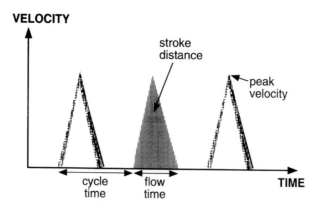

Fig. 5.1 Doppler velocity-flow waveform.

totally non-invasive and painless. However, up to 5% of patients cannot be readily measured due to either anatomical (e.g. short neck) or pathological (e.g. emphysema, mediastinal air postcardiothoracic surgery, aortic valve disease) factors.

Sufficient experience is a prerequisite for accurate measurement and there is an appreciable learning curve.[11] Furthermore, no adequate means has been found to tether the suprasternal probe in a correct position to enable continuous monitoring. In view of this, other approaches have been sought with varying success. A modified tracheal tube with a Doppler probe sited at the tip[12] was launched commercially with minimal validation and met an early demise. The oesophagus has proved the most promising route. Since first described in 1971,[13] a number of machines have been marketed though these have been of variable quality.[14–16] A personal preference is exercised for the ODM® device (Abbott Laboratories) which, importantly, has an integral monitor and loudspeaker displaying the spectral analysis to verify correct signal interrogation. Furthermore, this machine has undergone numerous single- and multi-centre validation studies which have shown reliable and reproducible results.[17,18] An important rider is the need for adequate training beforehand though the learning curve is steep.

A 6 mm diameter 4 MHz continuous wave Doppler transducer is inserted orally into the distal oesophagus to a depth of 35–40 cm. A characteristic blood flow signal from the descending thoracic aorta is readily distinguishable on the monitor. Insertion and correct positioning take a matter of minutes. The area of each velocity–time waveform – the **stroke distance** – is a representation of stroke volume flowing down the descending thoracic aorta. Applying a correction factor from a nomogram (incorporating the patient's age, height and weight) enables an estimate of total left ventricular stroke volume to be determined to 85–90% accuracy from the descending aortic flow measurement alone. Intra- and interobserver variability is low and trend-following is accurate despite wide variations in flow, blood pressure and body temperature. Trend-following has also been shown to be accurate in children[19] and a nomogram for cardiac output estimation is currently under development for this age group.

Only aortic coarctation, use of an intra-aortic balloon pump and, possibly, thoracic aortic aneurysms provide no meaningful signals. Moderate or severe aortic regurgitation produces a characteristic reverse flow throughout the whole of diastole. Caution should be observed in patients with oesophageal varices or other local pathology, and in those with marked coagulopathies. However, no serious adverse event has yet been reported.

The waveform shape also provides valuable information on left ventricular preload, afterload and resistance.[20,21] There are age-related normal ranges for peak velocity; values falling outside this range indicate hypo- or hyperdynamic circulations. The waveform base – the flow time – can be automatically corrected for heart rate by dividing the flow time by the square root of the cycle time. This corrected flow time (FTc) is inversely proportional to systemic vascular resistance. A dilated circulation is reflected by a prolonged FTc (usual range 0.33–0.36 s) and vice versa with vasoconstriction. This latter situation arises from hypovolemia, flow obstruction (e.g. pulmonary embolus, pericardial tamponade) and excess arterial constriction (e.g. excessive norepinephrine). Challenging the circulation with fluid or nitrate boluses is a useful and rapid means of distinguishing between these causes. Starling-like curves can be constructed to optimise fluid and dilator therapy. Whereas preload changes predominantly affect the FTc, inotropic changes mainly affect the peak velocity while afterload changes have an intermediate effect. The effects of therapy can thus be readily appreciated on a beat-by-beat basis.

ECHOCARDIOGRAPHIC EVALUATION

Echocardiographic techniques (either transthoracic or transoesophageal) can be used to estimate cardiac output[22-29] in one of two ways:

Combined use of imaging with Doppler signal derivation

Two steps are required. The Doppler flow velocity is measured as described above though, with the echocardiographic technique, the flow being interrogated is usually in or close to the heart, e.g. across the mitral valve or, commonly, in the aortic root. Echocardiographic measurement of cross-sectional area at this point will allow calculation of cardiac output as the product of blood velocity averaged over a minute and cross-sectional area. For the Doppler flow velocity profile, signal sampling of as little as 10% of the cross-sectional area allows mean velocity to be estimated. However, the non-uniform cross-sectional distribution of flow (especially in the presence of turbulence) at the aortic root may make this measurement unreliable. Further error derives from the difficulty in orientating the Doppler signal to that of the blood flow direction, and from beat-to-beat variation in stroke volume. Aortic vessel area at the valve ring (or just distal to the sinuses of Valsalva) is calculated from aortic root diameters from 2-dimensional images, assuming a circular shape. However, the aorta and main pulmonary trunk are more ellipsoid than circular, and root area varies with timing in the cardiac cycle, and with changes in preload, afterload and cardiac dynamics. Planimetric measurement, enhanced by recently-developed edge-detection technology, may improve the accuracy of calculated cardiac outputs although it may still prove difficult to obtain accurate short-axis views.

A similar methodology has been applied in measuring flow across a measured left ventricular outflow tract, pulmonary artery or mitral valve (at the level of the annulus) cross-sectional area. The use of transmitral flow seems particularly useful, with the valve area being measured by planimetry, or estimated from diameters obtained in two- and four-chamber views assuming an elliptical shape.

The use of combined transoesophageal echocardiographic imaging and Doppler probes allows estimation of cardiac output in the critically ill more readily than transthoracic imaging techniques.

Calculation from ventricular volumes

If ventricular volume at end-systole and end-diastole are measured, stroke volume can be calculated as the difference between these two values, and cardiac output as the product of this stroke volume and heart rate.

Recently developed technology allows 3-dimensional reconstruction of images of the left ventricle. Routinely, however, ventricular volumes will still be calculated from 2-D and M-Mode images although these often rely upon assumptions about LV shape, namely:

- The cube method assumes that $V = D^3$, where D = the LV short-axis diameter. This method assumes symmetrical wall motion.

- The Teichholz method better corrects for ventricular shape, and states that $V = D^3(7.0/[2.4 + D])$.

- The bullet method assumes that the LV cavity is bullet-shaped. Here, $V = 5AL/6$ where A is the area of the short axis in cross-section and L the cavity length.

- Area–length calculations assume that the ventricle is an elongated ellipse. Images in two planes (best obtained using biplanar transoesophageal images) are derived, length (L) and orthogonal short-axis diameters (D_1 and D_2, respectively) are measured, and LV volume calculated as $0.524 \times D_1 \times D_2 \times L$.

- Simpson's method involves obtaining multiple short-axis images of known spacing. The volume of each 'slice' is then calculated from its dimensions (or measured by planimetry), and the volumes summed to yield a total ventricular volume. Irregular ventricular shape entails deriving more slices, good endocardial imaging and accurate timing of images in the cardiac cycle.

- Automated quantitation of cavity size using sophisticated real-time edge-detection technology has recently been demonstrated, and has the advantage that continuous measures can be made, with little operator-dependence.

TRANSTHORACIC IMPEDANCE

In 1966, Kubicek described the thorax as a cylinder evenly perfused with blood of specific resistivity 'p', itself related to the haematocrit.[30] Pulsatile thoracic aortic blood flow caused negative impedance changes (measured from a steady state mean base impedance (Z), with a maximum rate of change $[(dZ/dt)_{max}]$ of Z_m during systole between pairs of electrodes placed around the neck and upper abdomen.

$$SV = p(L^2/Z^2)Z_m \qquad \text{Eq. 2}$$

where SV = stroke volume; p = electrical resistivity of the blood; L = mean separation of the inner pair of electrodes; Z_m = maximum rate of change of impedence $(dZ/dt)_{max}$ during systole; and Z = basic impedance between the inner electrodes.

The original Kubicek equation consistently overestimated SV. Furthermore, it was subsequently shown that the thorax behaves electrically more as a truncated cone rather than as a cylinder. Correction factors have been advanced, most notably by assuming that blood resistivity is a trivial component of total thoracic resistivity, and the original equation thus much refined, notably by Sramek[31] and Bernstein.[32] This, and the application of new technology, renders transthoracic impedance of potential clinical use and the new equations have been incorporated into commercial systems such as the NCCOM-3® (Biomed Medical Manufacturing Ltd, Irvine, CA, USA). Common systems have involved the application of a sensing electrode to either side of the neck root and to opposite sides of the body in a mid-coronal plain at xiphisternum level. Two pairs of transmitting electrodes are placed 5 cm above the neck sensors and 5 cm below the thoracic sensors, respectively. Accurate electrode placement is crucial using such systems. The use of oesophageal electrodes may overcome some of these problems, and may improve the reliability of data accrued on the ICU.[33] A clear ECG trace is required in order to allow gating of data acquisition, and displacement of a single lead will falsely reduce cardiac output.

Much of the systolic changes seen in bioimpedance relate to pulsatile descending aortic blood flow. Cardiac output measures derived in this way correlate reasonably with those derived by thermodilution and Doppler methodology (r values 0.5–0.9).[34–36] Although reliability may be impaired by body movement or mechanical ventilation, computer analysis can eliminate the variations due to gross movement (which changes the shape of the electrical field, and can be recognised as artifact) and respiration (whose fluctuations are much less frequent than the cardiac cycles being assessed). Shivering, valvular regurgitation, pacemaker devices, atrial fibrillation, the use of positive end-expiratory pressure, marked tachycardia, different brands of electrode and possibly poor left ventricular function all impede reliability and are much harder to account for.[37–39] The technique may overestimate cardiac output in low-flow states, and underestimate cardiac output in the hyperdynamic state (where correlation of results with thermodilution yields r values of only 0.3) and early after cardiac surgery.

Although data derived from this system may, under some circumstances, correlate well with those derived from thermodilution (and even prove more reproducible in individual subjects), the varying impedance technologies and derived equations have yet to be validated in individuals of both sexes and of diverse age and habitus in varied clinical situations. Adoption of the technique in the ICU setting cannot yet be recommended. Its use in the Emergency Room (to allow rapid and non-invasive monitoring of responses to resuscitation) or on the operating table may prove more rapidly accepted.

PULSE CONTOUR ANALYSIS

Since the rate at which blood flows from arteries to veins is proportional to the rate of fall of arterial pressure, analysis of the contour of the aortic pulse-wave allows determination of cardiac output. The area of the arterial waveform (or pulse contour) was first described as a means of monitoring cardiac output by Frank in 1899. This pulse contour cardiac output technique (PCCO) can be performed non-invasively from a finger pressure waveform using a Finapres® device[40] or from an indwelling arterial cannula which is being pressure-transduced.[41–44] However, it cannot be used for quantitation of cardiac output unless a calibration tool such as thermodilution is used. Over the last two decades, various equations have been developed by different researchers for monitoring stroke volume. Essentially, all use the product of the area below the pressure contour, the heart rate and an individual calibration factor which accounts for the individually variable vascular impedance. Despite being a century old, sparse data exist in the literature regarding validation of PCCO against other techniques and recognition of any pitfalls. The effect of rapid changes in blood pressure, posture, body temperature and vasopressor agents are but a few factors which could potentially render the technique unreliable. Further studies are necessary before this technique can be recommended for routine usage.

COLD® TECHNIQUE

Depending on the desired measurement, this technique[45] utilises cannulae placed in either femoral or radial artery, pulmonary artery and/or a central vein. A bolus of cold fluid can be injected into any central vein and thermodilution cardiac output measured from a special 3 French gauge arterial catheter placed in a femoral or radial artery. The size of catheter also makes it applicable for use in children.[46] This catheter has an optional oximetry probe for continuous measurement of arterial oxygen saturation. A similar catheter can be placed in the pulmonary artery for cardiac output measurement and monitoring of mixed venous oxygen saturation. A new development allows continuous measurement of cardiac output by pulse contour analysis with automatic re-calibration being performed by intermittent thermodilution injections.

The device is also geared for measurement of indocyanine green concentrations in the blood; following a bolus of indocyanine green into (preferably) a central vein, cardiac output can be computed from the dye dilution curve produced at the arterial catheter site. A fibreoptic reflectance densitometer inbuilt into this catheter measures the indocyanine green concentration. An additional advantage is that elimination of this dye is almost entirely via the liver. The plasma disappearance rate can be used to assess hepatic function. With normal liver function only a tiny fraction of the injected indocyanine green is still detectable in the bloodstream after 10 min.

The device also purports to measure: (i) global end-diastolic volume, i.e. the sum of the end-diastolic volumes of both left and right atria and ventricles; (ii) intrathoracic blood volume; and (iii) extravascular lung water. It has been suggested that intrathoracic blood volume can be used as an indicator of cardiac preload. A further claim is that cardiac performance can be derived from the ratio of cardiac output and global end-diastolic volume and be used to direct vasoactive drug therapy. Confirmatory studies to support these marketing claims are scanty.

DIRECT FICK METHOD

The Fick principle states that oxygen consumption (VO_2) equals the product of cardiac output and the arterio-venous oxygen concentration difference. For cardiac output measurement, the arterial oxygen concentration is measured from a peripheral arterial blood sample, the venous oxygen concentration from pulmonary arterial blood, while VO_2 is derived from minute ventilation and inspired and expired gas analysis.[23,28,47,48] In a variation of this method, CO_2 production may be used instead of oxygen consumption,[49] utilising the equation cardiac output equals VCO_2 divided by $(Cvco_2 - Caco_2)$ where VCO_2 is CO_2 production, and $Cvco_2$ and $Caco_2$ are mixed venous and arterial CO_2 concentrations, respectively. $Cvco_2 - Caco_2$ can be calculated from measured partial pressures while VCO_2 can now be accurately measured using computerised dual beam infrared absorption analysers. Estimates of oxygen consumption, based on either standard equations or on expired carbon dioxide production measurements, were found to be poor substitutes for metabolic measurements of oxygen consumption in critically ill subjects and gave inaccurate estimates of cardiac output.[49] This may be related to excessive respiratory O_2 consumption and CO_2 production in critical illness affecting the lung.

THE BRADLEY METHOD

A clinical means for estimating cardiac output and peripheral vascular resistance was devised by Bradley.[50] In experienced hands, this has been shown to be a reliable technique, however, a validation study showing good agreement when compared against thermodilution has only been published in abstract form and it has yet to be shown to be readily transferable to novices.

It relies upon a version of Ohm's law where the voltage gradient across a circuit equals the product of current and resistance. In the systemic circulation, the pressure gradient across the circuit (mean arterial pressure minus central venous pressure) measured in mmHg equals the product of cardiac output (in l/min) and peripheral vascular resistance (in Wood units). Assessment is made over four stages:

1. Assessment of pressure gradient. Central venous pressure (estimated clinically or recorded from a central venous catheter) and mean arterial blood pressure (from invasive or non-invasive measurements) are recorded.

2. Assessment of peripheral vascular resistance. This is quantified in Wood units. The Wood unit is dimensionless. A dimensional value is obtained by multiplying by 80 to yield $dyne.s.cm^{-5}$. This assessment assumes that a progressive increase in peripheral vascular resistance is associated with a progressively proximal level of vasoconstriction. Thus, if the resistance is very high (> 40 Wood units), there will be a palpable 'cut-off' between 'warm' and 'cold' skin above the elbow. With progressive dilatation, this cut-off level will move distally, until the whole arm and fingers are warm (20 Wood units). With more advanced dilatation, the fingers (when lightly squeezed together as in a hand-shake) will have a palpable pulsatile feel (15 Wood units). When very vasodilated (< 10 Wood units), the forearms can be felt to pulsate when lightly gripped circumferentially in both hands.

3. Using the data thus derived, cardiac output (l/min) and stroke volume (ml) can be calculated.

4. Stroke volume (SV) is also estimated directly by palpation of the central arterial pulses. If SV derived in this way (SV_2) matches that derived from step 'c' (SV_1) then assessment is concluded. Otherwise, a back-calculation is performed using the new estimate of SV (i.e. SV_2) to provide new estimates of cardiac output (CO_2) and peripheral resistance (R_2). The original resistance value is now reassessed in the light of R_2. By repeated backward and forward adjustment of estimates, a final set of figures for estimated SV and resistance are obtained which are compatible with the blood pressure, central venous pressures, estimate of peripheral vasodilatation, and pulse character.

A confusing situation can arise where the stroke volume estimation from the pulse character predicts a very high cardiac output, yet this estimate cannot be resolved from that derived by direct assessment of peripheral vascular resistance, i.e. skin warmth and digit/forearm assessment which predict too high a resistance for the palpated pulse volume. In this circumstance a shunt must exist with very high flows going to areas other than the skin and forearm muscles. This occurs either in the septic circulation or when macrovascular shunts exist, e.g. aorto-caval fistula.

LITHIUM DILUTION

Though not yet commercially available, this technique, like indocyanine green, also employs the dye dilution principle but with lithium chloride as the indicator.[51,52] This is injected as a 0.15–0.3 ml bolus into a central vein. The arterial plasma [Li+] level is measured by a lithium-selective electrode in a flow-through cell connected by a three way tap to a standard arterial cannula. The sampling rate of blood is of the order of 4 ml/min. The voltage across the membrane of the electrode is related to the plasma [Li+] and a correction applied for the plasma sodium concentration which can cause some minor interference. The cardiac output is computed from the lithium concentration-time curve by the following equation:

$$\text{Cardiac output (l/min)} = \frac{\text{LiCl dose} \times 60}{\text{Area} \times (1 - \text{PCV})} \qquad \text{Eq. 3}$$

where LiCl is in mmol, area is the integral of the primary curve (mmol/s) and PCV is the packed cell volume. This may be estimated as hemoglobin concentration (g/dl) divided by 33 and is a necessary correction as lithium is only distributed in plasma and not in red blood cells. The primary curve is due to the initial circulation of lithium following injection. The integral of the primary curve is obtained from an equation deriving the integral of a log-normal from the first part of the curve. The secondary curve which is due to recirculation of the indicator is thus ignored. Early studies with this technique have shown good agreement with cardiac output measured by both continuous and bolus thermodilution techniques.[52]

Key points for clinical practice

- There are a number of cardiac output monitoring techniques that are either non- or minimally invasive.

- Cardiac output data derived from different methods do not necessarily correlate well, even against so-called gold standards.

- Many provide additional information on circulatory status, e.g. cardiac preload, ventricular contractility and extravascular lung water.

- These techniques facilitate early identification and prevention/faster correction of circulatory derangements before a significant tissue oxygen debt has been allowed to develop.

- The operator should be familiar with the theory and practice underlying a particular device, be aware of any limitations, and be able to recognise unreliable or erroneous signals.

References

1. Gore J M, Goldberg R J, Spodick D H, Alpert J S, Dalen J E. A community-wide assessment of the use of pulmonary artery catheters in patients with acute myocardial infarction. Chest 1987; 92: 721–727
2. Elliot C G, Zimmerman G A, Clemmer T P. Complications of pulmonary artery catheterisation in the care of critically ill patients. A prospective study. Chest 1979; 76: 647–652
3. Slung H B, Scher K S. Complications of the Swan-Ganz catheter. World J Surg 1984; 8: 76–81
4. Report of the National Confidential Enquiry into Perioperative Deaths (NCEPOD) 1993/1994, London 1996
5. Connors Jr A F, Speroff T, Dawson N V et al. The effectiveness of right heart catheterization in the initial care of critically ill patients. SUPPORT Investigators. JAMA 1996; 276: 889–897
6. Mythen M G, Webb A R. Perioperative plasma volume expansion reduces the incidence of gut mucosal hypoperfusion during cardiac surgery. Arch Surg 1995; 130: 423–429
7. Sinclair S, James S, Singer M. Intraoperative intravascular volume optimisation reduces hospital stay following repair of proximal femoral fracture. BMJ 1997; In press
8. Light L H. Non-injurious ultrasonic technique for observing flow in the human aorta. Nature 1969; 224: 1119–1121
9. Huntsman L L, Stewart D K, Barnes S R, Franklin S B, Colocousis J S, Hessel E A. Non-invasive Doppler determination of cardiac output in man. Circulation 1983; 67: 593–602
10. Chandraratna P A, Nanna M, McKay C et al. Determination of cardiac output by transcutaneous continuous-wave ultrasonic Doppler computer. Am J Cardiol 1984; 53: 234–237
11. Gardin J M, Dabestani A, Matin K, Allfie A, Russell D, Henry W L. Reproducibility of Doppler aortic flow measurements: studies on intra-observer, inter-observer and day-to-day variability in normal subjects. Am J Cardiol 1984; 54: 1092–1098
12. Abrams J H, Weber R E, Holmen K D. Continuous cardiac output determination using transtracheal Doppler: initial results in humans. Anesthesiology 1989; 71: 11–15
13. Side C D, Gosling R J. Non-surgical assessment of cardiac function. Nature 1971; 232: 335–336
14. Siegel L C, Shafer S L, Martinez G M, Ream A K, Scott J C. Simultaneous measurements of cardiac output by thermodilution, esophageal Doppler and electrical impedance in anesthetized patients. J Cardiothorac Anesth 1988; 2: 590–595

15. Lavandier B, Cathignol D, Muchada R, Bui Xuan B, Motin J. Noninvasive aortic blood flow measurement using an intraesophageal probe. Ultrasound Med Biol 1985; 11: 451–460

16. Singer M, Clarke J, Bennett E D. continuous hemodynamic monitoring by esophageal Doppler. Crit Care Med 1989; 17: 447–452

17. Belot J P, Valtier B, de la Coussaye J E, Mottin D, Payen D. Continuous estimation of cardiac output in critically ill mechanically ventilated patients by a new transoesophageal Doppler probe. Intensive Care Med 1992; 18 (Suppl.2): P241

18. Klotz K-F, Klingsiek S, Singer M et al. Continuous measurement of cardiac output during aortic cross-clamping by the oesophageal Doppler monitor ODM 1. Br J Anaesth 1995; 74: 655–660

19. Murdoch I A, Marsh M J, Tibby S M, McLuckie A. Continuous haemodynamic monitoring in children: use of transoesophageal Doppler. Acta Paediatr 1995; 84: 761–764

20. Singer M, Bennett E D. Non-invasive optimization of left ventricular filling by esophageal Doppler. Crit Care Med 1991; 19: 1132–1137

21. Singer M, Allen M J, Webb A R, Bennett E D. Effects of alterations in left ventricular filling, contractility and systemic vascular resistance on the ascending aortic blood velocity waveform of normal subjects. Crit Care Med 1991; 19: 1138–1145

22. Wilson A F. Noninvasive measurement of cardiac output. Cardiologia 1995; 40: 551–559

23. Christie J, Sheldahl L M, Tristani F E, Sagar K B, Ptacin M J, Wann S. Determination of stroke volume and cardiac output during exercise: comparison of two-dimensional and Doppler echocardiography, Fick oximetry, and thermodilution. Circulation 1987; 76: 539–547

24. Flachskampf F. Recent progress in quantitative echocardiography. Curr Opin Cardiol 1995; 10: 634–639

25. Uehara Y, Koga M, Takahashi M. Determination of cardiac output by echocardiography. J Vet Med Sci 1995; 57: 401–407

26. Pai R G, Shah P M. Echocardiographic and other noninvasive measurements of cardiac hemodynamics and ventricular function. Curr Probl Cardiol 1995; 20: 681–770

27. Troianos C A, Porembka D T. Assessment of left ventricular function and hemodynamics with *transesophageal echocardiography. Crit Care Clin 1996; 12: 253–272

28. Axler O, Tousignant C, Thompson C R et al. Comparison of *transesophageal echocardiographic, Fick, and thermodilution cardiac output in critically ill patients. J Crit Care 1996; 11: 109–116

29. Darmon P L, Hillel Z, Mogtader A, Mindich B, Thys D. Cardiac output by *transesophageal echocardiography using continuous-wave Doppler across the aortic valve. Anesthesiology 1994; 80: 796–805

30. Kubicek W G, Karnegis J N, Patterson R P, Witsoe D A, Mattson R H. Development and evaluation of an impedance cardiac output system. Aerospace Med 1966; 37: 1208–1212

31. Sramek B B. Thoracic electrical bioimpedance measurement of cardiac output. Crit Care Med 1994; 22: 1337–1339

32. Bernstein D P. A new stroke volume equation for thoracic electrical bioimpedance. Theory and rationale. Crit Care Med 1986; 14: 902–904

33. Balestra B, Malacrida R, Leonardi L, Suter P, Marone C. Esophageal electrodes allow assessment of cardiac output by bioimpedance. Crit Care Med 1992; 20; 62–67

34. de May C, Matthews J, Butzer R, Schroeter V, Belz G G. Agreement and reproducibility of the estimates of cardiovascular function by impedance cardiography and M-mode echocardiography in healthy subjects Br J Clin Pharmacol 1992, 34: 88–92

35. Appel P, Kram H B, Mackabee J, Fleming A W, Shoemaker W C. Comparison of measurements of cardiac output by bioimpedance and thermodilution in severely ill surgical patients. Crit Care Med 1986; 14: 933–935

36. Tremper K. Transthoracic electrical bioimpedance versus thermodilution technique for cardiac output measurement during mechanical ventilation Intensive Care Med 1989; 15: 219–220

37. Preiser J C, Daper A, Parquier J N, Contempre B, Vincent J L. Transthoracic electrical bioimpedance versus thermodilution technique for cardiac output measurement during mechanical ventilation. Intensive Care Med 1989; 15: 221–223

38. Sageman W S, Amundson D E. Thoracic electrical bioimpedance measurement of cardiac output in postaortocoronary bypass patients. Crit Care Med 1993; 21: 1139–1142

39. Young J D, McQuillan P. Comparison of thoracic electrical bioimpedance and thermodilution for the measurement of cardiac index in patients with severe sepsis. Br J Anaesth 1993; 70: 58–62

40. Gratz I, Kraidin J, Jacobi A G, deCastro N G, Spagna P, Larijani G E. Continuous noninvasive cardiac output as estimated from the pulse contour curve. J Clin Monit 1992; 8: 20–27

41. English J B, Hodges M R, Sentker C et al. Comparison of aortic pulse-wave contour analysis and thermodilution methods of measuring cardiac output during anaesthesia in the dog. Anesthesiology 1980; 52: 56–61

42. Tannenbaum G A, Mathews, Weissman C. Pulse contour cardiac output in surgical intensive care unit patients. J Clin Anesth 1993; 5: 471–478

43. Dos Santos P, Coste P, Bernadet P, Durrieu-Jais C, Besse P. Continuous monitoring of cardiac output by analysis of the pulse contour. Arch Mal Coeur Vaiss 1994; 87: 65–74

44. Irlbeck M, Forst H, Briegel J, Haller M, Peter K. Continuous measurement of cardiac output with pulse contour analysis. Anaesthesist 1995; 44: 493–500

45. von Spiegel T, Wietasch G, Bursch J, Hoeft A. Cardiac output determination with transpulmonary thermodilution. An alternative to pulmonary catheterization? Anaesthesist 1996; 45: 1045–1050

46. McLuckie A, Murdoch I A, Marsh M J, Anderson D. A comparison of pulmonary and femoral artery thermodilution cardiac indices in paediatric intensive care patients. Acta Paediatr 1996; 85: 336–338

47. Neuhoff H, Wolf H. Method for continuously measured oxygen consumption and cardiac output for use in critically ill patients. Crit Care Med 1978; 6: 155–161

48. Espersen K, Jensen E W, Rosenborg D et al. Comparison of cardiac output measurement techniques: thermodilution, Doppler, CO_2-rebreathing and the direct Fick method. Acta Anaesthesiol Scand 1995: 39; 245–251

49. Sherman M S, Kosinski R, Paz H L, Campbell D. Measuring cardiac output in critically ill patients: disagreement between thermodilution-, calculated-, expired gas-, and oxygen consumption-based methods. Cardiology 1997; 88: 19–25

50. Thomson G, Baker L, Mawby E, Leach R M. Simultaneous comparison of five techniques of cardiac output measurement [Abstract]. Intensive Care Med 1996; 22: S354

51. Linton R A F, Band D M, Haire K M. A new method of measuring cardiac output in man using lithium dilution. Br J Anaesth 1993; 71: 262–266

52. Linton R, Band D, O'Brien T, Jonas M, Leach R. Lithium dilution cardiac output measurement: a comparison with thermodilution. Crit Care Med 1998; In press

Ian S. Grant Graham R. Nimmo

Inotropic support in the critically ill patient

A successful outcome in the critically ill patient depends upon normalisation of physiological function, which in turn depends upon the re-establishment of adequate tissue oxygen delivery. In the last 15 years, a more systematic approach to this objective has evolved based upon the clinical measurement and subsequent therapeutic manipulation of the patient's haemodynamic and oxygen transport variables. Invasive monitoring in the form of an arterial line and pulmonary artery catheter (PAC) allow measurement of mean arterial pressure (MAP), cardiac output (CO) and oxygen content in both arterial (CaO_2) and mixed venous ($C\bar{v}O_2$) blood, from which other parameters of cardiovascular function and global oxygen transport can be derived.

The complexities of regional perfusion are such that monitoring of local and regional oxygen delivery is much more difficult to achieve, and overall adequacy of tissue oxygen delivery can only be assessed in clinical practice by surrogate markers such as hydrogen ion (H^+) concentration, base deficit, blood lactate concentration and gastric intramucosal pH (pH_i).

Inotropic agents are a crucial component of the management strategy in most areas of critical illness; this review attempts to discuss the role of the various inotropic agents in the context of a variety of critical illness states, and in relation to the objective of optimising tissue oxygen delivery (DO_2).

AIMS OF INOTROPIC THERAPY

Tissue oxygen delivery and normal organ function

The function of the circulation is to deliver oxygen and nutrients to the metabolically active tissues, whilst removing carbon dioxide and waste products,

Dr Ian S. Grant FRCP FFARCSI, Consultant Anaesthetist and Director of Intensive Care, Western General Hospital, Crewe Road, Edinburgh EH4 2XU, UK

Dr Graham R. Nimmo MD MRCP FFARCSI, Consultant Physician, Acute Receiving Unit, Intensive Care Unit, Western General Hospital, Crewe Road, Edinburgh EH4 2XU, UK

allowing the organs to function normally. Initial resuscitation of the critically ill patient involves correction of hypoxaemia with oxygen therapy and ventilatory support, and optimisation of intravascular volume. If, after these interventions, there are ongoing signs of tissue hypoxia or organ dysfunction with inadequate blood pressure and/or cardiac output, then vasoactive drug treatment is indicated.

In general terms, the aim is to achieve an appropriate level of tissue DO_2 for each patient. Critical illness comprises a heterogeneous group of conditions with different metabolic demands, while the patients have varying physiological reserve (ischaemic heart disease, chronic obstructive pulmonary disease etc), and hence precise therapeutic end-points must be tailored to the individual situation. The goals of treatment will, therefore, depend on: (i) the disease process, (ii) the patient's acute physiological derangement, and (iii) chronic disease and prior treatment, e.g. drugs for cardiac disease. In all patients, the aim is for a blood pressure, cardiac output and oxygen delivery which will result in the restoration of normal end-organ function with normalisation of arterial blood lactate and improvement in base deficit as markers of this.

MONITORING OF THERAPY

Haemodynamics and oxygen transport

Systemic haemodynamics and whole body oxygen transport are widely used to guide resuscitation of critically ill patients. Since the most flow dependent function of the circulation is the bulk transport of oxygen, it is clear that 'haemodynamic' monitoring must involve consideration of the adequacy of oxygen transport.

Standard monitoring in the critically ill involves systemic arterial and central venous pressure measurement. The use of a balloon-tipped, flow-directed PAC allows measurement of central venous, pulmonary artery and wedge pressure, cardiac output and mixed venous oxy-haemoglobin saturation ($S\bar{v}O_2$). The PAC allows optimal volume loading with titration of fluids against wedge pressure to achieve optimal left ventricular function.

Until recently, the PAC has been accepted as standard monitoring in the critically ill patient.[1] However, results of one multi-centre study have led the authors to state that ICU patients with PACs inserted in the first 24 h of admission have a higher mortality than those without.[2] Detailed analysis of this paper, and the ensuing debate, is outwith the scope of this chapter, but a balanced viewpoint is presented in the statement by the Society of Critical Care Medicine on the use of the PAC.[3] A comprehensive review of haemodynamic and oxygen transport monitoring is provided by Nightingale.[4]

Since vaso-active drugs can affect oxygen transport by altering cardiac output, regional perfusion and metabolic rate, comprehensive monitoring of these would be ideal (*vide infra*). Since VO_2 reflects the balance between supply and requirements it cannot be used on its own as a marker of the adequacy of oxygen transport.

Acid–base status: H+, lactate and base deficit

The search for indicators of the adequacy of tissue perfusion and oxygenation is long-running, and continues. In the light of the complex pathophysiology of tissue hypoxia in critical illness, it is unlikely that any one single marker will monitor all situations, and an approach which combines a group of variables may be most valuable.

Lactate

Lactate is formed from pyruvate as the product of anaerobic oxidation of glucose. Arterial blood lactate (ABL) concentration has been proposed as an indicator of anaerobic respiration but reflects the balance between production (which is increased by factors other than tissue hypoxia, e.g. hyperglycaemia) and removal, thus complicating its interpretation. The response of elevated blood lactate concentrations to resuscitation may be more useful since a falling lactate usually reflects improvement.[5] In contrast, vasoconstrictors may worsen tissue hypoxia, and some catecholamines may raise lactate concentrations by increasing intracellular lactate production.[6] Adrenaline is more likely to raise lactate concentrations than noradrenaline, and metabolic acidosis can occur (*vide infra*).

Base deficit and H⁺

The metabolic acidosis in shock is not solely a lactic acidosis. Some investigators have used base deficit to guide resuscitation, since metabolic acidosis may reflect altered cellular metabolism without tissue hypoxia.[7] In clinical practice, the achievement of improving base deficit and/or falling ABL are useful, if crude, guides to resuscitation. Central or mixed venous acid–base status may better reflect tissue hypoxia than arterial acid–base status.[8]

Hepatosplanchnic oxygenation

It has been suggested that gut mucosal hypoxia leads to loss of the mucosal barrier, and paves the way for endotoxaemia, sepsis syndrome and multiple organ failure. The ability to measure the adequacy of splanchnic oxygenation is thus important as a guide to the adequacy of resuscitation. Hypoperfusion of the gastrointestinal tract is associated with intramucosal acidosis, and gastric pH_i can be measured using a saline filled balloon tonometer.[9] The clinical usefulness of these measurements to guide resuscitation has yet to be confirmed. This type of monitoring may be most useful when other indicators of adequacy of resuscitation are normal, e.g. during ICU stay rather than during initial resuscitation.[10]

Organ function

Renal function

The quantity of urine produced is used as a marker of the adequacy of resuscitation, whilst urine quality is frequently not measured.[11] If urinary sodium is low and osmolality high there is a pre-renal element to oliguria which will often respond to improvements in the circulation. Urine output temporally lags behind the achievement of adequate renal oxygen delivery,

Table 10.1 Activity of inotropes at adrenoreceptors and other sites

Agents	Sites of action				
	α_1	β_1	β_2	DA	PDE
Noradrenaline	++++	++	0	0	0
Adrenaline	+++	+++	++	0	0
Dopamine	+++	+++	+	+++	0
Dobutamine	(+)	+++	+++	0	0
Dopexamine	0	+	++++	++	0
Milrinone	0	0	0	0	+++
Enoximone	0	0	0	0	+++

DA, dopamine; PDE, phosphodiesterase; α_1, alpha-1-adrenoreceptor; β_1, beta-1-adrenoreceptor; β_2, beta-2-adrenoreceptor.

and time should be allowed for improvement. Creatinine clearance is a good indicator of renal function but is not a real time monitor, and loss of 50% of renal function occurs before plasma creatinine rises. Once diuretics (including dopamine) have been administered, urine output is even less useful as a guide to the adequacy of resuscitation.

CATEGORIES OF INOTROPIC DRUG

The three main groups of drugs with inotropic actions are catecholamines, phosphodiesterase inhibitors and digitalis glycosides. Most of the agents which we use have additional, and clinically important, vasoconstrictor or vasodilator effects mediated through α_1 or β_2 effects. The activity profiles for the commonly used inotropes are shown in Table 10.1 and a practical classification of vasoactive drugs according to effects is presented in Table 10.2. Differences in the response of individuals to these drugs are related to the heterogeneity of patients and the specific conditions which are present. Many of the clinical studies have been, by necessity, conducted on small numbers of patients and generalisation to larger populations is difficult. In both septic and low flow shock, the relationship between oxygen delivery and consumption is extremely finely balanced and this balance may be affected either beneficially or detrimentally by vasoactive drug therapy. Several important practical points regarding the initiation of inotropic treatment are listed in Table 10.3.

Catecholamines

Sympathomimetic amines are used extensively in the management of the critically ill patient. The classification set out in Table 10.1 takes account of the effects of the drugs on the cardiovascular system, mediated via the α- and β-adrenoreceptors. These effects often differ in the critically ill patient from those seen in physiologically normal subjects. The effect of inotropes on cardiac contractility is reduced in certain disease states, e.g. left ventricular failure or severe sepsis where the numbers and function of β-adrenoceptors may be

Table 10.2 Functional classification of vasoactive drugs

Vasoconstrictors	Inoconstrictors	Inodilators	Vasodilators
Methoxamine	Adrenaline	Dobutamine	GTN
Phenylephrine	Dopamine	Dopexamine	SNP
Noradrenaline		Milrinone	
		Enoximone	

GTN, glyceryl trinitrate; SNP, sodium nitroprusside.

subnormal, the phenomenon of receptor down-regulation.[12] The same phenomenon may involve α-adrenoreceptors in septic shock.

The naturally occurring catecholamines (adrenaline, dopamine, noradrenaline) are the mainstay of the normally functioning human sympathetic nervous system with effects on heart rate, vascular tone and myocardial function. In the presence of circulatory dysfunction, these agents are used in pharmacological amounts to improve haemodynamics. The synthetic sympathomimetic amines (isoprenaline, dobutamine, dopexamine, ephedrine, phenylephrine, methoxamine) are all used in various areas of anaesthesia, but, apart from dobutamine and dopexamine, are of limited use in the critically ill.

Phosphodiesterase inhibitors

These agents increase myocardial contractility and cause vasodilatation by increasing intracellular cAMP concentrations via inhibition of the enzyme phosphodiesterase (PDE). PDE is present as a number of different enzymes and inhibitors, such as theophylline, which act on several of these will have some effect on haemodynamics. However, those agents which are specific for PDE-III (enoximone, milrinone, amrinone) have clinically useful inodilator effects with reduction in preload and afterload in addition to increased cardiac output (Table 10.2).[13] Their principal clinical indications are in severe left ventricular failure and in cardiogenic shock compounded by left ventricular failure, where their profile of haemodynamic effects results in improved left ventricular function and reduction in cardiac filling pressures (*vide infra*). In low cardiac output septic shock refractory to catecholamines, PDEs have been shown to improve left ventricular function and CO.[14]

Table 10.3 Practical points regarding the use of catecholamines

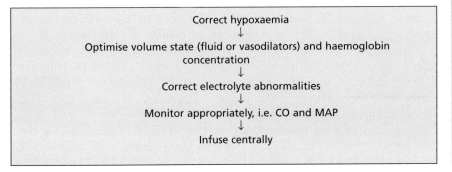

Correct hypoxaemia
↓
Optimise volume state (fluid or vasodilators) and haemoglobin concentration
↓
Correct electrolyte abnormalities
↓
Monitor appropriately, i.e. CO and MAP
↓
Infuse centrally

Digoxin

Digoxin and the other digitalis glycosides have long been used in the treatment of heart failure complicated by atrial fibrillation, for the combination of inotropic effect and control of heart rate. Despite having been in common use for over 200 years, the exact mechanisms of action of digoxin on myocardial contractility are still debated. The use of digoxin in the ICU is limited, and has not been systematically investigated. However, it can contribute to the management of the patient with impaired cardiac function who will require continued inotropic therapy when weaned from ventilation and intravenous agents.[15]

Vasodilators

In order to optimise cardiac filling pressures and haemodynamics, particularly in low flow states (*vide infra*), vasodilators are used in conjunction with inotropes. Intravenous nitrates, such as glyceryl trinitrate, at low doses are venodilators acting through the nitric oxide pathway. At higher doses, arterial vasodilatation may be achieved.

Angiotensin converting enzyme inhibitors (ACEI) are also used in patients with poor myocardial function and high cardiac filling pressures and, like nitrates, may form part of the medium and long term treatment for these patients. Caution must be exercised in the introduction of ACEIs, as the ICU patient may be at risk of severe hypotension or renal dysfunction with their administration. Further discussion on these and other vasodilators is outwith the scope of this chapter.

Catecholamines: individual agents

Adrenaline

In health, adrenaline is the most abundant endogenous circulating catecholamine, and its plasma concentrations increase 50-fold in severe haemorrhagic shock. It produces a combination of α-, β_1- and β_2-receptor activation with a tendency to predominance of α activity at higher concentrations, e.g. with bolus administration. Its effects include positive inotropism and chronotropism (β_1), peripheral vasodilatation especially in skeletal muscle and bronchodilator effects (β_2) and peripheral vasoconstriction (α). Metabolic effects mediated by β_1- and β_3-adrenoreceptors include hyperglycaemia, lipolysis and lactate and ketone production.

By bolus injection, adrenaline 1 mg (10 ml of 1:10 000 solution) has long been a mainstay in the management of cardiac arrest, largely for its vasopressor action. Its balance of vasoconstrictor, inotropic and bronchodilator effects make it the ideal agent for anaphylactic shock (1–2 ml i.v. boluses of 1:10 000 solution), and theoretically beneficial by infusion for patients with shock of various aetiologies. This usage of adrenaline has lessened in the face of newer agents, such as dopamine and dobutamine, but its role in the intensive care unit has recently been re-examined both in the context of first-line treatment of septic shock[16–18] and in high dosage as a treatment for unresponsive shock.[19,20]

As a first-line agent, adrenaline in a dosage range of 0.05–0.4 µg/kg/min consistently improves MAP and CO in fluid resuscitated patients with septic shock. Heart rate change is small, and left ventricular stroke work index (LVSWI) rises markedly (70–100%). The balance of effects on systemic vascular resistance (SVR) appears to depend on the pattern of shock present. Those patients with low CO tend to vasodilate in response to the rise in CO, while those with hyperdynamic septic shock tend to vasoconstrict.[16] Wilson et al[17] demonstrated a rise in ABL in some patients following adrenaline infusion with associated poor outcome. The hyperlactataemia may reflect local vasoconstriction and ischaemia, hyperglycaemia causing increased lactate production, or lactate washout from re-perfused tissues. Nevertheless, adrenaline's balance of beneficial α and β agonist effects make it a useful first-line therapy in shock.

Other workers have examined its role as a vasoconstrictor in patients with hyperdynamic septic shock already treated with dopamine[19] or dobutamine.[20] Much larger doses were employed (0.11–1 µg/kg/min) and the predominant effect was one of vasoconstriction with a rise in MAP but minimal effect on CO. Bollaert and colleagues again demonstrated an increase in ABL level in all patients, although it subsequently decreased in survivors.[19]

A number of groups have compared the effects of adrenaline in septic shock with other catecholamines, either a combination of dobutamine and noradrenaline[21,22] or dopamine alone,[23] with particular focus on ABL concentrations, splanchnic blood flow[22] and gastric pH_i.[21,22] In randomised prospective trials, all three groups[21–23] demonstrated an adrenaline-induced lactic acidosis, which resolved when adrenaline was discontinued. In those studies with the dobutamine/noradrenaline combination as comparator, the adrenaline-induced lactic acidosis was shown to be associated with splanchnic ischaemia as assessed by gastric intramucosal acidosis, and ICG-measured splanchnic blood flow. Furthermore, splanchnic oxygen delivery and consumption were significantly reduced during adrenaline infusion.[22] The results of these studies provide evidence that the hyperlactataemia seen with adrenaline in septic shock patients may be in part the result of splanchnic ischaemia, which is at the very least potentially harmful to the patient. It is unclear why adrenaline should be more detrimental than the noradrenaline/dobutamine combination, which has similar receptor effects and pharmacological actions, and more work requires to be done to explain this. In the meantime, however, it would appear that adrenaline has no routine place in long-term vasoactive therapy in shock. However, it is still valuable and, indeed, may be the agent of choice in the resuscitation and stabilisation of the severely shocked patient.

Noradrenaline

Noradrenaline is the principal postganglionic sympathetic neurotransmitter in the body, as well as being secreted in small amounts by the adrenal medulla. Synthesised by hydroxylation of dopamine, its clinical effects are due to activation of α- and $β_1$-adrenoreceptors, the α effects predominating, especially at higher doses.

After a gap of around 15 years during which time noradrenaline was discarded as a therapeutic agent in shock, the clinical introduction of the PAC led to a better understanding of the haemodynamic picture in individual patients with septic shock, and paved the way for its re-introduction to correct otherwise intractable hypotension associated with systemic vasodilatation.[24,25] In a dose range of 0.5–5 µg/kg/min, it consistently raises SVR and MAP without significantly affecting CO in fluid resuscitated septic shock; LVSWI rises substantially, reflecting the effect of noradrenaline's cardiac β_1 agonist activity counteracting the α mediated vasoconstriction. It should be stressed that noradrenaline should, in general, be employed with pulmonary artery catheter monitoring to ensure adequate filling, and to follow changes in CO, and with sequential measurement of H^+, base excess and blood lactate levels.

Anxiety about the effect of noradrenaline on renal and splanchnic circulations is based on its α agonist activity profile, and observations in non-septic subjects.[26] Studies in critically ill septic patients provide strong evidence that noradrenaline improves urine production following restoration of MAP, and improves renal function as assessed by serum creatinine and creatinine clearance whether or not noradrenaline is given in combination with low dose dopamine.[27,28] There are few studies of renal blood flow in relation to noradrenaline, but what evidence there is suggests that, while noradrenaline increases renal vascular resistance, renal blood flow is maintained or increased.[29]

The effect of noradrenaline on the splanchnic circulation is possibly of greater importance given the postulated role of the gut and liver in the pathogenesis of sepsis and multiple organ failure.[30] Ruokonen and his colleagues[31] investigated the effects of both dopamine and noradrenaline in 10 patients with hyperdynamic septic shock using hepatic venous catheterisation to allow measurement of splanchnic blood flow from ICG clearance and calculation of splanchnic oxygen delivery and consumption from splanchnic blood flow and arterial and hepatic venous oxygen saturations. They found a variable effect on splanchnic blood flow, with either an increase or little change. Overall splanchnic blood flow rose by 34% while CI increased by 14%. Using gastric pH_i as a measure of splanchnic perfusion, a noradrenaline infusion increased pH_i in comparison to dopamine which led to a decrease in pH_i after 3 h infusion.[32] The combination of correction of gastric intramucosal acidosis, correction of lactic acidosis and improvement in urine production following administration of noradrenaline in septic shock patients[27,31,33] suggests reversal of hypotension is beneficial to regional perfusion. The finding that oxygen consumption (VO_2) may rise also in the absence of a rise in DO_2 further implies beneficial effects on tissue oxygenation.[34]

Noradrenaline may also be used beneficially in situations where an increase in MAP is required without otherwise unduly affecting systemic haemo-dynamics or regional perfusion, e.g. to increase cerebral perfusion pressure in acute brain injury (*vide infra*).

Dopexamine

Dopexamine is a relatively new synthetic dopamine analogue. Its spectrum of receptor activity includes a potent post-junctional DA-1 agonism, weaker DA-2 agonism, and β_2 agonism. There is only weak β_1 agonist activity and an absence of α receptor activity. Dopexamine does, however, have positive inotropic action by virtue of its inhibition of neuronal catecholamine re-uptake.

Its inodilator properties would appear ideally suited to low cardiac output cardiac failure, where its dopaminergic activity may, in addition, augment renal perfusion, diuresis and natriuresis. The diuresis is principally mediated by DA-1 receptors in the renal tubules rather than being solely due to renal vasodilatation.[35,36]

The presence of dopaminergic and β_2 receptors in the splanchnic circulation has prompted the clinical investigation of its use in critically ill surgical patients and patients with sepsis, where its potential effect of improving hepatosplanchnic blood flow may be considered important in preventing or treating multiple organ failure. Some of the studies relating to splanchnic perfusion are outlined below.

Dopexamine was the agent used by Boyd et al[37] in their study on optimising DO_2 in surgical patients. The benefits in terms of improved survival resulting from peri-operative achievement of a DO_2 of $\geq$ 600 ml/min/m² have been attributed to dopexamine, but it remains to be seen whether the fluid administered or another inodilator would have had a similar result.

Ephedrine

The haemodynamic effects of ephedrine can be likened to 'weak' adrenaline. It has direct and indirect α- and β-adrenoreceptor agonism, β predominating, with positive inotropic and chronotropic effects resulting in increased cardiac output, and with increased blood pressure. Although it is valuable in many anaesthetic settings, its relatively low potency and the potential for tachyphylaxis make it unsuitable for most intensive care situations.

Dopamine

This naturally occurring catecholamine has a fascinating range of actions (Table 10.3) due to the receptors with which it interacts, and its ability to trigger noradrenaline release when infused. Initial study of its effects led investigators to conclude that there was a simple linear dose response effect from renal vasodilatation through an inotropic range (β_1) to a vasoconstrictor dose (α_1).[38,39] The evidence for a selective increase in renal blood flow with 'low' or 'renal' dose dopamine in critically ill humans is scanty[40] and it is interesting to remember that the range for 'renal dose' dopamine (varying from 1–4 µg/kg/min depending on the author) includes doses which were used to improve CO and reverse hypotension in the original study of its use in human shock.[38] In clinical practice, the effects do not follow the dose-response pattern detailed above and, in a study of human septic shock,[41] Meier-Hellmann and colleagues showed an increase in CI of 1 l/min/m² (23%) with 3 µg/kg/min. The wide interpatient variation in response to dopamine (and dobutamine) may be partly explained by the findings of a study of catecholamine clearance in children.[42] These investigators found a wide spread of plasma clearance rates of free dopamine and dobutamine due to differences in renal excretion and liver metabolism.

Recent studies and commentary have highlighted the complexity of potentially detrimental effects of dopamine on splanchnic oxygenation.[31,43] Further information is required before it can be assumed that 'low dose' dopamine is beneficial.[31,43] Meier-Hellmann and colleagues suggested that the effects of 'low dose' dopamine (3 µg/kg/min) on splanchnic blood flow in septic shock are variable depending on initial fractional splanchnic flow.[41] In patients with lower fractional splanchnic flow, the overall splanchnic blood flow increased by 89% along with splanchnic DO_2 (72%) and splanchnic VO_2 (37%), while there were no significant changes in patients with higher fractional splanchnic perfusion.

There is increasing evidence to show that dopamine exhibits suppression of the majority of anterior pituitary-dependent hormones, an effect which is unlikely to be beneficial.[44] In addition dopamine may be involved in reducing the hypoxic ventilatory response, a potentially important effect in the spontaneously ventilating critically ill patient.[45]

Many clinicians use dopamine first line in septic shock because of its spectrum of activity, adding dobutamine or noradrenaline as appropriate. Like adrenaline, it will increase blood pressure whilst increasing or maintaining CO in many circumstances. In view of this we would recommend one of these agents for 'first aid' resuscitation, e.g. in theatre or during transfer when we are monitoring invasive BP and CVP but not CO, and until PAC insertion.[16] Dopamine has compared favourably to adrenaline in a study of septic shock,[26] where adrenaline use was associated with worsening lactic acidosis.

Dobutamine

Dobutamine is a synthesised derivative of isoprenaline and is a mixture of two isomers. It exhibits inodilator effects through its β_1- and β_2-adrenoreceptor activity (Table 10.3). It has less chronotropic effect than isoprenaline, and, in a small proportion of patients – notably those with β_1 adrenoreceptor down-regulation – increases blood pressure via α-adrenoreceptor stimulation.[46]

Dobutamine was originally used for low flow states, and is still widely used in severe left ventricular dysfunction and cardiogenic shock.[47] Its place in the management of septic shock, low flow shock and neurogenic pulmonary oedema are detailed below. Another potential indication is in the resuscitation of patients with low cardiac output secondary to negatively inotropic drugs taken as treatment or as self-poisoning.

As with all of the drugs reviewed here, the effects of dobutamine on systemic haemodynamics are well documented but the effects on regional blood flow are still being researched (*vide infra*). Ruokonen and colleagues have measured the effect of dobutamine infusion in acute pancreatitis,[48] showing that, as in studies of dopamine or noradrenaline infusion in sepsis, the effects on hepatosplanchnic perfusion vary and are unpredictable. In all patients, cardiac index and systemic DO_2 increased (DO_2 by 29.1%), with hepatosplanchnic blood flow increasing in 50% of patients but falling markedly in the rest. These studies used techniques to measure overall hepatosplanchnic perfusion, but the effects on the microcirculation are unknown.

Isoprenaline

Isoprenaline is an inodilator agent (Table 10.3), with significant chronotropic effect. It is not in current use as an inotrope, but may be useful in the immediate management of profound bradycardia especially complete heart block (pending cardiac pacing). It is also used to treat Torsades de Pointes, since it shortens the Q–T interval.[49]

EFFECTS OF INOTROPIC THERAPY ON REGIONAL PERFUSION

Splanchnic circulation

The hypothesis of goal directed therapy to increase global CO and DO_2 is that improved tissue DO_2 will lead to improved oxygen consumption and the clearance of oxygen debt. Increasingly it is realised that there are marked regional differences in blood flow and oxygen transport in certain disease states, not least in the splanchnic vascular bed.

Splanchnic blood flow and oxygen transport have been investigated in both sepsis and low cardiac output states. In sepsis, while splanchnic blood flow measured by indocyanine green (ICG) clearance is increased in comparison with non-septic patients, hepatic venous oxygen content is markedly reduced, indicating a substantially greater increase in hepatosplanchnic oxygen consumption indicative of hypermetabolism in the splanchnic vascular distribution.[50] In contrast, patients with low cardiac output states, e.g. following myocardial infarction or cardiac surgery, show a proportionate decrease in splanchnic blood flow which may also result in critically reduced hepatic venous oxygen saturation.

This has also been shown to be the case in relatively mild degrees of hypovolaemia. The compensatory mechanisms which are activated in acute illness with hypovolaemia, hypotension or low flow result in hepatosplanchnic vasoconstriction as documented by Edouard and colleagues.[51] In a study of normal human volunteers, these workers showed that, even when transient, hypovolaemia will cause prolonged splanchnic vasoconstriction.

The presence of α_1, β_2 and dopaminergic DA-1 receptors in the splanchnic bed indicates that dopexamine (β_2 and dopaminergic agonist), dopamine(α_1, β_2 and dopaminergic) and dobutamine (β_1 and β_2 agonist) should increase splanchnic blood flow and, hence, improve gut perfusion. Studies of vasoactive therapy on splanchnic flow and oxygen transport have been carried out in a number of disease states including sepsis, postcardiac surgery and pancreatitis. In addition, gastric pH_i and arterial-gastric mucosal PCO_2 difference provide further information on the gut microcirculation less invasively.

Initial studies of dopexamine infusions in critically ill patients suggested that it led to rapid clearance of intramucosal acidosis and improved liver blood flow as determined by ICG clearance and meg-x production, in contrast to dopamine which had no significant effect on these measurements.[52,53] These preliminary findings, however, appear to be refuted by more detailed randomised studies.[54,55] In a prospective placebo-controlled cross-over study involving a 3 h dopexamine infusion in stable ICU patients, Trinder and colleagues found that dopexamine failed to improve pH_i in comparison with placebo,[54] although there was a time related improvement in pH_i in both groups. In patients following cardiopulmonary bypass, Berendes and colleagues compared a number of doses of dopexamine with placebo in a randomised prospective trial.[55] While dopexamine was associated with an increase in DO_2, there was no change in hepatic venous oxygen saturation, but gastric pH_i fell, implying a deterioration in the gut microcirculation. In low doses (0.5–1 µg/kg/min), however, dopexamine did improve renal function and attenuated release of the pro-inflammatory mediators, endotoxin and interleukin-6 (IL-6). These rather negative findings have been confirmed by Uusaro et al,[56] who likewise found that dopexamine caused intramucosal acidosis despite increasing splanchnic blood flow in cardiac surgical patients.

Dopamine similarly failed to improve, or even decreased gastric pH_i in general intensive care patients[53] or septic patients.[32] The huge rise (65%) in splanchnic oxygen delivery following dopamine shown in septic patients by Ruokonen[31] may suggest an explanation for the apparent deterioration in mucosal oxygenation. The splanchnic vasodilatation may uncouple nutrient flow from tissue oxygen needs, with shunting through less metabolically active tissues.

Dobutamine in combination with colloid resuscitation has been recommended for the correction of mucosal acidosis in critically ill patients.[57] However, recent studies in cardiac surgical patients[58] and those suffering from acute pancreatitis[48] suggest that dobutamine does not have specific beneficial effects on splanchnic perfusion. In stable cardiac surgical patients, randomised either to dobutamine infusion or to serve as controls, Parviainen[58] demonstrated that dobutamine increased CO and global DO_2 but failed to alter splanchnic blood flow and splanchnic DO_2. Furthermore, pH_i fell in those patients with low CO indicating gut ischaemia. In pancreatitis, where splanchnic oxygen consumption is increased reflecting hypermetabolism, dobutamine likewise failed to increase splanchnic blood flow despite an increase in CO.[48]

The adverse effects of adrenaline on splanchnic perfusion have already been discussed, and must limit its use to initial resuscitation only.

Paradoxically, noradrenaline, without significant splanchnic vasodilator activity, appears, when used alone[33] or in combination with dobutamine,[21,22] to result in correction of gastric mucosal acidosis by improvement in splanchnic blood flow. It may be that its lesser degree of metabolic stimulation leads to an improved oxygen supply demand relationship and, hence, improved tissue oxygenation. Furthermore, studies of villous microcirculation stress the importance of maintenance of an adequate perfusion pressure to maintain flow.

Cerebral circulation

There are few studies of vasoactive agents on cerebral blood flow (CBF). Given the effect of autoregulatory control, it might appear unlikely that exogenous catecholamines would cause much change in CBF. Nevertheless, in acute brain injury, cerebral autoregulation is lost in some patients, and CBF is pressure dependent. Furthermore, in patients with high intra-cranial pressure (ICP), cerebral perfusion pressure (CPP) may be reduced below the limits of autoregulation and hence CBF would also be affected. After major trauma, a systemic inflammatory response occurs and, indeed, an inflammatory cytokine gradient has been demonstrated across the brain.[59] Our experience in head injured patients is that CO tends to be increased with a reduced SVR reflecting the systemic inflammation, and that low dose noradrenaline (0.05–0.25 µg/kg/min) satisfactorily restores MAP, CPP and CBF as reflected by measurement of the jugular bulb oxygen saturation. Dobutamine has been shown to increase CBF measured by a thermodilution catheter in the internal jugular vein in patients with sepsis.[60]

Renal circulation

The effects of inotropes on renal function are mainly due to improvements in systemic haemodynamics (MAP and CO). It has been one of the crucial rediscoveries of the last decade that, in hyperdynamic septic shock appropriately monitored, administration of vasopressors, notably noradrenaline, will improve renal function and urine output.[61,62] There is no evidence that dopamine improves renal function in shock unless it improves haemodynamics. The use of routine 'renal-dose' dopamine in surgery with a high risk of renal impairment cannot be supported on current evidence.[43,63] There may be an increase in urine output and sodium excretion due to the loop diuretic effects of dopamine. As in the hepatosplanchnic circulation, the effects of treatment on the renal microcirculation are most interesting and quite elusive.

THE CRITICALLY ILL SURGICAL PATIENT

Since the early 1970s, Shoemaker[64] has systematically studied the haemodynamic and oxygen transport patterns in groups of high-risk surgical patients. He initially documented the changes which occur peri-operatively and went on to examine the data in order to identify variables which were associated with survival. He found that those patients with higher CO, DO_2 and VO_2 had a better prognosis: MAP was also higher in this group. Prospective studies were then carried out using the median values of survivors as the endpoints for resuscitation with fluids and dobutamine. Mortality in the protocol (goal directed) group was 13% and in the control (standard therapy) group was 48%.[65]

Boyd and colleagues[37] have repeated the high-risk surgical studies with similar results to those of Shoemaker. In this elderly, British group of high risk surgical patients with an oxygen delivery of >600 ml/min/m² as the main therapeutic goal, there were 75% fewer deaths in the protocol group. Although the study designs are similar, the inherent differences in the actions of dobutamine and dopexamine (particularly the potential for specific beneficial effects on hepatosplanchnic oxygen delivery of dopexamine) make direct comparison difficult. In a small (16 patients) comparative study, dopexamine was better tolerated than dobutamine with regard to adverse cardiac effects.[66] A Canadian multi-centre, randomised, controlled, prospective study of pre-operative supranormalisation of DO_2 is currently underway.

Other investigators have extrapolated the above findings to different clinical situations, e.g. sepsis, ARDS and multiple organ failure, despite a lack of hard evidence to support this. This is discussed further in the next section.

Inotropic support in the critically ill patient

SEPTIC SHOCK AND ADULT RESPIRATORY DISTRESS SYNDROME (ARDS)

In contrast to shock states where vasoregulation is intact and the potential for increased oxygen extraction maintained, (e.g. early hypovolaemic or cardiogenic shock), septic shock and multiple organ failure may be associated with loss of vasoregulation, peripheral vasodilatation and failure of the regulation of oxygen extraction. In certain patients, at least, oxygen consumption tends to be related to oxygen delivery[67] and an increase in DO_2 is associated with an increase in VO_2. Those patients who respond positively to a DO_2 challenge, i.e. where VO_2 increases in parallel with DO_2 augmented by a dobutamine infusion, have a considerably improved outcome compared with patients whose VO_2 is fixed.[68] Likewise, survivors of septic shock tend to have supranormal VO_2 ($\geq$170 ml/min/m^2) and normal blood lactate in contrast to non-survivors who fail to generate a high VO_2 or to correct hyperlactataemia in response to a fluid and inotrope resuscitation.[69]

It was obvious that these findings, taken in conjunction with Shoemaker's observations in critically ill surgical patients, would prompt studies in septic shock based upon vasoactive therapy to try to achieve Shoemaker's 'optimal goals' of CI, DO_2 and VO_2. Hayes and colleagues,[70] using fluid and dobutamine to drive CO in combination with noradrenaline to maintain MAP, found in a randomised prospective trial that this regimen was associated with a higher mortality than a control group in whom normal haemodynamic values were aimed for. In some protocol patients who failed to mount a VO_2 response, they used very large doses of dobutamine in combination with substantial noradrenaline doses which would not appear to have been beneficial. Gattinoni and colleagues,[71] in an Italian multi-centre study, applied goal directed haemodynamic therapy to 762 heterogeneous patients in 56 ICUs. Diagnoses included septic shock, acute respiratory failure, multiple trauma and critical surgical illness. They found no difference in outcome between three groups of patients treated to achieve normal CI (2.5–3.5 l/min/m^2), supranormal CI ($\geq$4.5 l/min/m^2) or an S$\bar{v}O_2$ $\geq$70%. The failure in these studies of haemodynamic therapy to achieve supranormal goals of oxygen delivery and consumption, coupled with much recent controversy regarding the benefits or otherwise of pulmonary artery catheter monitoring, has led to a rather nihilistic attitude to haemodynamic monitoring and therapy. It has been suggested that goal directed haemodynamic therapy is only applicable as a prophylactic measure in peri-operative surgical patients, but is ineffective when organ dysfunction is established. It should be noted that both Hayes' and Gattinoni's studies comprised very heterogeneous groups of patients with presumably very varied physiological reserve. Their control groups were also aggressively managed with fluid and vasoactive agents, albeit to 'normal' haemodynamic goals, representing, in itself, goal directed intensive care. Furthermore, those who go on to survive have the capacity to increase their oxygen utilisation, in contrast to the high mortality of patients who fail to respond to an increase in CI and DO_2 with an increase in oxygen consumption.

It appears appropriate, therefore, to identify those patients with evidence of tissue hypoxia, restore fluid volume according to peripheral temperature and pulmonary artery wedge pressure measurements, measure CO, $S\bar{v}O_2$ and hence DO_2 and VO_2.[72] Where hypotension persists despite a greater than normal CO and DO_2, noradrenaline should be commenced as a vasopressor, while in those patients where CO and DO_2 are low or normal and VO_2 is reduced, a challenge with inotrope to assess the response of VO_2 is applicable. In general circumstances, dobutamine will be the most appropriate agent; additional volume and noradrenaline may be required to control the effects of its β_2 mediated vasodilatation. Failure to respond to doses of dobutamine up to 20 µg/kg/min should provoke a review of vasoactive therapy.

CARDIOGENIC SHOCK

The development of low flow shock in the setting of acute myocardial infarction identifies a group of patients with a 10-fold increase in mortality.[73] The treatment set out in Table 10.3 must have been initiated before using inotropes in cardiogenic shock (CS). The aim of inotropic therapy in CS is to achieve a cardiac output and oxygen delivery sufficient to meet the body's metabolic requirements and avert the development of MOF without worsening of myocardial ischaemia. This necessitates use of the PAC, and a cardiac index of 2.2 1/min/m² with an Sv^-O_2 >60% have been successfully used as therapeutic goals.[47] The haemodynamic target is based on Forrester's work,[73] and the prognostic importance of Sv^-O_2 in acute myocardial infarction (AMI) has been highlighted by Sumimoto and colleagues.[74]

The choice of inotrope in CS is determined by the haemodynamics, low stroke volume and high WP favouring the use of dobutamine. Enoximone or milrinone may have beneficial effects, especially if filling pressures are very high, and these agents can have synergistic effects with catecholamines.[75] This may be related to the finding that the reduced density of β-adrenoreceptors in the failing myocardium causes reduced cAMP production, a deficit which can be rectified due to the intracellular site of action of the PDEIs. In some patients with CS, hypotension is compounded by systemic vasodilatation secondary to the effects of inflammatory mediators released in response to tissue hypoxia. In these patients, noradrenaline is necessary to maintain MAP and thus coronary perfusion.

The practical approach is to secure oxygenation, treat the AMI with aspirin and thrombolysis as appropriate, and to start cardiovascular resuscitation whilst getting an echocardiogram to exclude a surgically remediable lesion. The decision to proceed to coronary angiography and balloon angioplasty, with or without stenting, will be made on the basis of response to initial therapy; the intra-aortic balloon pump may augment the effects of inotropic therapy during this period. There is increasing discussion about the place of early revascularisation and mechanical support of the circulation in these patients, with preliminary evidence in favour of these interventions.[76]

NEUROGENIC PULMONARY OEDEMA

Although first documented in 1908, the haemodynamic picture of neurogenic pulmonary oedema (NPO) was only described in a systematic manner in

1996.[77] A relatively common complication of severe subarachnoid haemorrhage, NPO is generally associated with an extremely low CO and LVSWI, systemic hypotension, pulmonary hypertension, and a raised pulmonary artery wedge pressure. Conventional treatment of NPO comprising ventilation with positive end-expiratory pressure and diuretic frequently fails to correct hypoxaemia. In contrast, administration of an inodilator, dobutamine, rapidly results in improved CO and LVSWI, corrects the high pulmonary artery wedge pressure

Key points for clinical practice

- The heterogeneity of the haemodynamic derangements, which occur in critical illness and which may be compounded by chronic intercurrent disease, necessitates an individual approach to the patient's haemodynamic management.

- This approach demands measurement of haemodynamic and oxygen transport variables, and continued monitoring and repeated assessment after each therapeutic intervention. Generally this will involve arterial and pulmonary artery catheterisation, and repeated measurement of indices of tissue oxygenation and organ function, such as hydrogen ion, base excess, blood lactate and urine output.

- Correction of hypoxaemia, anaemia, abnormalities of blood volume and electrolyte abnormalities (especially potassium) should ideally precede inotrope use.

- Adrenaline by small bolus and infusion is still the agent of choice for first-line emergency management of profound shock states, but its now well documented effects on splanchnic perfusion rule it out for longer term therapy.

- Dobutamine is generally the first agent of choice for low flow shock states (cardiogenic shock, low cardiac output septic shock and neurogenic pulmonary oedema) but safe usage demands appropriate monitoring of circulating volume, and ECG monitoring to detect ischaemia and dysrhythmias.

- Noradrenaline has been demonstrated to be a safe and effective agent to correct hypotension in sepsis and other states where organ perfusion is threatened. With adequate filling, splanchnic and renal perfusion and function appear to benefit.

- The role of dopaminergic agents has yet to be fully defined. While little evidence exists of deleterious effects, robust evidence of clinical benefit is lacking.

- As Talley pointed out in 1969, 'it seems reasonable that no single drug would be adequate to correct the hemodynamics in all cases of shock', then going on to say 'optimal drug or combination drug therapy appears to be obtainable only by sequential administration with serial hemodynamic and clinical evaluations of each drug's effects'.

and improves oxygenation. Dobutamine frequently requires to be administered in combination with noradrenaline which is required to stabilise the cerebral perfusion pressure in the face of a raised intracranial pressure.

References

1. Bennett E D, Boldt J, Brochard L et al. The use of the pulmonary artery catheter. Intensive Care Med 1991; 17: I–VIII
2. Connors A F, Speroff T, Dawson N V et al. The effectiveness of right heart catheterization in the initial care of critically ill patients. JAMA 1996; 276: 889
3. Taylor R W (ed). Controversies in pulmonary artery catheterization. New Horizons 1997; 5: 73–296
4. Nightingale P. Measurements, technical problems and inaccuracies. In: Edwards J D, Shoemaker W C, Vincent J-L. (eds) Oxygen Transport, Principles and Practice. London: Saunders, 1993; 41–69
5. Bakker J, Gris P, Coffernils M, Kahn R J, Vincent J L. Serial blood lactate levels can predict the development of multiple organ failure following septic shock. Am J Surg 1996; 171: 221–226
6. Schade D S. The role of catecholamines in metabolic acidosis. In: Ciba Foundation Symposium 87: Metabolic Acidosis. London: Pitman Books, 1982; 235–253
7. Botha A J, Moore F A, Moore E E et al. Base deficit after major trauma directly relates to neutrophil CD 11b expression: a proposed mechanism of shock-induced organ injury. Intensive Care Med 1997; 23: 504–509
8. Adrogue H J. Rashad N, Gorin A B et al. Assessing acid-base status in circulatory failure. Differences between arterial and central venous blood. N Engl J Med 1989; 320: 1312–1316
9. Fiddian-Green R G, McGough E, Pittenger G, Rothman E. Predictive value for intra-mural pH and other risk factors for massive bleeding from stress ulceration. Gastroenterology 1983; 85: 613–620
10. Trinder T J, Lavery G G, Fee J P H, Lowry K G. Low gastric intra-mucosal pH: incidence and significance in intensive care patients. Anaesth Intensive Care 1995; 23: 315–321
11. Dries D, Waxman K. Adequate resuscitation of burn patients may not be measured by urine output and vital signs. Crit Care Med 1991; 19: 327–329
12. Bristow M R, Ginsburg R, Minobe W. Decreased catecholamine sensitivity and β-adrenergic-receptor density in failing human hearts. N Engl J Med 1982; 307: 205–211
13. Boldt J, Moosdorf R, Hempelmann G. Enoximone treatment of impaired myocardial function following cardiac surgery. Combined effects with epinephrine. J Cardiothorac Vasc Anesth 1990; 4: 462–468
14. Grant I S, Mackenzie S J. Clinical observations on the use of phosphodiesterase inhibitors as second-line inotropes in septic shock. Clin Intensive Care 1996; 8: 10–13
15. Lewis R P. Digitalis. In: Leier C V. (ed). Cardiotonic Drugs. A Clinical Survey. New York: Dekker, 1986; 85–150
16. Mackenzie S J, Kapadia F, Nimmo G R, Armstrong I R, Grant I S. Adrenaline in treatment of septic shock: effects on haemodynamics and oxygen transport. Intensive Care Med 1991; 17: 36–39
17. Wilson W, Lipman J, Scribante J et al. Septic shock: does adrenaline have a role as a first-line inotropic agent? Anaesth Intensive Care 1992; 20: 470–474
18. Moran J L, O'Fathartaigh M S, Peisach A R, Chapman M J, Leppard P. Epinephrine as an inotropic agent in septic shock: a dose-profile analysis. Crit Care Med 1993; 21: 70–77
19. Bollaert P E, Bauer P, Audibert G, Lambert H, Larean A. Effects of epinephrine on hemodynamics and oxygen metabolism in dopamine-resistant septic shock. Chest 1990; 98: 949–953
20. Lipman J, Roux A, Kraus P. Vasoconstrictor effects of adrenaline in human septic shock. Anaesth Intensive Care 1991; 19: 61–65
21. Levy B, Bollaert P-E, Charpentier C et al. Comparison of norepinephrine and dobutamine to epinephrine for hemodynamics, lactate metabolism and gastric

tonometric variables in septic shock: a prospective, randomised study. Intensive Care Med 1997; 23: 282–287

22. Meier-Hellman A, Reinhart K, Bredle D L, Specht M, Spies C D, Hannemann L. Epinephrine impairs splanchnic perfusion in septic shock. Crit Care Med 1997; 25: 399–404

23. Day N P J, Phu N H, Bethell D P et al. The effects of dopamine and adrenaline infusions on acid-base balance and systemic haemodynamics in severe infection. Lancet 1996; 348: 219–223

24. Meadows D, Edwards J D, Wilkins R G, Nightingale P. Reversal of intractable septic shock with norepinephrine therapy. Crit Care Med 1988; 16: 663–666

25. Desjars P, Pinaud M, Potel G et al. A reappraisal of norepinephrine therapy in human septic shock. Crit Care Med 1987; 15: 134–137

26. Hoffman B B, Lefkowitz B. Catecholamines, sympathomimetic drugs and adrenergic receptor antagonists In: Hsardman J G, Limbird L E. (Eds) The Pharmacological Basis of Therapeutics, 9th Edn. New York: McGraw Hill, 1995; 199–263

27. Martin C, Eon B, Saux P, Aknin P, Gouin F. Renal effects of norepinephrine used to treat septic shock patients. Crit Care Med 1990; 18: 282–285

28. Redl-Wenzl E M, Armbruster C, Edelmann G et al. The effects of norepinephrine on hemodynamics and renal function in severe septic shock states. Intensive Care Med 1993; 19: 151–154

29. Schaer G L, Fink M P, Parrillo J E. Norepinephrine alone versus norepinephrine plus low-dose dopamine: enhanced renal blood flow with combination pressor therapy. Crit Care Med 1985; 13: 492–496

30. Meakins J L, Marshall J C. The gut as the motor of multiple system organ failure. In: Marston A, Bulkley G B, Fiddian-Green R G, Haglund U H (eds) Splanchnic Ischaemia and Multiple Organ Failure. London: Edward Arnold, 1989; 339–348

31. Ruokonen E, Takala J, Kari A, Saxen H, Mertsola J, Hausen EJ. Regional blood flow and oxygen transport in septic shock. Crit Care Med 1993; 21: 1296–1303

32. Marik P E, Mohedin M. The contrasting effects of dopamine and norepinephrine on systemic and splanchnic oxygen utilisation in hyperdynamic sepsis. JAMA 1994; 272: 1354–1357

33. Grant I S, Kelly K P, Mackenzie A F. Effects of catecholamine therapy on regional blood flow and tissue oxygenation in septic shock. In: Vincent J L. (Ed) Yearbook of Intensive Care and Emergency Medicine 1994. Berlin: Springer-Verlag, 1994; 179–188

34. Bernardin G, Pradier C. Tiger F. Deloffre P, Mattei M. Blood pressure and arterial lactate level are early indicators of short-term survival in human septic shock. Intensive Care Med 1996; 22: 17–25

35. Leier C V. Binkley P F, Carpenter J, Randolph P H, Unverferth D V. Cardiovascular pharmacology of dopexamine in low output congestive heart failure. Am J Cardiol 1988; 62: 94–99

36. Magrini F, Foulds R, Roberts N. Macchi G, Mondadori C, Zanchetti A. Human renovascular effects of dopexamine hydrochloride: a novel agonist of peripheral dopamine and beta 2 adreno-receptors. Eur J Clin Pharmacol 1987; 32: 1–4

37. Boyd O. Grounds R M, Bennett E D. A randomised clinical trial of the effect of deliberate peri-operative increase of oxygen delivery on mortality in high risk surgical patients. JAMA 1993; 270: 2699–2707

38. Goldberg L I. Cardiovascular and renal actions of dopamine. Potential clinical applications. Pharmacol Rev 1972; 24: 1–29

39. Talley R C, Goldberg L I, Johnson C E, McNay J L. A hemodynamic comparison of dopamine and isoproterenol in patients in shock. Circulation 1969; 36: 361–378

40. Stevens P E, Bolsin S, Gwyther S J et al. Practical use of duplex Doppler analysis of the renal vasculature in critically ill patients. Lancet 1989; 1: 240–242

41. Meier-Hellmann A, Bredle D L, Specht M et al. The effects of low-dose dopamine on splanchnic blood flow and oxygen uptake in patients with septic shock. Intensive Care Med 1997; 23: 31–37.

42. Berg R A, Padbury J F. Sulfconjugation and renal excretion contribute to interpatient variation of exogenous catecholamine clearance in critically ill children. Crit Care Med 1997; 25: 1247–1251

43. Balwin L, Henderson A, Hickman P. Effect of low dose dopamine on renal function after elective major vascular surgery. Ann Intern Med 1994; 120: 744–747

44. Van den Berghe G, deZehger F. Anterior pituitary function during critical illness and dopamine treatment. Crit Care Med 1996; 24: 1580–1590

45. Llados F, Zapata P. Effects of dopamine analogues and antagonists on carotid body chemosensors in situ. J Physiol 1978; 274: 487–499

46. Ruffolo R R. Review: the pharmacology of dobutamine. Am J Med Sci 1987; 294: 244–248

47. Creamer J E, Edwards J D, Nightingale P. Hemodynamic and oxygen transport variables in cardiogenic shock secondary to acute myocardial infarction and response to treatment. Am J Cardiol 1990; 65: 1297–1300

48. Ruokonen E, Uusaro A, Alhara E, Takala J. The effect of dobutamine infusion on splanchnic blood flow and oxygen transport in patients with acute pancreatitis. Intensive Care Med 1997; 23: 732–737

49. Fontaine G, Frank R, Grosgogeat Y. Torsades de Pointes: definition and management. Mod Concepts Cardiovasc Dis 1982; 51: 103–106

50. Dahn M S, Lange M P, Wilson R F, Jacobs L A, Mitchell R A. Hepatic blood flow and splanchnic oxygen consumption measurements in clinical sepsis. Surgery 1990; 107: 295–301

51. Edouard A R, Degrémont A-C, Duranteau J, Pussard E, Berdeaux A, Samii K. Heterogeneous regional vascular responses to simulated transient hypovolaemia in man. Intensive Care Med 1994; 20: 414–420

52. Smithies M, Yee T H, Jackson L, Beale R, Bihara D. Protecting the gut and the liver in the critically ill: effects of dopexamine. Crit Care Med 1994; 22: 789–795

53. Maynard N D, Bihari D J, Dalton R N, Smithies M N, Mason R C. Increasing splanchnic blood flow in the critically ill. Chest 1995; 108: 1648–1654

54. Trinder T J, Lavery G G, Fee J P H, Lowry K G. Correction of splanchnic oxygen deficit in the intensive care unit: dopexamine and colloid versus placebo. Anaesth Intensive Care 1995; 23: 178–182

55. Berendes E, Mollhoff T, Van Aken H et al. Effects of dopexamine on creatinine clearance, systemic inflammation and splanchnic oxygenation in patients undergoing coronary artery bypass grafting. Anesth Analg 1997; 84: 950–957

56. Uusaro A, Ruokonen E, Takala J. Dopexamine induces gastric mucosal acidosis despite increased splanchnic blood flow after cardiac surgery. Crit Care Med 1994; 22: 70

57. Guttuerez G, Palizas F, Doglio G et al. Gastric intramucosal pH as a therapeutic index of tissue oxygenation in critically ill patients. Lancet 1992; 339: 195–199

58. Parviainen I, Ruokonen E, Takala J. Dobutamine-induced dissociation between changes in splanchnic blood flow and gastric intramucosal pH after cardiac surgery. Br J Anaesth 1995; 74: 277–282

59. McKeating E G, Andrews P J D, Signorini D F S, Mascia L. Transcranial cytokine gradients in patients requiring intensive care following acute brain injury. Br J Anaesth 1997; In press

60. Berre J, DeBacker D, Moraine J-J et al. Dobutamine increases cerebral blood flow velocity and jugular bulb hemoglobin saturation in septic patients. Crit Care Med 1997; 25: 393–398

61. Cumming A D. Renal function in septic shock. In: Vincent J L. (ed) Update in Intensive Care and Emergency Medicine, vol 8. Berlin: Springer-Verlag, 1989; 348–360

62. Hesselvik J F, Brodin B. Low dose norepinephrine in patients with septic shock and oliguria: effects on afterload, urine flow and oxygen transport. Crit Care Med 1989; 17: 179–180.

63. Myles P S, Buckland M R, Schenk N J et al. Effect of 'renal-dose' dopamine on renal function following cardiac surgery. Anaesth Intensive Care 1993; 21: 56–61

64. Shoemaker W C. Cardiorespiratory patterns of surviving and non-surviving post-operative surgical patients. Surg Gynecol Obstet 1972; 134: 810–814

65. Shoemaker W C, Appel P L, Waxman K et al. Clinical trial of survivors' cardiorespiratory patterns as therapeutic goals in critically ill post-operative patients. Crit Care Med 1982; 10: 398–403

66. Boyd O, Lamb G, Mackay C J et al. A comparison of the efficacy of dopexamine and dobutamine for increasing oxygen delivery in high-risk surgical patients. Anaesth Intensive Care 1995; 23: 478–484

67. Danek S J, Lynch J P, Weg J G, Dautzker D R. The dependence of oxygen uptake on oxygen delivery in adult respiratory distress syndrome. Am J Respir Crit Care Med 1980; 122: 387–395

68. Vallet B, Chopin C, Curtis J E et al. Prognostic value of dobutamine test in patients with sepsis syndrome and normal lactate values: a prospective, multicenter study. Crit Care Med 1993; 21: 1868–1875

69. Hayes M A, Yau E H S, Timmins A C et al. Response of critically ill patients to treatment aimed at achieving supranormal oxygen delivery and consumption. Chest 1993; 103: 886–895

70. Hayes M A, Timmins A C, Yau E H S, Palazzo M, Hinds C J, Watson D. Elevation of systemic oxygen delivery in the treatment of critically ill patients. N Engl J Med 1994; 330: 1717–1722

71. Gattinoni L. Brazzi L. Pelosi P et al. A trial of goal-oriented hemodynamic therapy in critically ill patients. N Engl J Med 1995; 333: 1025–1032

72. Nimmo G R, Mackenzie S J, Walker S W et al. The relationship of blood lactate concentrations, oxygen delivery and oxygen consumption in septic shock and ARDS. Anaesthesia 1992; 47: 1023–1028

73. Forrester J E, Diamond G, Chatterjee K, Swan H J C. Medical therapy of acute myocardial infarction by application of hemodynamic subsets. N Engl J Med 1976; 295: 1356–1362

74. Sumimoto T, Takayama Y, Iwasaka T et al. Mixed venous oxygen saturation as a guide to tissue oxygenation and prognosis in patients with acute myocardial infarction. Am Heart J 1991; 122: 27–33

75. Vincent J-L, Carlier E, Berre J et al. Administration of enoximone in cardiogenic shock. Am J Cardiol 1988; 62: 419–423

76. Hochman J S, Boland J, Sleeper L A et al. Current spectrum of cardiogenic shock and effect of early revascularization on mortality. Results of an international registry. Circulation 1995; 91: 873–881

77. Deehan S C, Grant I S. Haemodynamic changes in neurogenic pulmonary oedema: effect of dobutamine. Intensive Care Med 1996; 22: 672–676

Suveer Singh Timothy W. Evans

Nitric oxide in ARDS: uses and abuses

Since the first description of acute respiratory distress syndrome (ARDS) by Ashbaugh and coworkers[1] in 12 patients with distinctive clinical, physiological, radiographical and pathological abnormalities,[2] considerable progress has been made in understanding the epidemiology and pathophysiology of the condition. Further, new supportive strategies, such as volume-recruitment ventilation, permissive hypercarbia, prone positioning and the use of inhaled nitric oxide (NO), have been adopted widely, although evidence of their benefit from formal randomised controlled trials is lacking. Thus, many questions remain to be answered in the research and clinical setting if inhaled NO is to become established as a therapeutic intervention of proven benefit in the management of ARDS.

L-ARGININE–NITRIC OXIDE PATHWAY AND INTERACTIONS

In 1987, the chemical and pharmacological properties of an endothelium-derived relaxant factor (EDRF), responsible for the vascular relaxation induced by acetylcholine,[3] were shown to be virtually identical to those of NO.[4] Nitric oxide is synthesized from the amino acid, L-arginine, by a group of flavin-containing oxygenase enzymes commonly termed nitric oxide synthase (NOS) (Fig. 11.1).[5] Endothelial cells were the first mammalian cells shown to release NO, a potent vasodilator. It is now accepted that various cell types can release NO and that at least three distinct isoforms of NOS exist. Endothelial NOS (eNOS) and neuronal NOS (nNOS) are constitutive and calcium-dependent enzymes, but a third isoform is induced (iNOS) by endotoxin (lipopolysacharride, LPS) and inflammatory cytokines. Although differences exist in the

Timothy W. Evans BSc MD PhD FRCP EDICM, Professor of Intensive Care Medicine, Unit of Critical Care Medicine, Imperial College School of Medicine, Royal Brompton Hospital, London SW3 6NP, UK

Suveer Singh BSc MB MRCP, British Heart Foundation Clinical Training Fellow, Unit of Critical Care Medicine, Imperial College School of Medicine, Royal Brompton Hospital, London SW3 6NP, UK

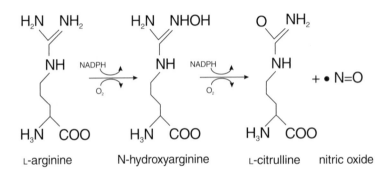

Fig 11.1 Chemical reactions involved in the synthesis of nitric oxide. L-arginine is converted to L-citrulline and nitric oxide. The reaction is catalysed by nitric oxide synthase (NOS) in the presence of oxygen and the co-substrate nicotinamide adenine dinucleotide diphosphate (NADPH). NOS requires several cofactors including flavones and tetrahydrobiopterin.

biochemistry of the three NOS isoforms, the basic pathway of metabolism of L-arginine to NO and L-citrulline is well conserved and all are inhibited by the L-arginine analogs N^G-monomethyl-L-arginine (L-NMMA), N^G-nitro-L-arginine (L-NNA) and/or N^G-nitro-L-arginine methyl ester (L-NAME).[6,7] Such inhibitors cause a rapid increase in blood pressure in animals and in man, suggesting that, in health, NO is required in order to maintain systemic vascular tone.

Appropriate agonists or stimulation by shear stress activate cNOS via a rapid increase in intracellular calcium concentration, resulting in NO release within seconds or minutes. After a stimulus such as interferon gamma (IFN-γ), interleukin-1 beta (IL-1β), tumour necrosis factor alpha (TNFα), endotoxin or exotoxin, iNOS is induced in the relevant cell type by gene transcription, via transcription factors like nuclear factor kappa beta (NF-κB). This process can be inhibited by glucocorticoids.[8] iNOS generates up to 1000 times more NO than cNOS and cellular production continues for a number of hours.

The biological actions of NO are, in the main, attributable to activation of guanylyl cyclase after binding to its haem moiety (Fig. 11.2). This enzyme catalyzes the conversion of guanylate triphosphate (GTP) to cyclic guanylate 3′5′-monophosphate (cGMP). The rise in cGMP, which is an intracellular messenger, causes a reduction in the intracellular concentration of calcium, resulting in smooth muscle relaxation in vascular and nonvascular tissues, inhibition of platelet adherence and aggregation, inhibition of polymorpho-nuclear leukocyte chemotaxis and signal transduction in the nervous system, as reviewed elsewhere.[9] NO also has cGMP-independent actions, including cytotoxic effects due to the inhibition of mitochondrial Fe–S enzymes and cyclooxygenase activation in macrophages.[10,11] Other intracellular second messenger systems, such as protein kinase activation and inositol triphosphate inhibition, have been proposed as effectors of NO function at the cellular level. Indeed, NO is thought to form intermediary complexes with thiols such as cysteine; and the formation of sulphydryl complexes may prolong the half life of extracellular NO promoting its role in cell–cell communication prior to inactivation.[12]

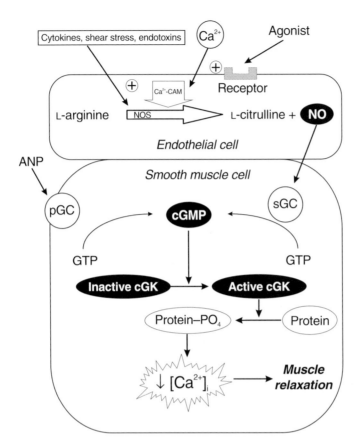

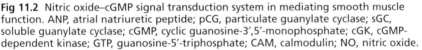

Fig 11.2 Nitric oxide–cGMP signal transduction system in mediating smooth muscle function. ANP, atrial natriuretic peptide; pCG, particulate guanylate cyclase; sGC, soluble guanylate cyclase; cGMP, cyclic guanosine-3′,5′-monophosphate; cGK, cGMP-dependent kinase; GTP, guanosine-5′-triphosphate; CAM, calmodulin; NO, nitric oxide.

The interaction of the NO and other biologically relevant pathways, such as the cyclooxygenase-prostaglandin (COX) and endothelin (ET) systems, adds another regulatory dimension at the cellular level during inflammation; cyclooxygenase is a key enzyme in inflammation and catalyses the metabolism of arachidonic acid to vasoactive and inflammatory mediators such as prostaglandins (PG), thromboxanes (TX) and prostacyclin (PGI$_2$). COX may be modulated through the action of NO at a haem moiety on the enzyme's active site.[13] Indeed, peroxynitrite, the coupling product of NO and superoxide, has been shown to activate the peroxidase activity of COX in vitro, further defining the link.[14] The role of NO as a free radical with its potentially detrimental interactions is discussed later.

ACUTE LUNG INJURY

There has been considerable debate concerning the exact definition of ARDS and a variety of diagnostic criteria have evolved to incorporate clinical and

Table 11.1 Definitions: ALI and ARDS (adapted from Bernard et al[16])

Timing	Oxygenation	Chest radiograph	Pulmonary artery occlusion pressure
ALI Acute onset	PaO_2/FiO_2 <300 mmHg (39.5 kPa) (regardless of PEEP level)	Bilateral infiltrates seen on frontal CXR	<18 mmHg (2.5 kPa) when measured, or no clinical evidence of left atrial hypertension
ARDS Acute onset	PaO_2/FiO_2 < 200 mmHg (26.3 kPa) (regardless of PEEP level)	Bilateral infiltrates seen on frontal CXR	<18 mmHg (2.5 kPa) when measured, or no clinical evidence of left atrial hypertension

radiographic features, characteristic lung/chest wall compliance, oxygen and ventilatory requirements. Currently, most investigating authorities accept that ARDS probably represents only the pulmonary manifestation of a pan-endothelial insult resulting from a systemic inflammatory insult.[15] An American-European Consensus Conference defined ARDS recently as non-cardiogenic pulmonary oedema with refractory hypoxaemia (PaO_2/FiO_2 < 26.3 kPa [200 mmHg]), associated with bilateral infiltrates on chest radiography[16] (Table 11.1). The recognition of its occurrence in children as well as adults necessitated a reversion to the term '**acute** respiratory distress syndrome' from the widely adopted '**adult**' prefix. Acute lung injury (ALI) was also defined as a distinct clinical entity in recognition of the spectrum of severity of lung injury that may occur as a result of these precipitating conditions, although it is generally accepted that ARDS represents the extreme end of this spectrum (Fig. 11.3). Nevertheless, in terms of recognising the incidence, epidemiology, and histopathological evolution of lung injuries – and in carrying out trials of new therapeutic interventions – the distinction is important.

Epidemiology

The lack, until recently, of a unified definition of ALI/ARDS has made establishing the true incidence difficult. Estimates from recent studies range between 1.5 and 6 per 100 000 population or 2–3% of ICU admissions. Of the major precipitating conditions, sepsis is the commonest. Some 25–40% of patients with sepsis develop ARDS. The mortality from ARDS ranges from 40–70% and is undoubtedly dictated by the nature of the associated condition in a given patient population; many studies suggest that trauma related ARDS has a better outlook than sepsis. Further, the associated non-pulmonary organ dysfunction appears to be the major determinant of mortality in these patients rather than the severity of respiratory failure. For example, respiratory failure accounts for only 16% of deaths, the greatest part (~50%) being attributable to associated sepsis/multiple organ failure (MOF).[17–19] To date, however, no marker of sufficient sensitivity and specificity has been identified to predict

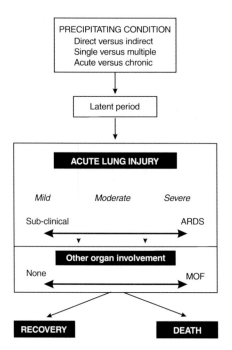

Fig. 11.3 Acute lung injury: the spectrum of disease.

reliably the development of ARDS in at-risk populations, although this is an area of active research.

Pathogenesis

It is recognised that ARDS may complicate a wide variety of direct pulmonary and non-pulmonary conditions through the activation of inflammatory vascular mediators (Table 11.2). Furthermore, it is assumed that the underlying pathophysiological mechanisms are the same, i.e. that ALI/ARDS represent the common endpoint of a wide variety of inflammatory pathways. Thus, the syndrome is characterised by high permeability alveolar oedema, pulmonary capillary microthrombosis, a loss of hypoxic pulmonary vasoconstriction and mismatching of alveolar perfusion (Q) with ventilation (V). These processes account, in the main, for the characteristic clinical features of pulmonary oedema – refractory hypoxaemia and pulmonary hypertension.

Alveolar-capillary membrane permeability

Injury to, and activation of, the endothelium is central to the inflammatory response in ALI/ARDS, resulting in damage to the alveolar/capillary barrier. This allows penetration of plasma into the alveolus leading to alveolar oedema. The presence of this fluid, rich in protein, impairs surfactant function, so increasing surface tension within alveoli; smaller alveoli, therefore, empty into larger neighbouring ones resulting in the characteristic dependent atelectasis. The alveolar/capillary complex may be injured by direct pulmonary insult or by a systemically mediated process involving humoral factors such as

Table 11.2 Clinical conditions associated with the development of ARDS

Respiratory	Non-respiratory
Pneumonia (bacterial/viral/fungal)	Sepsis syndrome
Aspiration of gastric contents	Major trauma/shock
Pulmonary contusion	Massive burns
Post-pneumonectomy	DIC
Inhalation of smoke or toxins	Transfusion reactions
Near-drowning	Fat embolism
Thoracic irradiation	Pregnancy-associated
	(e.g. amniotic fluid embolism)
Oxygen toxicity	Pancreatitis
Ischaemia-reperfusion	Drug/toxin reactions
	(e.g. paraquat, heroin)
Vasculitis (e.g. Goodpasture's)	Post-CP bypass
	Head injury/raised ICP
	Tumour lysis syndrome

DIC: disseminated intravascular coagulopathy; CP: cardiopulmonary; ICP: intracranial pressure.

endotoxin, TNFα and other cytokines such as interleukin-8 (IL-8) capable of inducing endothelial cell injury;[20] thereby stimulating ultrastructural changes within the cells leading to increased permeability.[21] Endothelial cell activation also facilitates the adherence and subsequent migration of activated neutrophils, crucial to the inflammatory process, from blood to tissue. This occurs principally in postcapillary venules, within which white cells marginate, become more adherent, and migrate through the basement membrane, between endothelial cells, into the interstitium. This process is mediated by specific cell surface adhesion molecules (CAM) on both the neutrophil and endothelial cell, as reviewed in detail elsewhere.[22] Thus, pulmonary endothelial disruption can lead to mild respiratory impairment or overwhelming alveolar oedema, although the extent of the increase in vascular permeability does not appear to predict outcome in ALI/ARDS.[23,24]

Moreover, the role of NO in ALI/ARDS-associated pulmonary vascular permeability is likely to be protective. This is based on a number of laboratory and clinical studies implicating the capillary–venous resistance vessels as the predominant site of vasodilatory action of inhaled NO, so reducing pulmonary capillary pressure, filtration pressure, transvascular protein flux and, hence, pulmonary oedema.[25] This is discussed further in the section on inhaled NO.

Hypoxic pulmonary vasoconstriction

Hypoxic pulmonary vasoconstriction (HPV) is the physiological response by which blood is diverted away from underventilated alveoli, thereby improving V/Q matching of perfusion and ventilation. Two possible mechanisms underlie HPV; firstly pulmonary vascular smooth muscle cells may sense hypoxia **directly** causing membrane depolarization, elevated intracellular calcium and vasoconstriction. Alternatively, or additionally, increased constrictor or decreased dilator release from adjacent oxygen sensing cells could **indirectly** account for vasoconstriction during alveolar hypoxaemia. The mechanism is, however, unclear.[26]

It has long been recognised that the endothelium has an inhibitory effect on HPV. The release of endothelially-derived constrictor agents, like prostaglandins, leukotrienes and endothelins, have all been studied as potential modulators of HPV with variable results. The endothelium may also remove such circulating vasoconstrictor substances and, importantly, releases a range of vasoactive agents locally, such as prostacyclin and NO. Any change in the dynamic balance of these factors could modulate the vascular tonic response.

In some species, HPV is dependent upon an intact pulmonary vascular endothelium, and hypoxia-induced contractions of pulmonary arteries in vitro are reduced by endothelial removal. Nevertheless, endothelial injury can also enhance HPV and, in the longer term, structural alterations in pulmonary vascular endothelial cells may also contribute to the development of chronic pulmonary hypertension.[27,28] A reduction in NO production or a decrease in its target receptor sensitivity could also theoretically explain HPV. Certainly, endothelium-dependent relaxation is impaired by hypoxia and NOS inhibitors in rabbit and rat pulmonary artery rings, although there is little consistency between such in vitro results and those obtained in human tissue or in isolated lung experiments.[29–31]

The homeostatic function of HPV is disrupted in ALI/ARDS. Using the multiple inert gas technique, investigators have demonstrated that the associated intra-pulmonary shunt is large enough to account for the observed arterial/alveolar PO_2 gradient, even without invoking a reduction in diffusion capacity.[32] In sepsis and inflammatory states, such as ALI/ARDS, substantial quantities of NO are produced through increased expression of iNOS. This may impair HPV by causing global pulmonary vasodilatation leading to V/Q mismatch. However, the role of NO in modulating HPV is by no means clear cut. Laboratory studies have shown that NOS inhibition, chronic hypoxia and TNF enhance pulmonary arterial vasoconstriction. However, sensitivity to vasopressors and hypoxia is increased or unchanged in endotoxin-treated rats despite increased iNOS activity.[33,34] Moreover, studies of inhaled NO in healthy volunteers have shown both improvements and deteriorations in oxygenation, suggesting that a degree of V/Q heterogeneity exists even in normal lungs.[35,36]

Pulmonary vascular resistance

Nitric oxide is as an important mediator of pulmonary blood flow and consequently of ventilation (V)–perfusion (Q) matching within the lungs. In health, the action of eNOS probably contributes to the maintenance of a low resting pulmonary vascular tone, although this is controversial. Indeed, although pulmonary vascular endothelial cells produce NO in response to agonists such as acetylcholine and bradykinin, this may have little or no effect on basal PVR. Nonetheless, hypoxia reduces this release.[37]

Clinical studies have identified elevated PVR as a universal finding in patients with acute respiratory failure.[38] In ARDS, PVR is increased via a combination of increased vascular tone and structural influences, such as extrinsic compression by oedema fluid, the application of positive pressure ventilation, thromboembolic phenomena and vascular remodelling.

The pulmonary hypertension in ARDS is characterized by thickening of the pulmonary arteries and narrowing of the pulmonary arterial luminal diameter.[39,40] Further, diminution of pulmonary eNOS mRNA expression has been shown to correlate inversely with total PVR and the morphological severity of pulmonary hypertension,[41] implicating diminished basal NO production as a mechanism of the pulmonary hypertension. However, whether endothelial dysfunction (i.e. diminished basal NO production) leads to the development of pulmonary hypertension as a result of subsequent vasoconstriction, *in situ* thrombosis and vascular smooth muscle proliferation or perturbed endothelial function is the consequence of secondarily elevated pulmonary artery pressure (Ppa) remains unresolved.[42] This recent work extends the findings of studies in patients with primary pulmonary hypertension and earlier in vitro studies that demonstrated a reduced vasodilator response to acetylcholine in human pulmonary arterial vessels in vitro following pretreatment with NOS inhibitors.[29,43]

Pulmonary hypertension (mean pulmonary artery pressure Ppa > 20 mmHg) in ALI/ARDS contributes to impaired right ventricular performance (as is discussed below) and has been identified as a poor prognostic indicator although not causally related to increased mortality.[44] Further, impaired gas transfer coefficient has been identified as being of adverse prognostic significance in ARDS and is inversely correlated with PVR.[45] Thus, in ALI/ARDS, endothelially-derived vasoactive factors, such as NO, mediate the vasomotor changes that account predominantly for early rises in PVR which give way to structural alterations with time.[46]

INHALED NO IN ARDS

With the discovery of NO as an endogenous vasodilator, and its delivery via the respiratory tract, this selective pulmonary vasodilator has emerged as a potentially important therapeutic strategy to the management of ARDS. However, its clinical application must be considered in parallel with potential toxic effects, both those that are measurable and those presumed interactions at the inflamed alveolar–capillary interface, which are currently undetectable.

The concept of NO administered by inhalation producing selective pulmonary vasodilatation is an attractive one. The use of conventional intravenous vasodilators to reduce PVR and improve hypoxaemia and right ventricular dysfunction in ALI/ARDS is limited by two problems. Firstly, the global vasodilator effect of intravenous agents may abolish the protective HPV in underventilated alveoli, causing further deterioration in V/Q mismatch and worsening hypoxaemia. Secondly, the doses required to produce a beneficial effect in the pulmonary vascular bed frequently cause systemic vasodilatation and cardiovascular instability. Inhaled NO, which is rapidly inactivated by haemoglobin, is theoretically restricted in action to its area of deposition, thereby recruiting blood to functional lung units to which the inspired gas has access, without deleterious systemic effects. This should lead to a simultaneous improvement in V/Q matching, a reduction in shunt fraction and a fall in PVR.[47]

Laboratory studies

The potential use of inhaled NO as a selective pulmonary vasodilator was first demonstrated in spontaneously breathing lambs; 40–80 ppm NO reversed acute pulmonary vasoconstriction induced by hypoxia and thromboxane endoperoxide without altering systemic haemodynamics.[48] This was attributed initially to rapid inactivation of NO by haemoglobin. Similar reductions in Ppa and PVR were identified using 40–80 ppm inhaled NO, in a spontaneously breathing sheep model of heparin-protamine-induced pulmonary hypertension, without a reduction in systemic blood pressure or impairment in gas exchange.[49,50] Subsequently, improvements in oxygenation and V/Q matching following inhaled NO were demonstrated in a swine model of sepsis,[51] findings since confirmed in other animal species. However, the effects of inhaled NO on endotoxin-induced acute pulmonary hypertension are complex. In porcine *Escherichia coli*-induced endotoxaemia, the early increase in Ppa within 30 min of endotoxin administration was not affected by 10 ppm inhaled NO, although the same dose subsequently improved Ppa, arterial oxygenation and pH.[52] Thromboxane is believed to be responsible for the early rise in Ppa following endotoxin infusion and high levels of NO are frequently required to overcome this, at least experimentally.[53] However, the reasons for varying dose–response relationships in different species and models of acute pulmonary hypertension are not fully understood. In healthy human volunteers with hypoxia-induced pulmonary hypertension, the addition of NO to the inhaled gas ($FiO_2 = 0.12$) reduced Ppa to baseline levels without affecting mean systemic arterial pressure.[54] Indeed, the effect occurred within a minute of NO administration at 10 ppm, and discontinuation of NO during hypoxia resulted in only a partial increase in Ppa. This and similar studies suggested an increased sensitivity to inhaled NO in pulmonary hypertension compared to animal models, and partial reversibility following discontinuation.

Clinical studies

Initial results in animal studies using inhaled NO as a selective pulmonary vasodilator for pulmonary hypertension gave rise to therapeutic trials in ALI/ARDS. The effects of NO inhalation (18 and 36 ppm) compared with intravenously infused prostacyclin (4 ng/kg/min) were first tested in 9 patients with ARDS. Both agents reduced PVR by up to 20%. NO at both concentrations selectively reduced mean Ppa from 37 to 30 mmHg and improved PaO_2/FiO_2 ratio from 152 mmHg to 199 mmHg without affecting systemic pressures. By contrast, prostacyclin reduced the mean arterial pressure as well as PaO_2/FiO_2 ratio. Using a standardised multiple inert gas elimination technique, the beneficial effects of NO on oxygenation were shown to be related to a reduction in intrapulmonary shunt.[55] Subsequent reports have documented the use of lower inhaled concentrations (< 20 ppm) of NO to effectively reduce Ppa and increase PaO_2/FiO_2 ratio.[56] Several groups worldwide have now published results confirming that inhaled NO significantly reduces Ppa and may improve oxygenation in ARDS (Table 11.3).

The time course of these NO-induced changes is variable. Thus, enhanced oxygenation can be achieved within 1–2 min after starting NO and baseline conditions were re-achieved within 5–8 min. A beneficial effect of low dose NO (60–230 ppb) was reported after 9–13 days use in ARDS patients by the same

Table 11.3 ARDS: clinical studies with inhaled NO

Author (year)	n	NO (ppm)	Duration of NO	PaO$_2$	Ppa	RVEF	Shunt	Notes
Rossaint et al (1993)[55]	10	5–36	40m–53d	↑	→	?	→	
Gerlach et al (1993)[56]	12	0.01–100	15m	↑	→	?	?	
Gerlach et al (1993)[57]	3	0.06–0.23	9–13d	↑	↔	?	?	
Bigatello et al (1994)[63]	7	2–20	2–27d	↑	→	?	→	
Ricou et al (1994)[64]	6	15–45	30m	↑	→	?	?	
Mira et al (1994)[65]	6	15	30m	↔	↔	?	?	Initially 0% response. 66% response on reintro after 2–40 d
Puybasset et al (1994)[81]	11	2	30m	↑	→	?	→	↓ PVR due to perm. hypercap.
Wysocki et al (1994)[78]	17	5–10	30m	↑	→	?	?	+ i.v. almitrine
Lu et al (1995)[79]	6	0.15–15	2d	↑	→	?	→	+ i.v. almitrine
Fierobe et al (1995)[61]	13	5	15m	↑	→	↑	?	RV function, CO ↔
Rossaint et al (1995)[68]	10	18–36	40m	↑	→	↑	?	RV function, CO ↔
Rossaint et al (1995)[75]	30	0.01–25	2–53d	↑	→	?	→	83% NO responders
Mcintyre et al (1995)[62]	16	20–40	30m	↑	→	?	?	70% NO responders
Krafft et al (1996)[74]	25	18–36	varied	↑	→	↑	?	40% NO responders

n, number of patients; PaO$_2$, partial pressure of arterial oxygen, ↑, increase; dndn, decrease; ↔, no change; ?: not assessed; Ppa, pulmonary arterial pressure (mean); RVEF, right ventricular ejection fraction; Shunt, measured intrapulmonary shunt; PVR, pulmonary vascular resistance; CO, cardiac output.

authors,[57] while longer-term studies of up to 53 days use in guinea pigs did not cause adverse effects such as methaemoglobinaemia.[58]

The optimal dose of inhaled NO for reversal of pulmonary hypertension may exceed that required for maximal achievable arterial oxygenation. Thus, the calculated median effective dose (ED_{50}) for statistically significant improvements in oxygenation could be as low as 100 ppb. The ED_{50} for a fall in Ppa was 2–3 ppm in 12 patients with ARDS. The optimal improvement for oxygenation occurred at 10 ppm NO (higher doses reversed the beneficial effect) whereas reductions in Ppa continued at concentrations up to 100 ppm NO.[56] Thus, theoretically, at lower concentrations NO acts locally on ventilated lung units causing vasodilatation and improved V/Q matching. However, at higher concentrations, induced diffusion of the lipophilic NO through lung tissue into nonventilated 'shunt' areas may take place creating a more global pulmonary effect. This would result in selective pulmonary vasodilatation with a further reduction in Ppa, but an increase in intrapulmonary shunt and worsening oxygenation.[59] Therefore, inhaled NO would appear to show selectivity at two levels: on well ventilated versus poorly ventilated lung vasculature (dose dependent); and on the pulmonary versus systemic circulations (dose independent).[60] Dose-response studies in animal models with acute lung injury have on the whole required higher concentrations of NO (10–80 ppm) to achieve similar improvements in systemic oxygenation and reductions in Ppa than those seen in the clinical setting.

Which effect of inhaled NO in ARDS is the more desirable, improvement in oxygenation alone or reduction in Ppa, remains unclear but depends on a large number of factors. These include: the degree of hypoxaemia; right ventricular dysfunction and its effect on overall cardiac performance; toxicity/dependence risks of higher NO doses; the aetiology of ALI/ARDS (and the potential effect of NO on the original pathophysiological insult); and the application of continually changing supportive strategies. Several groups have shown that improved systemic oxygenation can be achieved without significant falls in Ppa and that the degree of improvement is related to baseline PVR, although this is not invariable.[59,61]

Despite its short term clinical utility becoming evident from an expanding group of studies, a common feature is the variability in response to inhaled NO with around 30% of ARDS patients showing minimal or no response in any parameter.[62–64] Indeed, an initial lack of response was reported in all patients in one study, subsequent beneficial effects on oxygenation and pulmonary hypertension appearing in 60% following reintroduction of NO after 2–40 days.[65] The reason underlying this apparent lack of effect in a proportion of patients is not well understood. Theoretically, the failure of the target enzyme guanylate cyclase or its products, in pulmonary vascular smooth muscle, to respond to NO may be responsible. Indeed, recent work in an endotoxic rat model suggests that hyporesponsiveness to inhaled NO may be attributable to reduced cGMP levels through increased cGMP catabolism by a cGMP-phosphodiesterase.[66] Currently, the best predictor of a response to NO appears to be the baseline PVR,[67] perhaps reflecting those patients with the greatest intrapulmonary shunt. Thus, clinical prerequisites for a response to inhaled NO appear to be a tightened pulmonary vasculature and reversibility of constricted vessels. A lack of response may then be explained either due to a

Nitric oxide in ARDS: uses and abuses

small elevation in PVR (indeed, pulmonary hypertension is frequently not a major feature in ARDS studies as compared with hypoxaemia), or a lack of pulmonary vascular reversibility (e.g. due to pulmonary vascular remodelling in pre-existing lung disease).

Inhaled NO increases right ventricular ejection fraction (RVEF) by reducing Ppa without altering cardiac output/index.[61,68] Thus, the RV dysfunction that usually accompanies ARDS is frequently clinically insignificant. This suggests that modifying PVR to improve RV performance in ARDS is unnecessary, except in rare patients with RV dysfunction significant enough to cause a fall in cardiac output.

Inhaled NO may be partially protective against the formation of pulmonary oedema in ALI/ARDS by lowering pulmonary capillary pressure, thereby reducing transvascular albumin flux mainly through a vasodilating effect on pulmonary venous rather than arterial resistance vessels.[69] Another potential mechanism is the prevention of IL-1-induced neutrophil (PMN) accumulation and the resulting alveolar capillary membrane damage, as demonstrated in isolated rat lungs.[70] Attenuation of capillary permeability may, therefore, partly explain the resolution of bilateral pulmonary infiltrates reported in relation to NO inhalation in models of ARDS and other conditions, such as pneumonia. Indeed, the role of NO in attenuating PMN accumulation and function (as reflected by decreased hydrogen dioxide and IL-8/IL-6 production in BAL fluid) might reduce lung inflammation as well as oedema formation[71]. Nitric oxide may, however, have detrimental effects on LV dysfunction. Patients with advanced chronic LV failure (New York Heart Association grade 3–4) developed increased LV filling pressure and worse LV dysfunction despite a fall in PVR with 80 ppm inhaled NO.[72] Further, in patients with ALI/ARDS and high pre-inhalation cardiac output, NO can adversely affect gas exchange, as assessed by changes in venous admixture.[73]

As yet, no trial of inhaled NO for the treatment of ARDS has demonstrated a reduction in mortality. Nevertheless, a trend towards reduced mortality has been identified in a subgroup of fluid-resuscitated inotrope/vasopressor dependent patients with ARDS secondary to sepsis who responded to inhaled NO (> 20% rise in PaO_2 and/or > 15% fall in mean Ppa).[74] A positive response was associated with increased RV function, cardiac index and improved oxygen delivery (DO_2) while a lack of response and higher mortality were characteristic of patients with depressed cardiac reserves. A retrospective review of 87 patients with severe ARDS, of whom 30 were given inhaled NO (0.01–25 ppm) for at least 48 h showed no change in survival, but over 80% of the treated group demonstrated improved PaO_2/FiO_2 ratios and venous admixture, suggesting NO had a positive effect on $\dot{V}/\dot{Q}$ matching.[75] In a recent clinical study of 20 patients with severe ARDS, in which inhaled NO was used as only one means of therapeutic optimization, 5–10 ppm NO improved systemic oxygenation and pulmonary haemodynamics in all but one patient and reversal of ARDS occurred in 80% of whom 88% were discharged.[76]

Future trials need to address the issues of outcome and which patient subgroups with ALI/ARDS might benefit most from inhaled NO (e.g. those with pulmonary sepsis as the underlying cause), although death may be an insensitive trial endpoint due to the influence of associated conditions on mortality.[77] Indeed, given that the commonest cause of death in patients with

ARDS remains sepsis/multiple organ failure, whilst respiratory failure accounts for only 16%, it is, therefore, questionable if any improvements in oxygenation and pulmonary haemodynamics attributable to inhaled NO will be sufficient to improve survival. Improvements in outcome of ARDS may depend more on treatment of sepsis and further understanding/prevention of MOF.

Interaction of inhaled NO and complementary therapies

Although vasoconstrictors in patients with ALI/ARDS may have negative effects on Ppa and, thereby, induce RV dysfunction, they could theoretically improve gas exchange if HPV is restored. The peripheral chemoreceptor stimulant almitrine acts as a selective pulmonary vasoconstrictor and is thought to improve intrapulmonary shunt in patients with ARDS by vaso-constricting pulmonary vessels located in non-ventilated lung areas, thereby improving V/Q matching. However, almitrine increases Ppa and early studies in ARDS in the late 1980s were inconsistent in demonstrating benefit. Since then, investigations considering the combined effect of NO and intravenous almitrine have shown an additive effect on gas exchange with the maintenance of Ppa.[78] It may be that such a benefit will only be seen in those who respond to NO.[79] Despite its potential utility at infusion rates between 2 and 16 ng/kg/min, serious concerns regarding neurotoxicity need to be addressed and further studies are required prior to any recommendation for its clinical use in ARDS.

A greater understanding of lung function and mechanics in ALI/ARDS, particularly through the use of computed tomography (reviewed elsewhere[80]), the susceptibility of mechanically ventilated patients with ALI/ARDS to baro- or volutrauma and an appreciation of the importance of lung volume recruitment and protection has led to a change in thinking with regard to the way in which these patients should be supported. Thus, volume- and pressure-limited ventilation with permissive hypercapnia has been widely adopted. Although this is potentially beneficial, the hypercapnia induced can increase PVR and Ppa. Whether these rises are clinically relevant is questionable, although 2 ppm inhaled NO has been shown to reduce Ppa and PVR whilst improving oxygenation during both normocapnic and hypercapnic ventilation.[81] This effect has been confirmed by other groups, potentially expanding the adoption of this ventilatory strategy while limiting its detrimental effects in ALI/ARDS.

The use of NOS inhibition in inotrope-refractory septic shock remains experimental, although such an approach has been shown in isolated cases to improve systemic blood pressure in patients with inotrope-refractory septic shock,[82] possibly because endogenous NO impairs vasopressor-respon-siveness in sepsis.[83] However, there is preliminary evidence that the balance between constitutive and inducible NOS isoforms is an important determinant of local vascular tone in the septic circulation, and that a sweeping disruption of this balance may be disadvantageous.[84] In particular, the pulmonary arterial hypertension that is characteristically seen in ALI/ARDS may be exacerbated. To date, specific iNOS inhibitors have not been applicable in the clinical arena due to toxicity. Since ARDS is most frequently associated with sepsis, the pursuit and clinical application of selective iNOS inhibition in combination with exogenous NO or NO donors, to maintain the basal requirement of NO, is an area of ongoing study.

Interest in other short acting vasodilators such as nebulised prostacyclin (PGI_2) has developed; its familiar pharmacology, rapid onset of action, short half-life (2–3 min) and lack of known toxicity make PGI_2 an attractive agent for use in inhalational therapy and a number of case reports have demonstrated improved systemic oxygenation in ARDS due to amniotic fluid embolism or intra-abdominal sepsis without detrimental systemic effects. Indeed, a comparison of inhaled PGI_2 and inhaled NO in ARDS at doses of 10 or 25 ng/kg/min and 4 or 8 ppm, respectively, revealed that they were equally efficacious in improving oxygenation and reducing Ppa.[85]

TOXICITY AND SAFE USE

Perhaps the first documented 'abuse' of NO followed the investigations of its properties by Davy in the seventeenth century. As a result of his experiences inhaling nitrous oxide (N_2O) followed by NO, both NO and nitrogen dioxide (NO_2) were identified as poisonous gases.[86] The earliest quoted therapeutic use of an NO donor for respiratory disease is amyl nitrate for asthma in 1866.[87] However, the poisonous nature of the nitrogen oxide gases was highlighted in 1966 with the deaths of at least 3 patients on induction of anaesthesia; N_2O had become contaminated by NO and NO_2.[88] Hence, reports of the successful therapeutic application of inhaled NO must be considered in parallel with its potential toxicity.

Nonetheless, it should be noted that, within the atmosphere, NO exists at levels close to 10 ppb. It is present in cigarette smoke for short periods at concentrations between 400 and 1000 ppm.[53] Indeed, NO is present normally in the expired air of humans,[89] originating mainly from the paranasal sinus mucosa of the upper respiratory tract (URT). This exhaled NO appears to reflect host defence activity for the URT and lower respiratory tract (LRT), whilst auto-inhalation of NO may be important in V/Q matching.[90] Many groups have now reported elevated levels of NO in the breath of patients with inflammatory lung disease, such as asthma, suggesting its potential as a measurable marker of pulmonary disease activity, given accurate, easy-to-perform measurements.[91] However, further investigation is required to improve the available methodology, and in analysing NO from specific lung regions to define more clearly its roles as a byproduct of inflammation or in modulating airway physiology.[92] Although increased exhaled NO levels are present in a rodent model of endotoxic sepsis syndrome, it is not clear what, if any, relationship exists between endogenous airway NO, PVR and inflammatory activity in ALI/ARDS. Preliminary data, from our group, suggest that ventilated ARDS patients demonstrate lower levels of endogenous NO in the lower airways than appropriate controls. This may reflect a rapid reaction of the evolving NO with neighbouring ROS at the alveolar-capillary interface preventing NO reaching the proximal airways.[93]

The potential toxicity of NO is attributable to the formation of several cytotoxic products such as nitrogen dioxide (NO_2), peroxynitrite radicals (in the presence of superoxide anions) and methaemoglobinaemia (metHb, by the interaction of nitrate and haemoglobin, causing a reduced oxygen carrying capacity). The deleterious pro-oxidant outcome versus the cytoprotective anti-oxidant outcome seems critically dependent on relative concentrations of oxygen and individual reactive species. Thus, NO combines with oxygen to produce NO_2 at a rate dependent upon the oxygen concentration and the square of the NO concentration. NO_2 dissolves to nitric and nitrous acids in aqueous solution which initiate lipid peroxidation in cells, resulting in cell damage or death.

Fatality due to acute NO_2 toxicity appears to be due to pulmonary oedema in short term doses above 150 ppm, although it is almost inconceivable that such concentrations could be generated at clinically relevant levels of NO. However, the Health and Safety Executive specify worker exposure limits for NO and NO_2 of 25 and 3 ppm over an 8 h time-weighted average period (TWA).[94]

Despite evidence to suggest that NO is an effective scavenger of reactive oxygen species (ROS)[95] that may inhibit xanthine oxidase and, therefore, reduce the formation of damaging ROS,[96] under hypoxic conditions NO reacts with superoxide to form peroxynitrite, which damages lipids, surfactants, nucleic acids and proteins through its pro-oxidant capacity.[97] However, frequently quoted toxicity studies have been carried out principally in non diseased animals exposed to inhaled NO.[98] This lack of demonstrable pulmonary toxicity may have little relevance to the clinical setting in which the propensity of inflamed lungs to produce ROS in the presence of a high FiO_2 would appear to be great.

In the circulation, endogenous NO combines rapidly with haemoglobin to form an intermediary nitrosyl Fe(II)-haemoglobin and then metHb. Clinically significant concentrations are rare at therapeutic inhaled NO concentrations although reports of levels upto 13% are documented in cases where accurate NO level monitoring was questionable. In human studies, metHb remained below 0.7% in healthy volunteers[99] and less than 3.5% of patients inhaling NO had metHb levels above 5%; all responded well to dose reduction of NO.[100] Whilst emphasising the small chance of metHb, the last study highlights a need to be aware that some patients may have reduced metHb reductase activity (hereditary or in newborns) and are at risk of methaemoglobinaemia in the face of increased haemoglobin oxidation by NO. Plasma metHb levels should be performed after starting NO therapy and following any dose increase.

Prolonged NO administration has been shown to increase bleeding time in rabbits and healthy human volunteers through its platelet inhibitory effect although this was not clinically significant.[59]

Long term follow-up of patients exposed to therapeutic inhaled NO is desirable in view of its potential mutagenicity, and its unknown effects on pulmonary morphology and healing after the acute illness. Indeed, redistribution of pulmonary blood flow away from damaged, hypoxic regions of lung toward healthier lung segments may deprive the damaged lung parenchyma of the blood supply necessary for tissue repair and functional recovery. Thus, although NO can improve arterial oxygenation in ARDS, it may simultaneously worsen underlying lung injury and impair healing. Further, any potentially beneficial bacteriostatic and antiviral effect of URT-derived NO on the LRT is likely to be lost by endotracheal intubation of patients with ALI/ARDS.

The haemodynamic 'NO dependency' that develops in some patients inhaling NO and the possibility of severe arterial oxygen desaturation on sudden withdrawal of therapy is a potential cause for concern. This effect is probably due to feedback inhibition of eNOS by exogenously supplied NO. Thus, sudden removal of NO results in rebound vasoconstriction in ventilated lung units, increased intrapulmonary shunt and subsequently impaired gas exchange. Hence the recommendation of slow weaning of inhaled NO therapy in acute hypoxic pulmonary hypertension and the importance of having a 'back-up' delivery system at hand.

CURRENT RECOMMENDATIONS FOR DELIVERY AND SAFE USE

Until multicentre trials determine the efficacy and safety of inhaled NO in patients with ALI/ARDS, its use as a therapeutic agent should be based on local/regional guidelines for compassionate use. Variations in the design of modern mechanical ventilators and the awareness of potential risks of inhaled NO to the patient and providers have necessitated different methods of administration and improved accuracy in monitoring. To this end, a number of safety issues pertaining to the clinical use of NO have been drawn up recently,[101] although national/international guidelines are awaited (Table 11.4). Important factors for its use in ventilated patients include the provision to introduce and regulate an additional gas source into the system, whether an intermittent or continuous flow of NO is generated in the inspiratory limb and where, in relation to the entrained oxygen, NO is introduced. Furthermore, adjustment of positive pressure parameters and ventilatory flow rates are likely to alter NO concentration actually entering the lower respiratory tract. Of the commercially available methods of NO detection and monitoring, chemiluminescence is relatively specific and highly sensitive for NO concentrations less than 1 ppb; NO_2 can also be measured indirectly by reduction to NO prior to reaction in the sampling chamber. However, these analysers have to date been bulky, noisy and expensive with high maintenance requirements. Moreover, sampling accuracy requires the source gas to be delivered at ambient pressures, which is not the case in positive pressure ventilation. The alternative method of detection and monitoring, utilizing electrochemical (fuel cell) sensors, enables mainstream (as opposed to sidestream) gas sampling, direct NO_2 detection, quick response times to NO concentration changes and insensitivity to gas pressure fluctuations. Thus, although they are less accurate (sensitivity error ± 0.5 ppm) than chemiluminescence, the relative ease of use and low cost of these devices make them the current choice for ICU monitoring of NO therapy at levels above 1 ppm.

SUMMARY

Since the early experimental work demonstrated the efficacy of inhaled NO as a selective pulmonary vasodilator with the ability to reduce PVR and Ppa, its clinical application in ALI/ARDS has progressed to Phase 3 trials of efficacy and safety. There appears to be biselectivity between well- and under-ventilated lung units, as well as between pulmonary and systemic circulations.

Table 11.4 Recommendations for the use of inhaled nitric oxide in the ICU (from Cuthbertson et al,[101] with permission)

Delivery
>   Medical NO/N$_2$ gas mixture
>   Stainless steel pressure regulators, connectors and
>   flowmeter needle valves
>   Calibrated flowmeter
>   Stainless steel/PTFE tubing

Monitoring
>   Inspiratory NO and NO$_2$
>   Chemiluminescence or electrochemical monitor
>   Daily methaemoglobin concentrations

Exposure
>   Maximum inhaled NO < 80 ppm
>   Maximum inhaled NO$_2$ <3 ppm
>   Maximum environmental NO < 25 ppm for 8 h TWA
>   Maximum environmental NO$_2$ < 3 ppm for 8 h TWA

Scavenging
>   Not required in well ventilated unit
>   Required in units with less than 10–12 air changes per hour

Scavenging techniques
>   ABEK HgCONO-P3 filter
>   Active scavenging (i.e. soda lime, charcoal absorbers)
>   Passive scavenging (i.e. tubing to atmosphere)

PTFE, polytetrafluroethylene; TWA, time-weighted-average; ABEK HgCONO-P3 filter, industrial NO/NO$_2$ scavenger (Dräger Industrial Ltd, Hemel Hempstead, Herts, UK).

In general, lower doses (5–30 ppm) appear to improve arterial oxygenation, through an improvement in V/Q matching; while levels above this reduce the Ppa in a dose-dependent manner but may impair oxygenation. Potentially detrimental effects of NO and its byproducts within the injured lung and circulation, and possible adverse long term effects on healing and pulmonary morphology remain concerns despite the availability of accurate NO, NO$_2$ and metHb monitoring. There are currently no practical methods to assess directly the degree of local oxidant-NO interaction/damage at the inflamed alveolar-capillary interface.

However, the utility of inhaled NO in improving oxygenation and reducing Ppa is evident, although this has not translated into survival benefit. Questions remain regarding which ALI/ARDS patient subsets are likely to benefit from inhaled NO therapy, why only a proportion of patients show clinically apparent improvement and at what stage of the disease NO will be most beneficial. Until ongoing randomised controlled trials are complete, the principle of best clinical practice would suggest that it be used in ALI/ARDS patients with severe hypoxaemia refractory to appropriate ventilatory manipulation, in combination with other therapeutic strategies, at the lowest effective dose to achieve improvements in oxygenation, within the framework of local/regional consensus guidelines.

Key points for clinical practice

- The use of inhaled NO should be considered in ARDS patients with severe hypoxaemia (PaO_2 <12 kPA with an FiO_2 = 1.0), in whom deterioration in oxygenation continues despite adequate treatment of the underlying cause and appropriate ventilatory manipulation, or if pulmonary hypertension is affecting cardiac output detrimentally.

- It should be used only on compassionate grounds, and in conjunction with other therapeutic strategies of perceived benefit (e.g. prone positioning), until evidence of definite benefit emerges from randomised controlled trials.

- Careful benefit/risk analysis must be undertaken and assessment of factors that may prevent a useful response to NO, namely pre-existing pulmonary hypertension.

- Any inhaled NO delivery system must have a means of accurately measuring NO and NO_2 concentrations in the inspiratory limb of the mechanical ventilator. metHb levels from the patient should be monitored.

- A dose-response study, with full pulmonary and systemic haemodynamic monitoring, should be performed prior to its implementation. A positive response to NO may be defined as >20% improvement in PaO_2/FiO_2 ratio or > 20% reduction in PVR.

- A number of dosing strategies are acceptable: starting in the middle of the dose range (20 ppm), reduce the NO concentration sequentially to 10 and 5 ppm at 15 min intervals until a reduction in the response is seen, or start at low concentrations (5 ppm) and increase through 10, 20 to a maximum of 40 ppm , assessing the response after 15 min at each dose, for the lowest concentration that produces the desired response.

- A back up system should be available, and weaning should be slow with pulmonary haemodynamic monitoring to reduce the risk of rebound pulmonary vasoconstriction.

ACKNOWLEDGEMENT

SS is supported by a British Heart Foundation Fellowship.

References

1. Ashbaugh DG, Bigelow DB, Petty TL, Levine BE. Acute respiratory distress in adults. Lancet 1967; 2: 319–323
2. Petty TL, Ashbaugh DG. The adult respiratory distress syndrome: clinical features, factors influencing prognosis and principles of management. Chest 1971; 60: 233–239
3. Furchgott RF, Zawadski JV. The obligatory role of endothelial cells in the relaxation of arterial smooth muscle by acetylcholine. Nature 1980; 288: 373–362

4. Ignarro LJ, Buga GM, Wood KS, Byrns RE, Chaudhuri G. Endothelium-derived relaxing factor produced and released from artery and vein is nitric oxide. Proc Natl Acad Sci USA 1987; 84: 9265–9269

5. Palmer RM, Ferrige AG, Moncada S. Nitric oxide release accounts for the biological activity of endothelium-derived relaxing factor. Nature 1987; 327: 524–526

6. Moncada S, Higgs A. The L-arginine-nitric oxide pathway. N Engl J Med 1993; 329: 2002–2012

7. Salter M, Knowles RG, Moncada S. Widespread tissue distribution, species distribution and changes in activity of Ca^{2+}-dependent and Ca^{2+}-independent nitric oxide synthases. FEBS Lett 1991; 291: 145–149

8. Adcock IM, Brown CR, Kwon OJ, Barnes PJ. Oxidative stress induces NF-κB DNA binding and inducible NOS mRNA in human epithelial cells. Biochem Biophys Res Commun 1994; 199: 1518–1524

9. Singh S, Evans TW. Nitric oxide, the biological mediator of the decade: fact or fiction? Eur Respir J 1997; 10: 699–707

10. Beckman JS, Crow JP. Pathological implications of nitric oxide, superoxide and peroxynitrite formation. Biochem Soc Trans 1993; 21: 330–334

11. Van der Vliet A, Smith D, O'Neill CA et al. Interactions of peroxynitrite with human plasma and its constituents:oxidant damage and antioxidant depletion. Biochem J 1994; 303: 295–301

12. Myers PR, Minor RL, Guerra R, Bates JN, Harrison DB. Vasorelaxant properties of the endothelium-derived relaxing factor more closely resemble 5-nitrocysteine than nitric oxide. Nature 1990; 345: 161–163

13. Mitchell JA, Larkin S, Williams TJ. Cyclooxygenase-2: regulation and relevance in inflammation. Biochem Pharmacol 1995; 50: 1535–1542

14. Landino LM, Crews BC, Timmons MD et al. Peroxynitrite, the coupling product of nitric oxide and superoxide, activates prostaglandin biosynthesis. Proc Natl Acad Sci USA 1996; 93: 15069–15074

15. Bone RC, Balk R, Slotman G et al. Adult respiratory distress syndrome. Sequence and importance of development of multiple organ failure. The Prostaglandin E_1 Study Group. Chest 1992; 101: 320–326

16. Bernard GR, Artigas A, Brigham KL et al. The American-European consensus conference on ARDS: definitions, mechanisms, relevant outcomes and clinical trial co-ordination. Am J Respir Crit Care Med 1994; 149: 818–824

17. Bone RC, Fisher Jr CJ, Clemmer TP, Slotman GJ, Metz CA, Balk RA. Sepsis syndrome: a valid clinical entity. Methylprednisolone Severe Sepsis Study Group. Crit Care Med 1989; 17: 389–393

18. Montgomery B, Stager MA, Carrico CJ, Hudson LD. Causes of mortality in patients with the adult respiratory distress syndrome. Am Rev Respir Dis 1985; 132: 485–489

19. Ferring M, Vincent JL. Is outcome from ARDS related to the severity of respiratory failure? Eur Respir J 1997; 10: 1297–1300

20. Curzen NP, Griffiths MJD, Evans TW. The role of the endothelium in modulating the vascular response to sepsis. Clin Sci 1994; 86: 359–374

21. Phillips P, Tsan M. Cytoarchitectural aspects of endothelial barrier function in response to oxidants and inflammatory mediators. In: Johnson A, Ferro TJ (eds) Lung Vascular Injury. New York: Marcel Dekker, 1992

22. Hamacher J, Schaberg T. Adhesion molecules in lung diseases. Lung 1994; 172: 189–213

23. Ferrari-Baliviera E, Mealy K, Smith RJ, Wilmore DW. Tumor necrosis factor induces adult respiratory distress syndrome in rats. Arch Surg 1989; 124: 1400–1405

24. Vijaykumar E, Raziuddin S, Wardle EN. Plasma endotoxin in patients with trauma, sepsis and severe haemorrhage. Clin Int Care 1991; 2: 4–9

25. Rossetti M, Guenard H, Gabinski C. Effects of nitric oxide inhalation on pulmonary serial resistances in ARDS. Am J Respir Crit Care Med 1996; 154: 1375–1381

26. Paterson NAM, McCormack DG. Pulmonary vascular control mechanisms. In: Evans TW, Haslett C. (eds) ARDS Acute Respiratory Distress in Adults. London: Chapman Hall, 1996: 297–316

27. Rodman DM, Yamaguchi T, Hasunuma K, O'Brien RF, McMurtry IF. Effects of hypoxia on endothelium-dependent relaxation of rat pulmonary artery. Am J Physiol 1990; 258: L207–L214

28. Liu SF, Dewar A, Crawley DE, Barnes PJ, Evans TW. Effect of tumor necrosis factor on hypoxic pulmonary vasoconstriction. J Appl Physiol 1992; 72: 1044–1049

29. Crawley DF, Liu SF, Evans TW et al. Inhibitory role of endothelium-derived nitric oxide in rat and human pulmonary arteries. Br J Pharmacol 1990; 101: 166–170

30. Rodman DM, Yamaguchi T, O'Brien RF et al. Hypoxic contraction of isolated rat pulmonary artery. J Pharmacol Exp Ther 1989; 248: 952–959

31. Dinh-Xuan AT. Endothelial modulation of pulmonary vascular tone. Eur Respir J 1992; 5: 757–762

32. Dantzker DR, Brook CJ, Dehart P, Lynch JP, Weg JG. Ventilation-perfusion distributions in the adult respiratory distress syndrome. Am Rev Respir Dis 1979; 120: 1039–1052

33. Zelenkov P, McLoughlin T, Johns RA. Endotoxin enhances hypoxic constriction of rat aorta and pulmonary artery through induction of EDRF/NO synthase. Am J Physiol 1993; 9: 346–354

34. Griffiths MJD, Curzen NP, Mitchell J, Evans TW. In vivo treatment with endotoxin increases rat pulmonary vascular contractility despite NOS induction. Am J Respir Crit Care Med 1997; 157: 654–658

35. Sitbon O, Brenot F, Denjean A et al. Inhaled nitric oxide as a screening vasodilator agent in primary pulmonary hypertension. Am J Respir Crit Care Med 1995; 151: 384–389

36. Katayama Y, Higenbottam TW, Diaz de Atauri MJ et al. Inhaled nitric oxide and arterial oxygen tension in patients with chronic obstructive pulmonary disease and severe pulmonary hypertension. Thorax 1997; 52: 120–124

37. Liu SF, Crawley DE, Barnes PJ et al. Endothelium-derived nitric oxide inhibits pulmonary vasoconstriction in isolated blood perfused rat lungs. Am J Respir Rev 1991; 143: 32–37

38. Zapol WM, Snider MT. Pulmonary hypertension in severe acute respiratory failure. N Engl J Med 1977; 296: 476–480

39. Wagenvoort CA. Grading of pulmonary vascular lesions – a reappraisal. Histopathology 1981; 5: 595–598

40. Wood P. Pulmonary hypertension with special reference to the vasoconstrictive factor. Br Heart J 1958; 20: 557–570

41. Giaid A, Saleh D. Reduced expression of endothelial nitric oxide synthase in the lungs of patients with pulmonary hypertension. N Eng J Med 1995; 333: 214–221

42. Loscalzo J. Endothelial dysfunction in pulmonary hypertension. N Engl J Med 1992; 327: 117–119

43. Dinh-Xuan AT. Endothelial modulation of pulmonary vascular tone. Eur Respir J 1992 ;5: 757–762

44. Bernard GR, Rinaldo J, Harris T et al. Early predictors of ARDS reversal in patients with established ARDS [Abstract]. Am Rev Respir Dis 1985; 131: A143

45. Pallares LCM, Evans TW. Oxygen transport in the critically ill. Respir Med 1992; 86: 289–295

46. Furchgott RF, Vanhoutte PM. Endothelium-derived relaxing and contracting factors. FASEB J 1989; 3: 2007–2018

47. Brett SJ, Evans TW. Nitric oxide: physiological roles and therapeutic implications in the lung. Br J Hosp Med 1995; Suppl. 5: 1–4

48. Frostell CG, Fratacci MD, Wain JC et al. Inhaled nitric oxide: a selective pulmonary vasodilator reversing hypoxic pulmonary vasoconstriction. Circulation 1991; 83: 2038–2047

49. Frattaci MD, Frostell CG, Chen TY et al. Inhaled nitric oxide: a selective pulmonary vasodilator of heparin-protamine vasoconstriction in sheep. Anesthesiology 1991; 75: 990–999

50. Pison U, Lopez FA, Heidelmeyer CF et al. Inhaled nitric oxide reverses hypoxic pulmonary vasoconstriction without impairing gas exchange. J Appl Physiol 1993; 74: 1287–1292

51. Ogura H, Cioffi WG, Offner PJ et al. Effect of inhaled nitric oxide on pulmonary function after sepsis in a swine model. Surgery 1994; 116: 313–321

52. Weitzberg E, Rudehill A, Lundberg JM. Nitric oxide inhalation attenuates pulmonary hypertension and improves gas exchange in endotoxin shock. Eur J Pharmacol 1993; 233: 85–94

53. Zapol WM, Hurford WE. Inhaled nitric oxide: a review. In: Fink MP, Payen D. (eds) Update in Intensive Care and Emergency Medicine, vol 24. Berlin: Springer, 1995; 323–341

54. Frostell CG, Blomquist H, Hedenstierna G et al. Inhaled nitric oxide selectively reverses human hypoxic pulmonary vasoconstriction without causing systemic vasodilation. Anesthesiology 1993; 78: 427–435

55. Rossaint R, Falke KJ, Lopez F et al. Inhaled nitric oxide for the adult respiratory distress syndrome. N Engl J Med 1993; 328: 399–405

56. Gerlach H, Rossaint R, Pappert D et al. Time-course and dose-response of nitric oxide inhalation for systemic oxygenation and pulmonary hypertension in patients with adult respiratory distress syndrome. Eur J Clin Invest 1993; 23: 499–502

57. Gerlach H, Pappert D, Lewandowski K et al. Long-term inhalation with evaluated low doses of nitric oxide for selective improvement of oxygenation in patients with adult respiratory distress syndrome. Intensive Care Med 1993; 19: 443–449

58. Dupuy PM, Shore SA, Drazen JM et al. Bronchodilator action of nitric oxide in guinea pigs. J Clin Invest 1992; 90: 421–428

59. Gerlach H, Rossaint R, Falke KJ. Nitric oxide inhalation in ARDS. In: Fink MP, Payen D. (eds) Update in Intensive Care and Emergency Medicine, vol 24. Berlin: Springer, 1995: 399–413

60. Grover ER, Bihari D. Inhaled nitric oxide therapy. In: Evans TW, Haslett C. (eds) ARDS Acute Respiratory Distress in Adults. London: Chapman and Hall, 1996; 495–506

61. Fierobe L, Brunet F, Dhainaut J-F. Effect of inhaled nitric oxide on right ventricular function in adult respiratory distress syndrome. Am J Respir Crit Care Med 1995; 151: 1414–1419

62. McIntyre RC, Moore FA, Moore EE et al. Inhaled nitric oxide variably improves oxygenation and pulmonary hypertension in patients with acute respiratory distress syndrome. J Trauma 1995; 39: 418–425

63. Bigatello LM, Hurford WE, Kacmarek RM, Roberts JD, Zapol WM. Prolonged inhalation of low concentrations of nitric oxide in patients with severe adult respiratory distress syndrome – effects on pulmonary haemodynamics and oxygenation. Anesthesiology 1994; 80; 761–770

64. Ricou B, Grandin S, Jolliet P, Chevrolet JC, Suter PM. Nitric oxide in the treatment of adult respiratory distress syndrome. Schweiz Med Wochenschr 1994; 124: 583–588

65. Mira JP, Monchi M, Brunet F, Fierobe L, Dhainaut JF, Dinh-Xuan AT. Lack of efficacy of inhaled nitric oxide in ARDS [letter]. Intensive Care Med 1994; 20; 532

66. Holzmann A, Bloch KD, Sanchez LS, Filippov G, Zapol WM. Hyporesponsiveness to inhaled nitric oxide in isolated, perfused lungs from endotoxin-challenged rats. Am J Physiol 1996; 271: L981–L986

67. Lowson SM, Rich GF, McArdle PA, Jaidev J, Morris GN. The response to varying concentrations of inhaled nitric oxide in patients with acute respiratory distress syndrome. Anesth Analg 1996; 82: 574–581

68. Rossaint R, Slama K, Steudel W et al. Effects of inhaled nitric oxide on right ventricular function in severe acute respiratory distress syndrome. Intensive Care Med 1995; 21: 197–203

69. Benzing A, Brautigam P, Geiger K et al. Inhaled nitric oxide reduces pulmonary trans-vascular albumin flux in patients with acute lung injury. Anesthesiology 1995; 83: 1153–1161

70. Guidot DM, Hybertson BM, Kitlowski RP et al. Inhaled nitric oxide prevents IL-1-induced neutrophil accumulation and associated acute Oedema in isolated rat lungs. Am J Physiol 1996; 271: L225–L229

71. Chollet-Martin S, Gatechal C, Kermarrec N, Gougerot-Pocidalo MA, Payen DM. Alveolar neutrophil functions and cytokine levels in patients with the adult respiratory distress syndrome during nitric oxide inhalation. Am J Respir Crit Care Med 1996; 153: 985–990

72. Loh EL, Stamler JS, Hare JM et al. Cardiovascular effects of inhaled nitric oxide in patients with left ventricular dysfunction. Circulation 1994; 90: 2780–2785

73. Benzing A, Loop T, Mols G et al. Effect of inhaled nitric oxide on venous admixture depends on cardiac output in patients with acute lung injury and acute respiratory distress syndrome. Acta Anaesth Scand 1996; 40: 466–474

74. Krafft P, Freidrich P, Fitzgerald RD et al. Effectiveness of nitric oxide inhalation in septic ARDS Chest 1996; 109: 486–493

75. Rossaint R, Gerlach H, Schmidt-Ruhnke H et al. Efficacy of inhaled nitric oxide in patients with severe ARDS. Chest 1995; 107: 1107–1115

76. Ley B, Bollaert PE, Bauer P et al. Therapeutic optimization including inhaled nitric oxide in adult respiratory distress syndrome in a polyvalent intensive care unit. J Trauma 1995; 38: 370–374

77. Brett SJ, Evans TW. Inhaled vasodilator therapy in acute lung injury: first, do NO harm? Thorax 1995; 50: 821–823

78. Wysocki M, Delclaux C, Roupie E et al. Additive effect on gas exchange of inhaled nitric oxide and intravenous almitrine bismesylate in the adult respiratory distress syndrome. Intensive Care Med 1994; 20: 254–259

79. Lu Q, Mourgeon E, Law-Koune JD et al. Dose-response curves of inhaled nitric oxide with and without intravenous almitrine in nitric oxide-responding patients with acute respiratory distress syndrome. Anesthesiology 1995; 83: 929–943

80. Bone RC. The ARDS lung. New insights from computed tomography. JAMA 1993; 269: 2134–2135

81. Puybasset L, Stewart T, Rouby J-J et al. Inhaled nitric oxide reverses the increase in pulmonary vascular resistance induced by permissive hypercapnia in patients with acute respiratory distress syndrome. Anesthesiology 1994; 80: 1254–1267

82. Petros A, Bennett D, Vallance P. Effect of nitric oxide inhibitors on hypotension in patients with septic shock. Lancet 1991; 338: 1557–1558

83. Hollenberg SM, Cunnion RE, Zimmerberg J. Nitric oxide synthase inhibition reverses arteriolar hyporesponsiveness to catecholamines in septic rats. Am J Physiol 1993; 264: H660–H663

84. Liu S, Adcock IM, Barnes PJ, Evans TW. Differential regulation of the constitutive and inducible NO synthase mRNA by endotoxin in vivo in the rat [Abstract]. Am J Respir Crit Care Med 1995; 151: A15

85. Walmrath D, Schneider T, Schermuly R et al. Direct comparison of inhaled nitric oxide and aerosolized prostacyclin in acute respiratory distress syndrome. Am J Respir Crit Care Med 1996; 153: 991–996

86. Davy H. Researches, Chemical and Philosophical; Chiefly concerning Nitrous Oxide, or Dephllogisticated Nitrous air, and its Respiration. London: J. Johnson, 1800

87. Riegel F. Diseases of the trachea and bronchi. In: Ziemssen HV. (ed.) Cyclopaedia of the Practice of Medicine, Vol 4. London: Sampson, Low, Martson, Saerle and Rivington, 1976; 275–586

88. Clutton-Brock J.Two cases of poisoning by contamination of nitrous oxide with higher oxides of nitrogen during anaesthesia. Br J Anaesth 1967; 39: 388–392

89. Gustaffson LE, Leone AM, Persson MG et al. Endogenous nitric oxide is present in the exhaled air of rabbits, guinea pigs and humans. Biochem Biophys Res Commun 1991; 181: 852–857

90. Gerlach H, Rossaint R, Pappert D et al. Autoinhalation of nitric oxide after endogenous synthesis in the nasopharynx. Lancet 1994; 343: 518–519

91. Lundberg JON, Weitzberg E, Lundberg JM et al. Nitric oxide in exhaled air. Eur Respir J 1996; 9: 2671–2680.

92. Barnes PJ, Kharitonov SA. Exhaled nitric oxide: a new lung function test. Thorax 1996; 51: 233–237

93. Brett SJ, Evans TW. Pulmonary production of nitric oxide in patients with the acute respiratory distress syndrome [Abstract]. Am J Respir Crit Care Med 1997; 155: A93

94. Health and Safety Executive. EH40/96 Occupational Exposure Limits for use with the Control of Substances Hazardous to Health Regulations 1996. ISBN 07176 10217. London: HMSO, 1996

95. Rubanyi GM, Ho EH, Cantor EH et al. Cytoprotective function of nitric oxide: inactivation of superoxide radicals produced by human leukocytes. Biochem Biophys Res Commun 1991; 181: 1392–1397

96. Fukahori M, Ichimori K, Ishida H et al. Nitric oxide reversibly suppresses xanthine oxidase activity. Free Rad Res 1994; 21: 203–212

97. Beckman JS, Beckman TW, Chen J et al. Apparent hydroxyl radical protection by peroxynitrite: implications for endothelial injury from nitric oxide and superoxide. Proc Natl Acad Sci USA 1990; 87: 1620–1624

98. Kooy NW, Royall JA, Kelly DR et al. Evidence for in vivo perooxynitrite production in human acute lung injury. Am J Respir Crit Care Med 1995; 151: 1250–1254

99. Von Neiding G, Wagner H, Kockeler H. Investigation of the acute effects of nitrogen monoxide on lung function in man. Staub-Reinhalt Luft 1975; 35: 175–178

100. Wessel DL, Adatia I, Thompson JE et al. Delivery and monitoring of inhaled nitric oxide in patients with pulmonary hypertension. Crit Care Med 1994; 22: 930–938

101. Cuthbertson BH, Stott S, Webster NR. Use of inhaled nitric oxide in British intensive therapy units. Br J Anaesth 1997; 78: 696–700

Christopher P. Leng   Andrew D. Lawson

Pain management in intensive care

Critically ill patients in the Intensive Care Unit (ITU) are a unique patient group often combining a high requirement for pain relief, such as occurs after major surgery or trauma, with a reduced tolerance to side effects of analgesic drugs and techniques. Understandably, in the initial stages of intensive care, pain relief may be a low priority as resuscitation takes place. However, although many patients receive adequate analgesia, 40–60% of patients have been reported as having recollection of moderate to severe pain whilst in the ITU.[1,2] The issue of pain relief has received minimal attention in the medical literature. The majority of references produced by a literature search combining pain with Intensive Care and Critical Care were from nursing journals. Increasing the awareness of untreated pain in intensive care units, the understanding of the pathophysiology of pain and of therapeutic and technical advances should lead to a demonstrable reduction in the incidence of pain in the ITU.

Relief from pain is indicated on humanitarian, ethical, medical and, possibly, financial grounds. The first step in providing good analgesia for patients in the ITU is to recognise that they **are** in pain. The cause of the pain should be identified, investigated and, where appropriate, treated at the same time as providing specific therapy for the pain itself. The nature of the pain should be elucidated. For example, simple measures such as immobilising a fractured bone, supporting a painful back or identifying and treating mouth ulcers may bring benefits as great as changing the analgesic drug used. Pre-existing conditions such as rheumatic or vascular disease, which may be painful in themselves, should not be forgotten and should be treated.

Dr Christopher P. Leng FRCA, Senior Registrar, Magill Department of Anaesthetics, Chelsea and Westminster Hospital, 369 Fulham Road, London SW10 9NH, UK

Dr Andrew D. Lawson FFARCSI FANZCA, Consultant in Pain Management, Magill Department of Anaesthetics, Chelsea and Westminster Hospital, London, UK

If pain is to be adequately treated then it must be appropriately diagnosed. Not all pain is due to tissue trauma and not all pain will be new when the patient is admitted to the ITU. Pain may be broadly divided on a functional basis into nociceptive and neuropathic pain. Nociceptive pain is pain produced by activation of nociceptors which are stimulated by chemical, mechanical or thermal energy. This is the pain of tissue damage and trauma. Pain may also be initiated or caused by a primary lesion or dysfunction in the nervous system – this is termed neuropathic pain.[3] This pain, which has a different character than nociceptive pain, is often not well treated by standard analgesics and may be quite unresponsive to systemic opioids.

WHY IS PAIN UNDERTREATED IN THE ITU?

Patients in the ITU often present with life threatening conditions and it is understandable that pain relief becomes of secondary importance compared with immediate resuscitation.[4] However, given the high nurse-to-patient ratio, familiarity with technical devices, such as infusion pumps, and the presence of continuous cardio-respiratory monitoring, one might expect pain relief in the ITU to be superior to that obtained elsewhere, yet this does not seem to be the case.

The same myths and prejudices that surround pain relief in general and morphine in particular may be equally prevalent in Intensive Care Units. Opioids given appropriately can provide effective analgesia for most kinds of pain, yet there is still resistance to the prescribing of strong opioids amongst both staff and patients. A 1994 Gallup poll revealed that 50% of adults would not want to take opioids for pain relief, even if they were in severe pain, because of the adverse connotations associated with morphine.[5] All opioids are respiratory depressants and concerns regarding respiratory function and weaning from artificial ventilation affect prescribing habits. Short acting opioids, such as alfentanil and remifentanil, may be indicated partly on the basis of the lack of prolonged respiratory depression in the absence of accumulation. Opioids also tend to have a hypotensive effect which may be considered a relative contra-indication to their usage.

Difficulties in assessing pain in the unconscious, sedated or paralysed patient will often lead to undertreatment. Inappropriate fears about addiction still persist. Fears about masking important clinical signs by providing effective early analgesia are largely unfounded.[6] Terminally ill patients may be denied analgesia through fear of being seen to hasten death and the possibility of facing prosecution. This emotive issue, especially in the light of recent controversy regarding euthanasia and assisted suicide, must not detract from the fundamental aim of relief from pain. British law is clear following the 1957 Bolam case. A doctor 'is not guilty of negligence if he has acted in accordance with the practice accepted as proper by a reasonable body of medical men'. The 'Bolam' Test[7] should ensure that no patient dies in pain in the ITU. Law in the USA and Australia has a different emphasis and the Bolam test has been rejected.[8] Discussion from the USA[9] centres around the 'double effect'. As long as the primary motivation in giving analgesia was pain relief, then actions are ethically justified despite any secondary effect of the drug.[10]

The successful management of pain initially depends on identifying the pain, assessing its severity and then re-assessing after therapeutic intervention. Whilst both simple and complex tools have evolved to measure pain in both the acute postoperative and chronic setting, none have adequately addressed the unique problems associated with the intubated, unconscious, non-communicating patient. Communication with heavily sedated patients or those with toxic confusional states is equally fraught. A common and well validated measure of pain intensity is based on a zero-to-ten visual or analogue scale.[11] Whilst there may be some patients in the ITU able to use such measures, it is of little use to the majority of intubated or sedated patients.[12] Other assessment tools such as the *McGill Pain Questionnaire*[13] or the *Wisconsin Brief Pain Inventory*[14] also depend fundamentally on communication. Tracheal intubation does not necessarily equate with inability to communicate and pen and paper or word cards can be helpful. There is some evidence, however, to suggest that greater pain is attributed to those who can verbalise their pain compared to those who cannot.[15]

As it is often not possible to ask the patient about their pain, other clues have to be sought. Physiological parameters, such as heart rate and blood pressure, give an indication of sympathetic stimulation which may be due to pain. However, other factors, such as the use of inotropic agents, may be responsible for this sympathetic stimulation. Patients with poor myocardial function may not be able to mount such a response, as will those patients prescribed beta blocking drugs.

A study from Wisconsin,[4] involving extubated patients, asked physicians what they had observed that made them think that their patients had obtained adequate analgesia: 47% said that they had asked the patient, whilst other reports included that the patient appeared comfortable, the patient did not complain, the patient was asleep, the patient was not tachycardic or hypertensive, and that the patient was able to cough and move around. One reported asking the nurse. The same study asked nurses what clues they used to assess pain. Asking the patient and vital signs were the most used, but facial expression, body language, sleep pattern and a decreased ability to cough were also cited.

Patients who have left Intensive Care have been asked how they communicated their pain.[1] Those who were able to talk merely asked for pain relief and responded positively when a nurse asked about their pain. Others who could not talk described how they would make signals with their eyes, use facial expressions or hand signals and try moving their legs up and down the bed. One patient reported 'I would try to grab the nurse and not let go because I was hurting so much'.

Pain assessment is not easy. If there is any reason to assume the patient is in pain, we should perhaps assume they are until they tell us otherwise.

CAUSES OF PAIN

Postoperative and trauma patients have obvious reasons for pain. However, there are other more subtle causes of pain and discomfort and the boundary between pain and discomfort is often blurred. When does discomfort become pain? Tracheal intubation and ventilation are uncomfortable, probably worse so with the use of techniques such as inverse ratio ventilation. Arterial, central venous or peripheral venous cannulation will all cause pain as will urinary catheterisation and the placement of nasogastric tubes. Predictable and intermittent sources of discomfort include physiotherapy and nursing procedures such as tracheal suctioning, dressing changes and turning.[16] Patients have described vividly the pain associated with chest drain removal: 'it felt like they were pulling my guts out'.[1] Peripheral intravenous potassium is painful, as are some anaesthetic drugs.

Pain control does not merely equate to administering analgesic drugs. In 1986 The International Association for the Study of Pain (IAPS) defined pain as: 'an unpleasant sensory and emotional experience associated with actual or potential tissue damage or described in terms of such damage'.[17] Whilst this has not met with universal acceptance, it does emphasise two concepts that are particularly relevant to intensive care. Firstly, the activation of the sensory input into the central nervous system which is experienced as pain is nociception. This is caused by thermal, chemical or mechanical damage that stimulate specific receptors called nociceptors. However, over periods of time, other apparently harmless sensations may become interpreted as painful. Lying in bed relatively immobile for any length of time can lead to joint stiffening or myalgia. A patient's head not adequately supported may lead to neck pain, and constipation may lead to abdominal discomfort.

Secondly, emotion plays an important role in patients' perception of pain. Indeed, pain itself may be considered to be an emotional response. There is, in all painful states, a significant emotional component that will be affected by degrees of anxiety related in part to the meaning of the pain. Does the pain mean that I am going to die? Will it ever get better? Have I got cancer? Anxiety alone can lead to the same stimulation of the stress response that is traditionally thought of as deriving from some physical injury. Hence pain not only causes anxiety, but may itself be exacerbated by anxiety. Altered mental state is common after prolonged ITU stay, and depression is another factor that adversely effects a patient's perception of pain. A patient's pre-morbid personality is important, as existing psychiatric disturbances render patients more prone to developing further mental disturbances during their stay in the ITU.[18] Age, type of procedure and concurrent drug therapy were also found to be risk factors for developing significant mental disturbance whilst in the ITU. In any situation, pain has a strong emotional component; alleviation of suffering involves treating that component of pain as well.

CONSEQUENCES OF PAIN

The relationship between quality of analgesia and outcome is controversial, although there is no doubt that good analgesia leads to greater patient comfort and is a desirable goal. There are many deleterious effects of pain (Table 12.1) which may secondary to sympathetic stimulation and the stress response. Sympathetic blockade *per se* may have a role in decreasing peri-operative morbidity through mechanisms that can be explained physiologically and, in some cases, demonstrated clinically.

Table 12.1 Adverse physiological effects of acute pain

System	Physiological effect	Clinical consequence
Respiratory	↓ Ventilation ↓ FRC ↓ FVC	Atelectasis Lobar collapse Pneumonia Hypoxaemia Hypercapnia
Cardiovascular	Tachycardia Hypertension ↑ SVR	Myocardial ischaemia/infarction
Gastrointestinal	Ileus Gastric stasis/distension	Nausea and vomiting Third space loss Aspiration
Urological	Retention	Hypertension Agitation Pain
Endocrine	↑ ADH ↑ Aldosterone ↑ Cortisol	Water retention Sodium retention Hyperglycaemia
Haematological	Venous stasis Platelet aggregation	Pulmonary embolism Deep vein thrombosis
Musculoskeletal	Immobilisation	Muscle wasting
CNS	Altered sleep pattern Depression	Acute anxiety states Depression Psychoses

FRC, functional residual capacity; FVC, forced vital capacity; SVR, systemic vascular resistance; ADH, antidiuretic hormone.

Psychological

Pain causes lack of sleep. Poor sleep patterns are recognised as a feature of ITU and pain is only one causative factor. Whilst the effect of sleep deprivation on outcome is controversial, there is some evidence to suggest that it is detrimental to the healing process as well as effecting mental state and is responsible for the so called 'ITU psychosis'.[19] Sleep deprivation in chronic pain states is associated with increased pain scores and increased levels of anxiety.

Cardiovascular system

Stimulation of the sympathetic nervous system by pain leads to an increase in blood pressure, heart rate and inotropy. The resultant increase in oxygen demand may lead to ischaemia if their is no matched increase in supply. Sympathetic activation leads to coronary vasoconstriction, in particular poststenotic vasoconstriction and a paradoxical vasoconstrictive response to vasodilators. These changes are possible without a change in heart rate or blood pressure and may be responsible for silent ischaemia. Once ischaemia develops, a secondary sympathetically mediated rise in heart rate and blood pressure may exacerbate the problem. These changes, coupled with the postoperative hypercoaguable state that may also be induced by the sympathetic nervous system, may influence peri-operative cardiac morbidity[20] as ischaemia that occurs postoperatively is more frequent, more severe, and more prolonged than ischaemia occurring pre- or peroperatively.[21]

Respiratory function

Pain after thoracic and abdominal surgery or trauma may lead to diaphragmatic splinting and reduced functional residual capacity.[22,23] Resulting impaired respiratory function may lead to hypoxaemia, atelectasis, lobar collapse and pneumonia. Postoperative altered respiratory function in these cases is not only due to pain but is also a consequence of abnormal diaphragmatic function[24] and increased abdominal and lower intercostal muscle tone during expiration.[25] Patients especially at risk include those with pre-existing respiratory disease,[26] obesity[27] and old age.[28]

Coagulation

Surgery and trauma result in a hypercoaguable state that is thought to be mediated, at least in part, by the stress response and increased sympathetic activity.[29] The site at which pain is blocked may have some significance in this respect, as the reduction in hypercoaguable state related morbidity associated with the use of epidural analgesia has not been demonstrated with analgesia provided by parenteral opioids.[30]

Gastrointestinal system

Pain leads to gastric stasis and may delay enteral feeding during an ITU admission. This has important consequences as early feeding has been demonstrated to improve wound healing[31] and reduce septic complications.[32] The reasons why pain leads to stasis are unclear, but it is possible that abdominal pain activates a spinal reflex arc. Also, increased sympathetic activity as part of the stress response to pain leads to inhibition of co-ordinated bowel activity.[33]

Immune function

Mediators of the stress response are known to also be potent immuno-suppressors.[34] Both cell mediated and humoral systems are affected.[35] Resultant immunosuppression can last for several days and is more severe in those patients with malignant disease or other immunosupressive diseases. This may increase the risk of infection or facilitate tumour growth or metastases.[36] Analgesia, by reducing the stress response, may attenuate these changes in immune function.

TREATMENT OF PAIN IN INTENSIVE CARE

The aetiology of the pain should be sought prior to initiating therapy. Whereas an opioid infusion might be adequate for a burns patient, a similar regimen

Table 12.2 Opioid infusions in intensive care

Drug	MEAC ng/ml	$t_{1/2}$ Terminal min	Dose μg/kg/h
Alfentanil	50–100	90	30–60
Fentanyl	1–3	185	1.0–5.0
Sufentanil	0.2–0.5	160–210	0.2–1.0
Remifentanil	n/a	10–20	30–60
Morphine	10–30	100–180	50–100

MEAC, minimum effective analgesic concentration.

might not be so appropriate for a patient with severe phantom pains. Systemic analgesics and local anaesthetic techniques should be used with an understanding of their advantages and limitations in critically ill patients. Attention should be given to administering appropriate sedation for anxious patients and ensuring as comfortable environment as possible. Minimising anxiety, calming and reassuring frightened patients, provides the optimum basis for treating pain.

Opioid analgesics

Opioid analgesic drugs remain the mainstay of analgesia in the ITU. All the available opioid drugs have been used at one time or another both by intermittent bolus and continuous infusion. In the setting of critical care, the minimum effective analgesic concentration (MEAC) for each individual

Table 12.3 Choice of opioid drugs in organ system failure

Drug	Elimination	Active metabolite	Renal failure	Liver failure
Fentanyl	90% Hepatic	None	No significant alteration of pharmacokinetics	Reduce dose up to 75%
Alfentanil	Predominantly hepatic	None	No significant alteration of pharmacokinetics	Reduce dose up to 75%
Sufentanil	Predominantly hepatic	Desmethyl-sufentanil	No significant alteration of pharmacokinetics	Reduce dose up to 75%
Remifentanil	Plasma	None	No significant alteration of pharmacokinetics	Reduce dose up to 75%
Morphine	77% Hepatic	Morphine-3-glucuronide 75–85% Morphine-6-glucuronide 5–15%	Reduce accumulation of active metabolites	Reduce dose up to 75%
Pethidine	90% Hepatic	Norpethidine	Accumulation of norpethidine, convulsions have been reported	Reduce dose up to 75%

Table 12.4 Side effects of opioids

	Effect	Receptor type mediated by
CNS	Euphoria	mu-1 (μ_1)
	Dysphoria	kappa (κ)
	Miosis	mu-1 (μ_1) & kappa (κ)
	Hypothermia	mu-1 (μ_1)
	Nausea	mu-1 (μ_1) & delta (δ)
Cardiovascular	Bradycardia	mu-1 (μ_1)
Gastrointestinal	Constipation	mu-2 (μ_2) & delta (δ) ? gut wall
Genitourinary	Retention	mu-1 (μ_1) & delta (δ)
	Diuresis	kappa (κ)
Respiratory	Depression	mu-2 (μ_2) & delta (δ)
Immune	Suppression?	

patient will vary widely. Consequently, the dosage regimen will need to be tailored to each patient. Table 12.2 summarises dosage regimens commonly used. There is no evidence that the choice of opioid drug used for analgesia alters outcome in critically sick patients. However, in the presence of different organ system failure, individual opioids might be indicated due to differences in metabolic pathways (Table 12.3). Aside from analgesia, principally mediated at μ receptors, opioids may have deleterious effects (Table 12.4).

The intravenous route is still the best method of delivering opioids in the critically ill. Fentanyl is available in a transdermal formulation. However, from a pharmacokinetic standpoint, the time to steady state levels of 12–14 h and the slow fall in plasma levels over 36 h following removal would seem inappropriate in the ITU setting. Inhaled opioids now exist in experimental settings and may have some role to play in patients with normal lungs. Transmucosal opioid administration, e.g. fentanyl 'lollipops', are inappropriate for use in the ITU. The future of continuous opioid therapy in intensive care probably is not that of variation of route of administration but rather through better appreciation of pharmacokinetic concepts. For example, usage of context sensitive half-time rather than elimination half-life may lead to better tailored infusion regimens.

Patient controlled analgesia is widely used in the management of postoperative pain. It requires a fully conscious patient with whom one can easily communicate. As such, many patients in ITUs would not benefit from its application. Attentive nursing staff will probably be more effective at administering doses of analgesics when appropriate.

Non steroidal anti-inflammatory drugs (NSAIDs)

NSAIDs are commonly used in the management of postoperative pain. This class of drug, a heterogeneous group mainly consisting of organic acids, has an opioid sparing effect and has both central and peripheral sites of analgesic activity. The use of such drugs in the critically ill is controversial. The majority of these drugs are metabolised by the liver and excreted by the kidney, both of which pathways may be affected in the critically ill. NSAIDs decrease prostaglandin dependent renal blood flow which may be critical in the elderly, in diabetic patients, following major surgery and trauma and in patients with cardiac failure. These groups of patients represent a significant proportion of ITU patients. Gastric ulceration may also occur due to reduction in gastric prostaglandins. The most recently released NSAID, ketorolac, has been associated with 20 deaths due to renal impairment and 47 deaths due to gastro-intestinal bleeding. Whilst this is a tiny fraction of the 16 million prescriptions world-wide, it would seem prudent to avoid this class of drug in the absence of any definitive gain to be had in the critically ill.

Non conventional analgesia

In patients with continuing pain and altered sleeping patterns tricyclic anti-depressants have been used extensively, particularly where the pain is thought to be neuropathic in aetiology. There might be a rationale for using these drugs in the medium-to-long stay ITU patient where pain, anxiety and depression co-exist with a disturbed sleeping pattern.

Alternative therapies

No evidence exists to support the use of alternative therapies in the critically ill. However, in the absence of any untoward effects, the use of TENS, acupuncture, aromatherapy, etc., should not be withheld. Anecdotal evidence has reported benefit from acupuncture in neuropathic pain and reduced sedative and analgesic requirements following aromatherapy.

Regional analgesia in the ITU

Local anaesthetic can be administered topically, by local infiltration, in specific nerve or plexus by intrathecal or extradural administration. Neural blockade can provide analgesia, sympathetic autonomic blockade, attenuation of the stress response, improved respiratory function, skeletal muscle relaxation, haemodynamic stability and avoids the risks of alternative therapy.[37]

Some techniques that are useful peroperatively are not useful in the ITU population because of specific contra-indications, inappropriate short duration of action, or practical difficulties in siting the local anaesthetic. However, local anaesthetic can be used to improve patient comfort as well as potentially decreasing morbidity in the ITU. Simple practical steps, such as the use of lignocaine gel for urinary catheter placement and local anaesthetic infiltration for peripheral and central venous cannulation, reduces patient discomfort.

Extradural analgesia

In specific groups of patients, the use of lumbar extradural analgesia (LEA) or thoracic extradural analgesia (TEA) with or without opioids has been shown to improve outcome. Generally, those studies that have used epidural analgesia per- and postoperatively in sick patients undergoing high risk procedures have been able to demonstrate a decrease in postoperative complications. Those studies looking at fit patients undergoing low risk procedures or with poorly controlled peri-operative analgesia have failed to show any improvement in outcome.[20]

The sympathetic innervation of the heart is derived from T1 to T5. TEA with local anaesthetic can block the cardiac sympathetic supply. In the absence of hypovolaemia, sympathetic blockade stabilises the cardiovascular system by attenuating increases in heart rate and blood pressure associated with movement or pain from unblocked areas. Vasodilatation leads to a decrease in afterload. These effects lead to a reduction in myocardial work and may decrease the risk of cardiovascular morbidity.

In patients with coronary artery disease, TEA has been shown to increase blood flow to ischaemic areas of myocardium whilst leaving total coronary blood flow unchanged. Poststenotic vasoconstriction is inhibited and the endocardial-to-epicardial blood flow ratio is improved. Therefore, TEA may improve myocardial oxygen supply as long as the systemic blood pressure is maintained.[20] Beneficial effects of TEA on cardiac segmental wall motion during vascular surgery have been reported, although interestingly these effects were reversed by the use of ephedrine.[38] However, there is only limited evidence to suggest a possible decrease in postoperative myocardial infarction rate associated with the use of TEA.[39] However, most cardiac events occur 3–4 days postoperatively[40] and investigation of the continuation of TEA well into the postoperative phase during the ITU stay may demonstrate, more readily, a decrease in cardiac morbidity. TEA been shown to be of use in the management of refractory cardiac ischaemic pain.[41]

Blomberg and his colleagues investigated the effect of thoracic epidural block on diseased coronary arteries and arterioles. By using quantitative angiography, they showed an increase in luminal diameter in stenosed segments whilst there was no change in the nonstenotic segments. Previously, Blomberg's group had used thoracic extradural anaesthesia to control pain in 9 patients with unstable angina pectoris.[42] These patients were monitored with pulmonary artery catheters and were receiving therapy of a combination of β-adrenoceptor antagonists, calcium channel antagonists, nitrates, salicylates and even low dose heparin. During ischaemic pain, both pulmonary artery and pulmonary capillary wedge pressures were increased. TEA provided good analgesia and significantly decreased these pressures as well as the systolic arterial blood pressure and heart rate. There was no decrease in coronary perfusion pressure, cardiac output or systemic vascular resistance. They concluded that TEA may favourably alter the oxygen supply–demand ratio within ischaemic myocardial areas.

In the spontaneously breathing patient, the incidence of respiratory complications such as atelectasis, hypoxia and infection should, theoretically, be reduced as the improved analgesia allows increased chest expansion and effective coughing. Respiratory function indices, such as peak expiratory flow rate (PEFR) and functional residual capacity (FRC), have been shown to improve faster postoperatively with epidural analgesia.[43] Extradural local anaesthetic has been shown to have a greater effect than both extradural and systemic opioids despite no difference between pain scores. One theory is that local anaesthetic inhibits the segmental spinal reflexes that lead to skeletal muscle splinting and allows greater chest movement for the same degree of effort.[44]

The role of extradural analgesia in postoperative pain relief is now well established. There exists equivocal evidence for improved outcome in otherwise fit patients,[23,45] despite much improved analgesia.[46] However, high risk surgical patients provided with extradural analgesia do have an improved outcome. Yaeger and colleagues[47] found, overall, significantly lower complication rates in high risk patients undergoing abdominal surgery who received extradural analgesia compared with those who did not. The group of 28 patients who received extradural analgesia had significantly lower mortality, a lower incidence of cardiovascular failure and major infections compared with controls that received opioids per- and postoperatively. Their reported incidence of respiratory complications was not significantly lower, but, in two cases, the epidural catheter was not working. If these two are discounted, the incidence of pulmonary complications was significantly lower.

Thoracic epidural blocks have been shown to reduce the incidence of fatal and non-fatal respiratory complications following thoraco-abdominal oesophagogastrectomy for oesophageal cancer.[48] This retrospective review of 156 patients reported a 5% 30 day mortality in the non-epidural group compared with a zero 30 day mortality in the epidural group. Watson and Allen suggested that a decrease in the incidence of anastamotic dehiscence may be one factor involved. A recent randomised double-blind study[49] reported early extubation, good analgesia and no side effects associated with the use of TEA. Blass and colleagues[50] suggested that thoracic epidurals allowed early extubation and, hence, a decrease in respiratory complications. Their mean extubation time, in a group of 20 patients undergoing thoraco-abdominal resection of the oesophagus, was 190 min. Good analgesia was provided by epidural morphine and local anaesthetic together with NSAIDs. This regimen allowed early extubation together with effective coughing and physiotherapy. Regular continuous positive airway pressure (CPAP) was used as part of their intensive respiratory therapy.

Postoperative epidural analgesia may reduce the overall incidence of major infection by a number of mechanisms. Firstly, critically ill patients appropriately provided with epidural analgesia spend a shorter time ventilated post-operatively than controls.[47,49,51] Endotracheal intubation bypasses natural defence mechanisms and early extubation may, therefore, reduce the risk of chest infection.[52] Secondly, by obtunding the stress response, patients retain, to some extent, their immunocompetence. Thirdly, the overall time spent in the ITU is reduced and so the risks of nosocomial infection and line sepsis is reduced. Early extubation also reduces the risks associated with ventilation.

Extradural analgesia has beneficial effects on the postoperative and trauma induced hypercoaguable state and the resultant vaso-occlusive and thrombotic postoperative morbidity and mortality.[53] General anaesthesia, surgery and immobility during ITU admission lead to a decrease in blood flow in the deep veins of the pelvis and lower limbs. Extradural local anaesthetic increase blood flow through the lower limbs,[54] enhances fibrinolytic activity[55] and, due to systemic absorption of the local anaesthetic, produces plasma concentrations sufficient to directly impair platelet aggregation.[56]

Problems with extradurals in the ITU

Epidural analgesia is certainly not a panacea of ITU pain control. The three main contra-indications to extradural catheter placement of systemic infection, local infection and coagulopathy are common in the critically ill and prevent their use. There has been much debate about the placement of catheters in patients with potential coagulopathy including those taking aspirin. The bleeding time has been advocated as the decisive factor,[57] but this test may not readily be available and is subject to user error both in carrying out the test and in its interpretation. Most would err on the side of caution.

Local and systemic infection are regarded as contra-indications because of the fear of epidural abscess formation. Barker in 1975 reviewed 37 patients with epidural abscesses but only one was thought to be secondary to catheter placement.[58] In a prospective study of 1620 paediatric catheter placements, Striffer[59] confirmed one epidural abscess. This was a 10-year-old girl with metastatic osteosarcoma who received two thoracic catheters over a period of 28 days for terminal pain relief. *Candida* was isolated from the catheter tip, and a necrotic mass seen at CT. Three other children who were considered clinically to have an abscess were found on scanning to have none.

The use of extradural analgesia in the multiple injured patient may not be appropriate. In the presence of dense neural blockade, relatively minor injuries, not apparent immediately on admission, may be missed. Delayed diagnosis of a compartment syndrome involving the lower limb has been reported.[60] Although the use of extradural analgesia for postlaparotomy head injured patients would seem ideal, raised intracranial pressure must be excluded as inadvertent dural puncture could prove fatal. Any neurological sequaelae from the injury may be blamed on the epidural. Perhaps most fundamentally of all, the practical difficulties of positioning a fully monitored, unstable, ventilated patient should not be underestimated. Sympathetic blockade in the hypovolaemic, or cardiovascularly compromised patient is contra-indicated.

Peripheral nerve blocks

Specific nerve blocks in the ITU can be used to alleviate pain, reduce the need for systemic analgesics which may be poorly tolerated in the critically ill, attenuate the stress response, treat peripheral vascular disorders and allow minor operative procedures without general anaesthesia. Nerve blocks are an integral part of many anaesthetic techniques and provide good postoperative analgesia, but their role in the critically ill is less well defined. There is little in the literature to show nerve blocks improve outcome in the ITU setting. The contra-indications of infection and coagulopathy exist, as with extradural blockade, and the positioning of patients to perform the block may prove difficult. The duration of block may be a limiting factor. Although repeat injections at the same site are possible, ideally, a catheter should be placed and local anaesthetic given by infusion or intermittent bolus. This minimises the risk of complications of performing the block, is much more tolerable to the patient and provides constant analgesia. Local anaesthetics encapsulated in liposomes may provide a slow release form of analgesia,[61] although the potential for toxicity exists.

Interpleural analgesia

The techniques, uses and literature on interpleural blocks have been well reviewed by Murphy.[62] Interestingly, whilst excellent analgesia has been reported for fractured ribs[63] and postoperative cholecystectomy pain,[64] post-thoracotomy pain was poorly controlled.[65] Potential problems include the leakage of local anaesthetic into chest drains, interference with diaphragmatic function, and high plasma levels of local anaesthetic, although clinical signs of toxicity are uncommon. Apart from improved analgesia, which is valuable in itself, there is little to suggest improved outcome in critically ill patients provided with interpleural blockade. Murphy[64] described significantly improved PEFR 40 min after top up of postoperative cholecystectomy patients.

Intercostal catheterisation and infusion of local anaesthetic has been used successfully in a patient with a head injury and multiple rib fractures.[63] There exists several different ways of inserting the catheter and much discussion as to where it ends up and the site of action of the local anaesthetic. The advantage over TEA was the avoidance of possible dural puncture in a patient with raised intracranial pressure.

Continuous femoral nerve block following femur fracture has been reported.[66] Four multiply injured children with closed head trauma were provided with excellent analgesia by this method. They avoided the use of systemic opioids and, by not using extradural analgesia, overcame the practical difficulties of positioning a child with a fractured femur.

Continuous brachial plexus blockade can provide analgesia, decrease vasospasm and promote collateral circulation in upper limb injury. Manriquez and colleagues[67] used continuous interscalene brachial plexus block in 3 patients with upper extremity vascular accidents. They reported good analgesia, improvement in peripheral colour and temperature and no problems with haematoma formation despite heparinisation.

CONCLUSIONS

This review has limited itself to discussion of analgesic techniques rather than sedation. Infusions of opioids are commonly used for sedation of ventilated patients, the analgesic properties being of secondary importance except where pain is a problem. Opioids are often combined with other sedating drugs, such as midazolam, either by bolus or infusion. There is no doubt that such regimens are effective, have passed the test of time and are also cheap. However, such regimens as these do not provide effective pain relief for all patients. What is needed to avoid patients experiencing pain whilst in the ITU is individualised, goal-directed, analgesic regimens, where the source of the pain is identified and treated, not as a side effect of the sedation used, but as an aim in itself. All modalities of pain therapy have their uses in the critically ill. In concert with analgesia, attention should be given to anxiety, the physical environment of the patient and the patient's sleeping pattern – all of which can mitigate against effective pain relief.

Key points for clinical practice

- Poorly controlled pain may prolong stay in the Intensive Care Unit.

- Many procedures carried out in Intensive Care cause pain, patients report simple procedures, such as suctioning and change of ET tubes, as painful.

- Pain is not homogeneous and not always responsive to standard opioid infusions. Neuropathic pain, in particular, may not be well treated in this manner.

- Assessment of pain is complex in the ITU setting: if no direct evidence is available that the patient is in pain then assume they are if a source of pain is identifiable.

- Anxiety, depression and sleep disturbance all exacerbate pain: in long-term ITU patients, psychoses may occur.

- Restricting analgesic techniques to opioid infusions will not ensure that most patients are pain free.

- In selected patients, regional analgesia may shorten stay in Intensive Care and improve postoperative haemodynamic stability.

- NSAIDs should be used with extreme caution in the critically ill.

- Complementary therapies may sometimes help.

References

1. Puntillo A P. Pain experiences of intensive care patients. Heart Lung 1990; 19: 526–533
2. Bion J F. Sedation and analgesia in the intensive care unit. Hosp Update 1988; 14: 1272–1286
3. Hamman W. Neuropathic pain: a condition which is not always well appreciated. Br J Anaesth 1993; 71: 779–781
4. Whipple J K, Lewis K S, Quebbeman E J et al. Analysis of pain management in critically ill patients. Pharmacotherapy 1995; 15: 592–599
5. Carter R. Give a drug a bad name. New Scientist 1996; 6 April: 14–15
6. Attard A, Corlett M, Kidner N, Apsara L, Fraser I. Safety of early pain relief for acute abdominal pain. BMJ 1992; 305: 554–556
7. Bolam v Friern Hospital Management Committee (1957) 1 WLR 582 (QBD)
8. Kirby M. Patients' rights – why the Australian courts have rejected Bolam. J Med Ethics 1995; 21: 5–8
9. Hooyman T, Veremakis C. Relief from pain and the double effect [letter]. JAMA 1992; 268: 1857–1858
10. Wilson W, Smedira N, Fink C, McDowell J, Luce J. Ordering and administration of sedatives and analgesics during the withholding and withdrawal of life support from critically ill patients. JAMA 1992; 267: 949–953
11. Revill S, Robinson J, Rosen M, Hogg M. The reliability of a linear analogue for evaluating pain. Anaesthesia 1976; 31: 1191–1198
12. Lonsdale M. Pain relief in the intensive care unit. Part 1. ITCM 1991; 1: 10–13
13. Melzack R. The McGill Pain Questionnaire: major properties and scoring methods. Pain 1975; 8: 143–154
14. Daut R, Cleeland C, Flannery R. Development of the Wisconsin Brief Pain Questionnaire to assess pain in cancer and other diseases. Pain 1983; 17: 197–210
15. Baer E, Davitz L, Lieb R. Inferences of physical pain and psychological distress. 1. In relation to verbal and non-verbal patient communication. Nurs Res 1970; 19: 383–392

16. Aitkenhead A. Analgesia and sedation in intensive care. Br J Anaesth 1989; 63: 196–206
17. Bonica J. Definitions and taxonomy of pain. In: Bonica J. (ed.) The Management of Pain. Philadelphia: Lea and Febiger, 1990; 18–27
18. Sanders K, Cassem E. Psychiatric complications in the critically ill cardiac patient. Tex Heart Inst J 1993; 20: 180–187
19. Eveloff S. The disruptive ICU. An issue to lose sleep over? Chest 1995; 107: 1483–1484
20. Liu S, Carpenter R, Neal J. Epidural anesthesia and analgesia. Their role in postoperative outcome. Anesthesiology 1995; 82: 1474–1506
21. Mangano D, Hollenberg M, Fegert G, Meyer M, London M, Tubau J. Perioperative myocardial ischaemia in patients undergoing noncardiac surgery. 1. Incidence and severity during the four day perioperative period. J Am Coll Cardiol 1991; 17: 843–850
22. Craig D. Postoperative recovery of pulmonary function. Anesth Analg 1981; 60: 46–52
23. Cuschieri R, Morran C, Howie J, McArdle C. Postoperative pain and pulmonary complications: comparison of three analgesic regimens. Br J Surg 1985; 72: 495–498
24. Pansard J, Mankikian B, Bertrand M, Kieffer E, Clegue F, Viars P. Effects of thoracic extradural block on diaphragmatic electrical activity and contractility after upper abdominal surgery. Anesthesiology 1993; 78: 63–71
25. Duggan J, Drummond G. Activity of lower intercostal and abdominal muscle after upper abdominal surgery. Anesth Analg 1987; 66: 852–855
26. Tarhan S, Moffitt E, Sessler A, Douglas W, Taylor W. Risk of anesthesia and surgery in patients with chronic bronchitis and chronic obstructive pulmonary disease. Surgery 1973; 74: 720–726
27. Rawal N, Sjostrand U, Christoffersson E, Dahlstrom B, Arvill A, Rydman H. Comparison of intramuscular and epidural morphine for postoperative analgesia in the grossly obese: influence on postoperative ambulation and pulmonary function. Anesth Analg 1984; 63: 583–592.
28. Wahba W. Influence of ageing on lung function: clinical significance of changes from age twenty. Anesth Analg 1983; 62: 764–776
29. Rosenfield B, Faraday N, Campbell D, Dise K, Bell W, Goldschmidt P. Hemostatic effects of stress hormone infusion. Anesthesiology 1994; 81: 1116–1126
30. Lichtenfeld K, Schiffer D, Helrich M. Platelet aggregation during and after general anesthesia and surgery. Anesth Analg 1979; 58: 293–296
31. Saito H, Trocki O, Alexander J. The effect of route of nutrient administration on the nutritional state, catabolic hormone secretion and gut mucosal integrity after burn injury. J Parenter Enter Nutr 1987; 11: 1–7
32. Moore F, Moore E, Jones T, McCroskey B. TEN vs TPN following major abdominal trauma. J Trauma 1989; 29: 916–923
33. Smith J, Kelly K. Pathophysiology of postoperative ileus. Arch Surg 1977; 112: 203–209
34. Davis J, Albert J, Tracey K et al. Increased neutrophil mobilisation and decreased chemotaxis during cortisol and epinephrine infusions. J Trauma 1991; 31: 725–732
35. Salo M. Effects of anaesthesia and surgery on the immune response. Acta Anaesthesiol Scand 1992; 36: 201–220
36. Eggermont A, Steller E, Sugarbaker P. Laparotomy enhances intraperitoneal tumour growth and abrogates the anti-tumour effects of interleukin-2 and lymphocyte activated killer cells. Surgery 1987; 102: 71–78
37. Rung G, Marshall W. Nerve blocks in the critical care environment. Crit Care Clin 1990; 6: 343–367
38. Saada M, Catoire P, Bonnet F et al. Effect of thoracic epidural anesthesia combined with general anesthesia on segmental wall motion assessed by transesophageal echocardiography. Anesth Analg 1992; 75: 329–335
39. Leon-Casasola O, Lema M, Karabella D, Harrison P. Postoperative myocardial ischaemia: epidural versus intravenous patient-controlled analgesia. Reg Anesth 1995; 20: 105–112
40. Rao T, Jacobs K, EL-Etr A. Reinfarction following anesthesia in patients with myocardial infarction. Anesthesiology 1983; 59: 499–505
41. Blomberg S, Curelaru I, Emanuelsson H, Herlitz J, Ponten J, Ricksten S-E. Thoracic epidural anaesthesia in patients with unstable angina pectoris. Eur Heart J 1989; 10: 437–444
42. Blomberg S, Emanuelsson H, Ricksten S. Thoracic epidural anesthesia and central hemodynamics in patients with unstable angina pectoris. Anesth Analg 1989; 69: 558–562
43. Pflug A, Murphy T, Butler S. The effects of postoperative peridural analgesia on pulmonary therapy and pulmonary complications. Anesthesiology 1974; 41: 8–13

44. Pansard J, Mankikian B, Bertrand M, Kieffer E, Clergue F, Viras P. Effects of thoracic extradural block on diaphragmatic electrical activity and contractility after upper abdominal surgery. Anesthesiology 1993; 78: 63–71

45. Jayr C, Mollie A, Bourgain J et al. Postoperative pulmonary complications: general anesthesia with postoperative parenteral morphine compared with epidural analgesia. Surgery 1988; 104: 57–63

46. Cullen M, Staren E, El-Ganzouri A, Logas W, Ivankovich A, Economou S. Continuous epidural infusion for analgesia after major abdominal operations: a randomised, prospective, double-blind study. Surgery 1985; 98: 718–727

47. Yaeger M, Glass D, Neff R, Brinck-Johnsen T. Epidural anesthesia and analgesia in high-risk surgical patients. Anesthesiology 1987; 66: 729–736

48. Watson A, Allen P. Influence of thoracic epidural analgesia on outcome after resection for esophageal cancer. Surgery 1994; 115: 429–432

49. Terai T, Yukioka H, Fujimori M. Administration of epidural bupivicaine combined with epidural morphine after esophageal surgery. Surgery 1997; 121: 359–365

50. Blass J, Straender S, Moerlen J. Complication-free early extubation following abdomino-thoracic esophagectomy. Anaesthesist 1991; 40: 315–323

51. Caldwell M, Murphy P, Page R, Walsh T, Hennessy T. Timing of extubation after oesophagectomy. Br J Surg 1993; 80: 1537–1539

52. Sachner M, Hirsch J, Epstein S. Effect of cuffed endotracheal tubes on tracheal mucous velocity. Chest 1975; 68: 774-777

53. Christopherson R, Beattie C, Frank S et al. The Perioperative Ischemia Randomised Anesthesia Trial Study Group: perioperative morbidity in patients randomised to epidural or general anesthesia for lower extremity vascular surgery. Anesthesiology 1993; 79: 422–434

54. Modig J, Malmberg P, Karlstrom G. Effect of epidural versus general anaesthesia on calf blood flow. Acta Anaesthesiol Scand 1980; 24: 305–309

55. Donadoni R, Baele G, Devulder J, Rolly G. Coagulation and fibrinolytic parameters in patients undergoing total hip replacement: influence of anaesthetic technique. Acta Anaesthesiol Scand 1989; 33: 588–592

56. Henny C, Odoom J, Ten Cate H, Ten Cate J, Oosterhoff R. Effects of extradural bupivacaine on the haemostatic system, Br J Anaesth 1986; 58: 301–305

57. O'Kelly S, Lawes E, Luntley J. Bleeding time: is it a useful clinical tool? Br J Anaesth 1992; 68: 313–315

58. Baker A, Ojemann R, Swartz M, Richardson E. Spinal epidural abscess. N Engl J Med 1975; 293: 463–468

59. Strafford M, Wilder R, Berde C. The risk of infection from epidural analgesia in children: a review of 1620 cases. Anesth Analg 1995; 80: 234–238

60. Strecker W, Wood M, Bieber E. Compartment syndrome masked by epidural anesthesia for postoperative pain. J Bone Joint Surg 1986; 9: 1447–1448

61. Lafont N, Legros F, Boogaerts J. Use of liposome-associated bupivacaine in a cancer pain syndrome. Anaesthesia 1996; 51: 578–579

62. Murphy D. Interpleural analgesia. Br J Anaesth 1993; 71: 426–434

63. Graziotti P, Smith G. Multiple rib fractures and head injury – an indication for intercostal catheterisation and infusion of local anaesthetics. Anaesthesia 1988; 43: 964–966

64. Murphy D. Continuous intercostal nerve blockade for pain relief after cholecystectomy. Br J Anaesth 1983; 55: 521–524

65. Rosenberg P, Scheinen B, Lepantalo M, Lindfors O. Continuous intrapleural infusion of bupivacaine for analgesia after thoracotomy. Anesthesiology 1987; 67: 811–813.

66. Tobias J. Continuous femoral nerve block to provide analgesia following femur fracture in a paediatric ICU population. Anaesth Intensive Care 1994; 22: 616-618

67. Manriquez R, Pallares V. Continuous brachial plexus block for prolonged sympathectomy and control of pain. Anaesth Analg 1978; 57: 128–129

Mark Hitchcock

The economics of anaesthesia

No country can afford all the healthcare that is available to it.[1] The ability of modern healthcare systems to provide high quality care has also now outstripped the ability of their funding organisations to pay for it. Thus purchasers of healthcare cannot afford both all the quantity and quality in healthcare that is now possible. Indeed, as the general health of the population has improved, patients now live longer, have higher expectations concerning healthcare, and require more interventions, usually of an increasingly complex and thus expensive nature. Healthcare costs form an increasingly large proportion of the gross national product of many developed countries, typically 6–11%, and despite the close financial scrutiny that is now applied to all healthcare, this trend seems likely to continue.

Anaesthesia is unusual within the spectrum of healthcare in that it has little if any therapeutic benefit in its own right and is only of value in that it permits treatment, usually of a surgical nature. Edge and Morgan have highlighted the fact that, to managers, anaesthesia appears as a low profile, high intensity – and thus expensive – speciality.[2] This makes anaesthesia very easily targeted in terms of cost reductions. After all, on the face of it, costing anaesthesia is simply a matter of dividing the cost of drugs and gases used by the number of patients anaesthetised to produce a figure that can easily be reduced by the use of cheaper drugs.

Few would dispute that decisions regarding the choice of different anaesthetic drugs or techniques should be based primarily on the quality of care attainable, with cost as only a secondary consideration. Purchasers now also require evidence that the standard of service they are offered meets accepted criteria. However, there are problems in defining what level of quality is acceptable and measuring the quality of service provided is often difficult if not impossible.[3] If one takes the safety of anaesthesia as a measure

---

Dr Mark Hitchcock BSc MBBS DCH FRCA, Director of Day Surgery and Consultant Anaesthetist, Addenbrooke's NHS Trust, Hills Road, Cambridge CB2 2QQ, UK

of quality, then it is apparent that the standard of service provided at the present time is very high indeed and it could be argued that there seems little justification for the increased expenditure associated with newer drugs and techniques that may offer marginal or intangible benefits in the eyes of the purchasers of healthcare.[4] However, it is precisely because modern anaesthesia is very safe that the assessment of high quality anaesthesia must now focus on other means of delineating quality, such as the pleasantness of induction, the rapidity and completeness of recovery, or even patient satisfaction. It is also becoming clear that, all too often, the requirements of anaesthetic staff, patients and managers are not identical, with safety being a priority to the anaesthetist, pleasantness and freedom from side effects being important to the patient, and cost being the concern of the management.

In modern healthcare systems, the debate thus focuses on the importance of, and the willingness to pay for, the degree of quality in anaesthetic care that is now possible. This in turn means that some understanding both of the ways in which anaesthesia can be costed, and the assessment of quality, is required to ensure that quality, rather than cost, remains the overriding determinant in the choice of anaesthetic drugs, technique, or equipment, in spite of external managerial pressure to reduce spending.

IMPORTANCE OF ANAESTHETIC COST DATA

Some knowledge of the economics of anaesthesia is important to the modern anaesthetist. Most studies investigate the medical benefits and advantages of alternative anaesthetic drugs or techniques, but fail to include any assessment of their relative costs.[5] An appreciation of the ways in which the choice of anaesthetic affects overall costs, through both the obvious direct costs and those indirect costs that are not always so readily identifiable, will enable the use of drugs and techniques in the most cost efficient manner.

Most new anaesthetic drugs are expensive due to the research and development costs involved in bringing any new product to market.[6] Just as a range of new products are appearing on the anaesthetic market, so anaesthesia is coming under intense financial scrutiny. The very introduction of new drugs is becoming dependent on some form of cost justification and, if this is poorly undertaken, then potentially useful drugs may never reach the market because of cost considerations alone. This decision may, in addition, be made by administrators who have little understanding of the potential benefits and possible overall savings that may accompany such a drug. 'Cost effectiveness' data are already required in certain countries before the introduction of new drugs and this practice is becoming more widespread.[7] Anaesthetists must have a clear understanding of how such cost effectiveness studies are undertaken and be able to appraise critically the data produced in this way.

Anaesthetists must also be aware that their choice of anaesthetic drugs and techniques can affect more than just the patient's intra-operative course alone. Affects on postoperative morbidity, in terms of postoperative nausea and vomiting (PONV), and drowsiness can be related to the type of anaesthesia utilised.[8] This is especially true in day case anaesthesia where failure of the stated intention of admitting, treating and discharging the patient in the same day can have profound cost effects. Too many studies of the comparative costs of anaesthetics concentrate solely on the acquisition cost of the drugs used and fail to investigate any of the financial consequences of the anaesthetics compared. Thus, while cost minimisation studies are applicable in certain circumstances, their use must be limited to where outcomes are indeed identical.[9] Finally, some knowledge of costing methods is important to ensure that the quality of anaesthesia is maintained in the face of pressure for reduction in healthcare costs, and also that cuts in expenditure are carried out in those areas where they will be most advantageous.

METHODS OF COSTING

Assessing the cost of anaesthesia is not a simple mathematical exercise. Recording the number of patients anaesthetised, the drugs and consumables used, and the duration of anaesthesia allows the calculation of a figure for the costs incurred per case: however, is this really meaningful? Many factors contribute to the overall cost of an anaesthetic, including, drug expenditure, medical and ancillary staff costs, equipment costs and service costs.[10] The true economics of anaesthesia can only be explored if the differing consequences of alternate anaesthetic drugs or techniques are included in the overall cost analysis. Four measures for assessing the financial impact of drugs and techniques are now commonly utilised. These differ not only in the range of costs they include in their analyses, but also in how they quantify improvement in outcome.[11]

'Cost minimisation' analysis compares alternate treatment regimens only in terms of direct resource costs for supplies and personnel.[9] This often used, but over simplistic, approach assumes that the outcomes of each anaesthetic regimen are identical and, as such, can be ignored for costing purposes. This type of analysis can be extremely misleading as it does not consider any of the indirect costs to the patient and family that arise due to the anaesthetic used, e.g. treatment side effects.

Much of the assessment of modern anaesthesia is concerned with improving not only the quantity, but also the quality, of human life. When the outcome of any anaesthetic is measured in units that consider the utility of the subject, by placing a value on 'quality of human life', the analysis is termed a 'cost utility ratio'.[12] This approach attempts to include those intangible costs, such as pain, nausea and suffering, that significantly contribute to the quality of the patient's outcome but are difficult to cost with any degree of accuracy. The relative values in terms of outcome are often so highly subjective and arbitrary, that it is difficult to apply these principles rigorously to clinical practice.

A 'cost benefit' analysis attempts to provide a monetary estimate of the ratio of total costs to benefits. This form of analysis attempts to include direct, indirect and intangible costs and places monetary values on the theoretical benefits for each form of anaesthesia. A cost benefit analysis concentrates on the benefits of interventions in terms of the savings made in other direct anaesthetic costs, and also on the production gains from, for example, an earlier return to work (indirect benefits). Benefits are expressed in monetary terms to enable the comparison with input costs. As in the case of cost utility ratios, this concept is appealing but has major practical limitations.[13] Once again, assigning a monetary value to intangible costs and benefits is often subjective and impractical. The willingness of the patient to pay more for a new drug or service and the increased earnings in patients receiving a specific therapy are two methods employed in estimating such benefits. The latter approach discriminates against those patients who do not work for their living, whereas the former involves asking patients how much they are willing to pay to avoid a given outcome and assigning this benefit to the group as a whole in proportion to those who would be expected to achieve the desired outcome. One difficulty with this approach is the lack of consistency in what patients are willing to pay for the same outcome, and is further complicated by the need to adjust monetary values downward for future benefits, while maintaining the value for current costs. Also, most studies in the anaesthetic literature involve small study groups. The incidence of side effects noted in these clinical studies may, therefore, not apply to the population as a whole. A sensitivity analysis, is required in these circumstances in order to test the stability of the original analysis over the range of assumptions and values used.[14]

'Cost effectiveness' analysis also compares the total costs, direct, indirect and intangible, of a given clinical outcome measure for different therapeutic regimens. Clinical outcomes are measured in non-monetary units which must be identified for each alternative, such as 'life years gained'. This type of analysis attempts to determine either the maximum improvement in the health status of patients for a fixed amount of resources or the minimal amount of resources required to achieve a given improvement.[15]

It can be seen that the methods used to cost all healthcare interventions, with the exception of cost minimisation, attempt to include as many cost inputs as possible. In the specific case of anaesthesia, this is essential, for, as Bulpitt and Fletcher have pointed out, even if a given anaesthetic is associated with additional costs, it may be preferred if the improvement in outcome is adequate to decrease the unit cost.[16] Indirect and intangible costs are less obviously associated with the anaesthetic used and yet exert a profound effect on the overall quality of the anaesthetic service provided. The methods used to quantify outcome all suffer from lack of direct clinical relevance when applied to anaesthesia, and the subjectivity inherent in costing intangible benefits, such as the lack of pain postoperatively. In addition, most studies published to date have been conducted under inadequate experimental conditions, with sample sizes that are too small for meaningful statistical analysis, insufficient length of follow-up, and often comparing inappropriate alternatives.[17] Jolicoeur and his colleagues have made ten recommendations concerning the conduct of studies to investigate the economics of healthcare.[18] As more and more future studies of anaesthetic drugs and techniques include some assessment of the costs involved, it is apparent that anaesthetists need to form a consensus of opinion concerning which direct, indirect, and intangible costs should be included in any cost analysis and how anaesthetic outcomes should be quantified and assessed.

WHERE ARE COSTS?

As anaesthesia is so easily targeted for cost reduction initiatives, it is useful to consider its cost amongst all the determinants of the cost of a surgical episode.

If we are to reduce costs, this knowledge will help us to decide where we can have the greatest effect. Macario and his colleagues analysed the data from the financial information system of a large American University hospital.[19] They recorded the costs and charges generated for 715 patients having one of four common, intermediate complexity, in-patient operations. Total hospital costs were separated into eleven hospital departments, and they identified cost to charge ratios for each operation and each department. Hospital costs were also divided into variable and fixed, i.e. costs that do and do not change with patient volume, and further partitioned into direct and indirect, i.e. costs that can and cannot be linked directly to a patient.

Macario found that 49% of total costs were variable and that 57% of costs were direct. The largest hospital cost category was the operating room (33%) followed by the patient ward (31%). This study also showed that the overall cost to charge ratio was 0.42, and while this was constant between operative groups, it varied 3-fold among hospital departments, so that patient charges overestimated resource consumption in some hospital departments, e.g. anaesthesia, and underestimated it in others, e.g. ward area. Analysts often use patient charges to approximate costs. The rationale behind this is that hospital charges are more accessible and are believed to be related to costs by a constant correction factor, i.e. the cost-charge ratio. Thus, it can be seen that basing economic analysis on charges alone is misleading.

If we are anxious to minimise costs, it is reasonable to assume that hospital departments with the largest proportion of costs have the highest potential for cost reduction. Thus reduction of operating room costs is likely to yield the largest cost gains. However, anaesthetic agents account for a mere 6–10% of the total cost of a procedure and, furthermore, these costs have remained fairly constant over time in comparison to the other costs, such as staff salaries, equipment, etc., that go to make up the remaining 90%.[20] Macario also estimated that intra-operative anaesthesia costs constitute only 5.6% of the total cost of any in-patient procedure with an absolute minimum of only 3%. It might then appear that, as the contribution of anaesthesia to overall costs is small, it does not constitute an area where significant cost reductions can be achieved. However, Broadway & Jones have pointed out that while they also found that the anaesthetic costs per case are small, given the large volume of anaesthetics administered, small savings per case could represent far more substantial savings.[21] It must be remembered, however, that while most intra-operative anaesthetic costs are variable and direct, their reduction, by the use of cheaper drugs, will only result in an overall saving as long as the quality of anaesthetic care, as manifested by an increased proportion of indirect costs, is not diminished.

COST REDUCTION: HOW AND HOW MUCH?

Orkin has stated that the American healthcare system is undergoing nothing short of a revolution as competition has given rise to various cost reduction initiatives.[22] To some extent. the same is true in the UK and it is interesting to examine how anaesthetic cost reduction can be achieved and how much can be saved. Hawkes and his colleagues investigated the financial impact of a cost awareness programme on anaesthetic drug expenditure over a one year period.[23] They concluded that the implementation of simple measures, such as the education of anaesthetic personnel regarding drug costs and decreasing drug wastage by more cost-effective dosage preparations, could be an effective means of controlling drug expenditure at a time when new drugs and techniques were being introduced. However, both Johnstone and Greco have shown that cost savings are generally not sustainable in the absence of continuing effort to maintain altered practice patterns, despite a general improvement in the knowledge of anaesthetic costs on the part of anaesthetists.[24-26] Furthermore, Johnstone showed that an aggressive cost education initiative directed at cheaper substitutes for anaesthetic drugs among hospitals' 'top ten' drug expenditures, resulted in savings of 23% in the departments' drug budget.[24] If such direct cost savings could be extended to the other anaesthetic drugs and disposables, comprising the rest of the 3–5% of the total hospital costs allocated to the anaesthetic department, the decrease in total hospital costs would only be around 0.7%.

Rhodes & Ridley have highlighted several aspects of anaesthesia that lend themselves to the economic scrutiny of the direct costs involved.[27] These include the choice of drugs, breathing system and mode of ventilation, and regional versus general anaesthesia. Due to the high cost of new drugs, attention of those seeking to evaluate the economics of anaesthesia has focused on the i.v. induction agent propofol, the volatile agents sevoflurane and desflurane, and the 5-HT$_3$ group of antiemetics.

Propofol has become very popular due to the rapid and high quality of recovery and its association with a low incidence of side effects, most notably nausea and vomiting.[28,29] Its pharmacokinetics and dynamics are such that the drug has also gained widespread popularity for use in a total intravenous anaesthesia (TIVA) technique.[30] The acquisition price of propofol is several times that of other induction agents, such as thiopentone. When used for maintenance of anaesthesia, propofol is also commonly perceived to be more expensive than the commonly used volatile agents, enflurane and isoflurane. Such perceptions arise because simply comparing the acquisition cost of different anaesthetics is to examine only a small proportion of the total costs involved. Hitchcock & Rudkin carried out a comparative cost analysis of TIVA using propofol with the use of propofol for induction of anaesthesia and maintenance using nitrous oxide and either enflurane or isoflurane.[31] This study, of day case anaesthesia, included in its analysis not only the direct cost of the drugs used, but also the indirect cost engendered by their use, including the cost of treating associated morbidity, mostly nausea and vomiting, the costs of anaesthetic related use of healthcare resources post discharge (Accident and Emergency department and general practitioner visits), and the cost of unanticipated hospital admission. While the authors concluded that, overall, TIVA using propofol was indeed more expensive that the use of more traditional volatile agents, the difference was small. However, the use of propofol was associated with higher quality anaesthesia and, in the case of operations of less than 30 min duration, the overall costs associated with the use of TIVA were, in fact, less than for volatile agents. Several studies have found that TIVA using propofol is associated with an overall cost reduction when compared to the use of thiopentone/isoflurane anaesthesia.[32,33] This illustrates than a perception of expense based on acquisition cost alone is misleading and casts doubt on the belief that such a technique is more expensive. Furthermore, anaesthetists have to appreciate that several factors, including the duration of anaesthesia, can alter the relative costs of different anaesthetic techniques, making one drug or technique more or less cost effective in any given clinical situation.

Several investigators have examined the cost implications of preventing and treating postoperative nausea and vomiting (PONV).[34,35] The reasons for this are 2-fold. Firstly, nausea and vomiting are common forms of post-operative morbidity and, secondly, because the new class of antiemetics, the 5-HT$_3$ antagonists, ondansetron, granisetron etc., have high acquisition costs, when compared to older antiemetics, such as metoclopramide and droperidol. PONV studies of postoperative nausea and vomiting concentrate on the investigation of the efficacy and effectiveness of antiemetics.[36] Economic evaluation of any healthcare intervention, such the prevention and treatment of PONV, however, should also consider the issue of availability, that is, matching the supply of resources to locations where they are required. In addition, and of crucial importance, policy analysis of healthcare interventions must consider distribution, that is, an examination of who gains and who loses by choosing to allocate resources to one healthcare programme instead of another.[11] It is, therefore, insufficient to consider the differing cost effectiveness of antiemetics. Such comparisons must be related to the incidence of the morbidity for a particular operation, the associated incidence of side effects, and a distinction made between the use of these drugs for prevention and treatment of established symptoms. Further, in view of the importance patients attach to avoiding some forms of postoperative morbidity, particularly nausea and vomiting, the issue of how much an administration is willing to pay for an anaesthetic service that minimises what is often considered to be minor morbidity, must be examined.[37] Watcha & Smith have shown that ondansetron is a cost effective alternative to low dose droperidol when used for prophylaxis of nausea and vomiting, but that, for this to be the case, the incidence of nausea and vomiting must exceed 33%.[35] Droperidol, on the other hand, is the more cost effective drug to treat established symptoms, although the incidence of side effects, even at low dosage, must be borne in mind.[38] The difficulty of costing postoperative morbidity, such as nausea and vomiting, is further complicated in that the type of anaesthetic administered can affect the incidence of the problem itself. TIVA, using propofol, may either remove the need for antiemetics at all, or reduce the incidence and severity of PONV to levels that may alter the cost-effectiveness of the various antiemetics available.[39]

The introduction of two new volatile agents, sevoflurane and desflurane, has given rise to several cost comparison studies to determine their relative cost.[40,41] Such studies have to differentiate between the use of the agent for induction, maintenance, or both, and between the use of low flow and normal or high flow anaesthesia, but have again concentrated on only the direct acquisition costs involved. Factors that must be considered when studying the costs of these new volatile agents include high acquisition costs, although the use of a low fresh gas flow circle system may reduce the amount of this agent used. In addition, both agents have associated equipment costs in that they require designated vaporisers, in the case of desflurane, of some degree of sophistication. Both sevoflurane and desflurane have low blood gas solubility coefficients and, thus, are associated with both rapid onset and offset of effect.[42,43] This, in turn, may have cost implications in those situations where rapid recovery has financial implications, e.g. in day case surgery. However, while sevoflurane is rapidly establishing itself in the UK as an almost ideal inhalational induction agent, especially in children, the same is not true for desflurane which is associated with a significant incidence of problems.[42,44] Also, the whole issue of whether anaesthetic agents with rapid recovery profiles actually do decrease costs through an effect on recovery room stay is unclear. While some investigators have described substantial savings through reduced recovery stay following the use of anaesthetics with rapid offset of effect, others have failed to show a beneficial effect on turn-around time and thus improved operating theatre time utilisation, an area where most costs arise.[45-47] Furthermore, such savings are only achievable through the reduction in the number of recovery room staff, the exclusive use of such anaesthetics and the performance of operations that do not require any length of recovery stay to observe for immediate complications. Potential savings may, therefore, be difficult to achieve in practice. Similarly, while Eger has stated that desflurane may be used in low flow circle systems with cost advantages, this is not always practical and may be undesirable in the case of sevoflurane, due to its reaction with soda lime.[41,48] Low flow anaesthesia has, however, been shown to be associated with significant cost savings when used extensively, although there is the need for a capital outlay to provide suitable monitoring equipment.[49]

The cost effectiveness of some articles of anaesthetic equipment have also been investigated. Macario and colleagues investigated the cost efficiency of the laryngeal mask airway (LMA) in spontaneously breathing patients undergoing isoflurane, nitrous oxide and oxygen anaesthesia.[50] Their results suggest that the use of the LMA in cases of less than 40 min duration was more costly than the use of a facemask. However, when the duration of anaesthesia exceeded 40 min and the LMA re-use rate approached 40, then the LMA became the cheaper alternative. This analysis could not quantify the cost implications of the reduction in morbidity associated with the use of the LMA, e.g. through the absence of the need for muscle relaxant drugs and the reduced incidence of sore throat.[51,52] In this way, economic analysis of the various facets of anaesthesia often fails to cost the very advantages that make one anaesthetic drug or technique the more favourable option. Also, some debate continues regarding the cost implications of serious, but uncommon, events. Thus, while the tracheal tube protects the airway from aspiration of gastric contents, an event associated with very significant hospital costs, the extremely low incidence of this complication with the correct use of the LMA, means that overall costs may not be sensitive to this form of complication.[53] If, however, a wider perspective is adopted, including both the morbidity or even mortality of the patient, and the potential legal expenses of the healthcare system following litigation, such serious but uncommon events may profoundly alter the balance of costs. Such an approach illustrates the differing total costs generated by the inclusion of indirect cost factors.

In future, some degree of rationing of healthcare seems inevitable. Although anaesthesia contributes only a small proportion to the total cost of a surgical episode, anaesthetists must be aware of the cost of the drugs and techniques that they use. Most of the published work has examined only the direct costs incurred, and has ignored both indirect and intangible costs and benefits. The perceived quality of anaesthetic care, however, is often highly dependant on the latter. While Kantor & Chung found that anaesthetists believed that cheaper anaesthetic drugs could be used without compromising the quality of care, the relationship between the quality of anaesthesia and its cost has been largely ignored, frustrating any meaningful attempts to determine the real value of various drugs and techniques.[54] Studies of the economics of anaesthesia are further complicated by the lack of any consensus for quality indicators and standards of practice in relation to outcome. It will only be by the use of such indicators and standards, that the real cost of various anaesthetic techniques or drugs can be assessed, and a sensible cost value assigned to each aspect of outcome. Finally, future economic evaluations must be sensitive to the fact that the cost of any anaesthetic drug or technique is determined by the circumstances and methods in which they are used. The rapid recovery associated with the use of some newer anaesthetic agents may be economical, e.g. in day surgery, but possibly less so after cardiac surgery.

It is not surprising that attempts to reduce the cost of anaesthesia have also focused on the reduction of direct expenses. However, in order to make cost savings in those areas of anaesthetic practice where quality of service will not decline and the moneys saved may have a positive effect on patient care, consideration must also be given to how anaesthesia influences the use of other resources, e.g. the value of pre-operative blood tests and X-rays, policies for the crossmatching of blood, etc. In addition, the determinants of the time spent in the operating theatre and ward must be examined due to its high cost. While both ward and operating room time may be open to modification by the anaesthesia used, it is worth remembering that the cost to an institution of even a 30 min delay in starting an operating list is greater than the cost of a 2 h propofol infusion.[21,55] The realisation of any potential savings will require co-operation between anaesthetists, surgeons, nurses and administrators to find both clinical and managerial solutions. These must be based on an understanding of the way in which costs arise and may result both in improved quality as well as overall savings.

Finally, just as meaningful cost assessment requires a broad perspective, so too does the management of departmental budgets. Previously, there has been little incentive for achieving overall cost savings if such measures resulted in an overspend in one's own departmental budget. With the amalgamation of clinical entities into larger functional units, there is a need for more enlightened 'transdepartmental' budgeting. Indeed, the evolving guidelines for the economic evaluation of healthcare interventions recommend the broadest perspective possible.[22] For too long, both the economic assessment and control of anaesthesia has been limited to a small proportion of costs that are, in turn, a small part of a much larger whole. It appears that modern anaesthesia is, in fact, 'good value for money'. This should not be difficult to prove.

Key points for clinical practice

- Economic pressures make it likely that some degree of rationing of healthcare will be introduced.

- Anaesthesia contributes only a small proportion of the total costs of an operation, but is easily targeted in terms of costs and will be scrutinised closely for potential savings.

- Some knowledge of methods of costing of anaesthetic techniques and drugs is important for anaesthetists.

- Methods of assessing the quality of anaesthetic care must be agreed and the link with costs developed.

- When costing anaesthesia, all costs both direct and indirect must be included, and intangible benefits must be borne in mind.

- The cost of any anaesthetic drug or technique can be affected by several factors, including the duration of the operation, associated complication rates and wastage.

- Anaesthesia can affect costs significantly via pre-operative testing protocols, operating room delays and length of hospital stay.

- A more enlightened approach to budgetary control must be adopted so that high expenditures on one budget can be tolerated because they, in turn, produce savings in another, with an overall saving and increase in the quality of patient care.

References

1. Bevan D R. Anaesthesia pharmacoeconomics. Can J Anaesth 1993; 40: 693–695
2. Edge G, Morgan M. Anaesthesia – value for money. Anaesthesia 1996; 51: 105–106
3. Ryan M, Shackley P. Assessing the benefits of health care: how far should we go? Qual Health Care 1995; 4: 207–213
4. Kapur P A. Cost containment: at what expense? Anesth Analg 1995; 81: 897–899
5. Johnstone R E, Martinec C L. Costs of anaesthesia. Anesth Analg 1993; 76: 840–848
6. Gilron I. The introduction of new drugs into anaesthetic practice: a perspective in pharmaceutical development and regulation. Can J Anaesth 1995; 42: 516–522
7. Rovira J. Economic analysis and pharmaceutical policy. Anaesthesia 1995; 50: 49–51
8. Watcha M F, White P F. Postoperative nausea and vomiting: its aetiology, treatment, and prevention. Anesthesiology 1992; 77: 162-184
9. Robinson R. Costs and cost-minimisation analysis. BMJ 1993; 307: 726–728
10. Wetchler B V. Economic impact of anaesthesia decision making: they pay the money, we make the choice. J Clin Anesth 1992; 4 (Suppl 1): 205–245
11. Detsky A S, Naglie I G. A clinician's guide to cost-effectiveness analysis. Ann Intern Med 1990; 113: 147–154
12. Mehrez A, Gafni A. Quality-adjusted life-years, utility theory and healthy years equivalents. Med Decis Making 1989; 9: 142–149
13. White P F, Watcha M F. Are new drugs cost-effective for patients undergoing ambulatory surgery? Anesthesiology 1993; 78: 2–5
14. Briggs A, Sculpher M. Sensitivity analysis in economic evaluation: a review of published studies. Health Economics 1995; 4: 355–372
15. Drummond M F, Jefferson T O. Guidelines for authors and peer reviewers of economic submissions to the BMJ. BMJ 1996; 313: 275–283

16. Bulpitt C J, Fletcher A E. Measuring costs and financial benefits in randomised controlled trials. Am Heart J 1990; 119: 766–771

17. Drummond M F, Davies L M. Economic analysis alongside clinical trials: revisiting the methodological issues. Int J Technol Assess Health Care 1991; 7: 561–573

18. Jolicoeur L M, Jones-Grizzle A J, Boyer J G. Guidelines for performing a pharmacoeconomic analysis. Am J Hosp Pharm 1992; 49: 1741–1747

19. Macario A, Vitez T S, Dunn B, McDonald T. Where are the costs in perioperative care? Anesthesiology 1995; 83: 1138–1144

20. Lethbridge J R, Secker Walker J. Cost of anaesthetic drugs and clinical budgeting. BMJ 1986; 293: 1587–1588

21. Broadway P, Jones J. A method for costing anaesthetic practice. Anaesthesia 1995; 50: 56–63

22. Orkin F. Meaningful cost reduction. Anesthesiology 1995; 83: 1135–1137

23. Hawkes C, Miller D, Martineau R, Hull K, Hopkins H, Tierney M. Evaluation of cost minimisation strategies of anaesthetic drugs in a tertiary care hospital. Can J Anaesth 1994; 41: 894–901

24. Johnstone R E, Jozefczyk K G. Costs of anaesthetic drugs: experience with a cost education trial. Anesth Analg 1994; 78: 766–771

25. Greco P J, Eisenberg J M. Changing physicians' practices. N Engl J Med 1993; 329: 1271–1273

26. Bailey C R, Ruggier R, Cashman J N. Anaesthesia: cheap at twice the price? Anaesthesia 1993; 48: 906–909

27. Rhodes S P, Ridley S. Economic aspects of general anaesthesia. Pharmacoeconomics 1993; 3: 124–130

28. Siler J N, Horrow J C, Rosenberg H. Propofol reduces prolonged outpatient PACU stay. Anesthesiol Rev 1994; 11: 129–132

29. Weir P M, Munro H M, Reynolds P I et al. Propofol infusion and the incidence of emesis in paediatric outpatient strabismus surgery. Anesth Analg 1993; 76: 760–764

30. Apfelbaum J L, Lichtor J L, Lane B S et al. Awakening, clinical recovery, and psychomotor effects after desflurane and propofol anaesthesia. Anesth Analg 1996; 83: 721–725

31. Hitchcock M, Rudkin G. The real cost of total intravenous anaesthesia: cost versus price. Amb Surg 1995; 3: 43–48

32. Suver J, Arikian S R, Doyle J J, Sweeney S W, Hagan M. Use of anaesthesia selection in controlling surgery costs in an HMO hospital. Clin Ther 1995; 17: 561–571

33. Wagner B K, O'Hara D A. Cost analysis of propofol versus thiopental induction anaesthesia in outpatient laparoscopic gynaecologic surgery. Clin Ther 1995; 17: 770–776

34. Tang J, Watcha M F, White P F. A comparison of cost efficacy of ondansetron and droperidol as prophylactic therapy for elective outpatient gynecologic procedures. Anesth Analg 1996; 83: 304–313

35. Watcha M F, Smith I, Cost-effectiveness analysis of antiemetic therapy for ambulatory surgery. J Clin Anaesth 1994; 6: 370–377

36. Gan T J, Ginsberg B, Grant A P et al. Double-blind, randomised comparison of ondansetron and intraoperative propofol to prevent postoperative nausea and vomiting. Anesthesiology 1996; 85: 1036–1042

37. Orkin F K. What do patients really want? Preferences for immediate postoperative recovery. Anesth Analg 1992; 74: S225

38. Melnick B M. Extrapyramidal reactions to low-dose droperidol. Anesthesiology 1988; 69: 424–426

39. Hitchcock M, Ogg T W. Antiemetics in laparoscopic surgery. Br J Anaesth 1994; 72: 608

40. Weiskopf R B, Eger E. Comparing the costs of inhaled anesthetics. Anesthesiology 1993; 79: 1413–1418

41. Eger E I. Economic analysis and pharmaceutical policy: a consideration of the economics of the use of desflurane. Anaesthesia 1995; 50: 45–48

42. Smith I, Ding Y, White P F. Comparison of induction, maintenance, and recovery characteristics of sevoflurane–N_2O and propofol–isoflurane–N_2O anesthesia. Anesth Analg 1992; 74: 253–259

43. Davis P J, Cohen I T, McGowan F X, Latta K. Recovery characteristics of desflurane versus halothane for maintenance of anesthesia in pediatric ambulatory patients. Anesthesiology 1994; 80: 298–302

44. Van Hemelrijck J, Smith I, White P F. Use of desflurane for outpatient anaesthesia: a comparison with propofol and nitrous oxide. Anesthesiology 1991; 75: 197–203

45. Patel N, Smith C E, Pinchak A C et al. Desflurane is not associated with faster operating room exit times in outpatients. J Clin Anesth 1996; 8: 130–135

46. Marais L M, Maher M W, Wetchler B V, Kortilla K, Apfelbaum J L. Reduced demands on recovery room resources with propofol compared to thiopental-isoflurane. Anesthesiol Rev 1989; 16: 29–40

47. Sung Y F, Reiss N, Tillette T. The differential cost of anesthesia and recovery with propofol-nitrous oxide anesthesia versus thiopental-sodium-isoflurane-nitrous oxide anaesthesia. J Clin Anesth 1991; 3: 391–394

48. Bito H, Ikeda K. Degradation products of sevoflurane during low-flow anaesthesia. Br J Anaesth 1995; 74: 56–59

49. Cotter S M, Petros A J, Dore C J, Barber N D, White D C. Low-flow anaesthesia. Anaesthesia 1991; 46: 1009–1012

50. Macario A, Chang P C, Stempel D B, Brock-Utne J G. A cost analysis of the laryngeal mask airway for elective surgery in adult outpatients. Anesthesiology 1995; 83: 250–257

51. Alexander C A, Leach A B. Incidence of sore throats with the laryngeal mask. Anaesthesia 1989; 44: 791

52. Lee S K, Hong K H, Choe H et al. Comparison of the effects of the laryngeal mask airway and endotracheal intubation on vocal function. Br J Anaesth 1993; 71: 648–650

53. Brimacombe J R, Berry A. The incidence of aspiration associated with the laryngeal mask airway: a meta-analysis of published literature. J Clin Anesth 1995; 7: 297–305

54. Kantor G S A, Chung F. Anaesthesia drug cost, control and utilisation in Canada. Can J Anaesth 1996; 43: 9–16

55. Lui S S, Carpenter R L, Mackey D C et al. Effects of perioperative analgesia technique on rate of recovery after colon surgery. Anesthesiology 1995; 83: 757–765

Index

A

Abdomen, injuries, diagnosis, 71
Abortion
  anaesthetic practice, 117
  and fetal sentience, 107
Abscess, epidural, 228
Acetylcholine, 7, 22–3, 28, 35, 37
  receptors, 22
    muscarinic, 36
    nicotinic, subunits, 29
    postjunctional, 29–32
  receptor desensitization, 32–3
  release, 23–4
  transporter protein, 22
Acetylcholinesterase, 22–3, 28, 32, 34–5
Acid-base status, 176–7
Acupuncture, 225
Acute chest pain, therapeutic strategies, 44
Acute myocardial infarction, 189
  mortality, 43–4
Acute respiratory distress syndrome, 198
Adenosine, 26–7
Adrenaline, 178, 179, 180–1
Adrenergic agents, 50
Adult respiratory distress syndrome 188
  see also Lung, acute injury
  clinical conditions, 200
  definition, 198
  and nitric oxide, 195–216
Advanced life support, 144–7
  prehospital components, 145
Advanced Trauma Life Support, 143–4
Aeronox Transport System, 136
Agrin, 30–31
Air transport, 137–8
Airway and ventilation, indications in
  child transport, 132
Alcuronium, 35
Alfentanil, 72, 76, 92, 218
  in organ system failure (in ICU), 223

Almitrine, 207
Alpha–dystroglycan, 30
Alveolar–capillary membrane permeability,
  199–200
American Association of Neurological
  Surgeons, 154
Amino acids, nicotinic receptor subunits, 30
Aminosteroidal compounds, 36–7
Amiodarone, 48, 50
Amniotic fluid embolism, and ARDS, 200
AMPA receptors, 10–11
Amrinone, 179
Anaesthesia
  see also General anaesthesia
  cost and costing, 233–44
    assessment, 235–6
    benefit analysis, 235–6
    data importance, 234–5
    day case, 238
    effectiveness analysis, 236
    issues, 236–7
    methods of costing, 235–6
    minimisation, 235
    reduction, 237–40
    utility ratio, 235
  economics, 233–44
  epidural, 77
  fetal, 117
  ideo-motor suggestion effects, 89
  intra–operative costs, 237
  intravenous regional, 77–8
  neonatal, 108
  outcomes, 235
  positive suggestion effects, 84–6
  quality delineation, 234
  safety, 233–4
  spinal, 77
  total intravenous, 238–9
  verbal material learning, 96–9
Anaesthetics
  binding, 9

245